Essential Revision Notes in Medicine for Students

Edited by
Philip A Kalra MA MB BChir FRCP MD

**Consultant Nephrologist and Honorary Lecturer Hope Hospital, Salford
Royal Hospitals Trust and the University of Manchester**

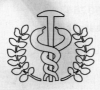
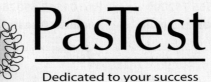

PasTest

Dedicated to your success

© 2006 PASTEST LTD
Egerton Court
Parkgate Estate
Knutsford
Cheshire
WA16 8DX

Telephone: 01565 752000

First Published 2006

ISBN: 190462720X

A catalogue record for this book is available from the British Library.

The information contained within this book was obtained by the author from reliable sources. However, while every effort has been made to ensure its accuracy, no responsibility for loss, damage or injury occasioned to any person acting or refraining from action as a result of information contained herein can be accepted by the publishers or author.

PasTest Revision Books and Intensive Courses

PasTest has been established in the field of postgraduate medical education since 1972, providing revision books and intensive study courses for doctors preparing for their professional examinations.

Books and courses are available for the following specialties:

MRCGP, MRCP Parts 1 and 2, MRCPCH Parts 1 and 2, MRCPsych, MRCS, MRCOG Parts 1 and 2, DRCOG, DCH, FRCA, PLAB Parts 1 and 2.

For further details contact:

PasTest, Freepost, Knutsford, Cheshire WA16 7BR

Tel: 01565 752000   **Fax: 01565 650264**
www.pastest.co.uk   **enquiries@pastest.co.uk**

Text prepared by Typestudy, Scarborough, UK

Printed and bound in the UK by Cambridge University Press, Cambridge, UK

Essential Revision Notes in Medicine for Students

 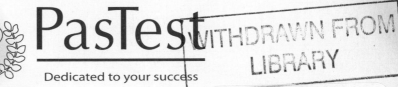

Dedicated to your success

Contents

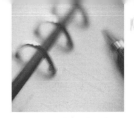

Contents

Contributors

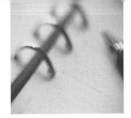

Masauso Chaponda MBBS MRCP DIPHIVMED
Specialist Registrar in Infectious Diseases and
Clinical Pharmacology, Honorary Lecturer
in Clinical Pharmacology, Royal Liverpool
University Hospital
Infectious Diseases

Colin Dayan MA MBBS FRCP PhD
Consultant Senior Lecturer in Medicine,
Head of Clinical Research, URCN, Henry Wellcome
Laboratories for Intergrative Neuroscience and
Endocrinology, University of Bristol
Endocrinology

Ben Goorney MBChB FRCP
Consultant Genito-Urinary Physician, Department
of Genito-Urinary Medicine, Hope Hospital, Salford
Genito-urinary medicine and AIDS

Philip A Kalra MA MB BChir FRCP MD
Consultant Nephrologist, Department of Renal
Medicine, Hope Hospital, Salford
Nephrology

Mike McMahon BSc MBChB FRCP
Consultant Physician and Rheumatologist,
Department of Medicine, Dumfries and Galloway
Royal Infirmary, Dumfries
Immunology and Rheumatology

Donal O'Donoghue BSc MBChB FRCP
Consultant Renal Physician, Department of Renal
Medicine, Hope Hospital, Salford
Metabolic diseases

John Paisey BM MRCP
Specialist Registrar, Cardiology, Wessex Region
Cardiology

Keith Patterson FRCP FRCPath
Consultant Haematologist, Department of
Haematology, University College London Hospitals,
London
Haematology

Geraint Rees BA BMBCh MRCP PhD
Wellcome Senior Clinical Fellow, Institute of
Cognitive Neuroscience, University College, London
Neurology

Helen Robertshaw BSc(Hons) MBBS MRCP
Consultant Dermatologist, The Royal Bournemouth
and Christchurch Hospitals NHS Foundation Trust
Dermatology

Andrew Robinson MA BM BCh FRCP PhD
Consultant Gastroenterologist, Honorary Clinical
Lecturer, Hope Hospital, Salford
Gastroenterology

Contributors

Katherine Smyth MBChB MRCP FRCOpth
Consultant Ophthalmologist, Royal Bolton
Hospital, Bolton
Ophthalmology

Deborah Wales MBChB FRCP FRCA
Consultant Respiratory Physician, Nevill Hall
Hospital, Brecon Road, Abergavenny,
Monmouthshire
Respiratory Medicine

Anne Garden MBChB FRCOG ILTM
Head of School of Medical Education,
University of Liverpool
Undergraduate Advisor

W Stephen Waring MRCP(UK) PhD
Consultant Physician and Honorary Senior
Lecturer, The Royal Infirmary of Edinburgh
Clinical Pharmacology, Toxicology and Poisoning

Louise C Wilson BSc MBChB MRCP
Consultant in Clinical Genetics, Clinical and
Molecular Genetics Unit, Institute of Child Health,
London
Genetics

Acknowledgement
The publishers would like to thank William R C Weir
FRCP FRCP (Edin) for his contribution to the
Infectious Diseases chapter.

Editor's Preface

There are numerous textbooks of medicine, some aimed specifically at medical undergraduates and others at the practising physician. Until now, there have been few texts that bridge the gap between student and doctor.

Essential Revision Notes in Medicine for Students follows the style of the PasTest *Essential Revision Notes* series, providing sufficiently detailed summary notes in all of the major specialities within medicine. It is designed for both the student and the doctor – bridging the gap between the comprehensive textbook and the short notes style text.

Each chapter has been written by an expert in their subject, and although all important topics have been covered, authors have been asked to concentrate upon those aspects of their subjects which are most important or poorly understood. Key points are emphasised as 'Essential notes' at various points in the text, whilst each chapter is concluded with a 'Revision summary'. Throughout the text, bulleted lists, tables and images are used to present information to the reader.

We anticipate the readership of this title to be wide and varied. It is ideal as an accompaniment to the 4th and 5th year medical syllabus, and its concise style makes it an excellent revision aid for final year examinations. It will be useful, also, to doctors embarking on the new Foundation Year programme.

I would like to thank all of the chapter authors for their efforts in ensuring that the book could be completed in timely fashion, and special thanks goes to Amy Smith and her colleagues at PasTest, who have energetically co-ordinated the development and production process.

Philip A Kalra
January 2006

About this book

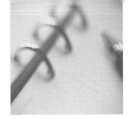

Essential Revision Notes in Medicine for Students is designed as a revision aid for medical undergraduates. It is an ideal accompaniment to the 4th and 5th year medical syllabus – the clinical years. The book has been developed by the team responsible for the bestselling *Essential Revision Notes for MRCP* – drawing on a wealth of medical knowledge.

Medical training within hospitals has undergone a radical change in recent years. The new Foundation Programmes for junior doctors present medical students with a new challenge to prepare for. *Essential Revision Notes in Medicine for Students* aims to equip students with a sound knowledge of a wide breadth of subject areas – giving them the confidence to deal with clinical cases encountered on the wards.

There are many books on the market for medical students. It can be hard to work out what essential knowledge is required for your examinations. Through this book, we have taken the time to work out what is essential for you and have condensed the information into one medical volume.

Essential Revision Notes in Medicine for Students:

- Helps you focus your revision
- Takes a succinct but detailed look at each specialty
- Draws on a wealth of knowledge from a list of experienced authors
- Incorporates figures and images to illustrate revision notes.

This title incorporates a number of features designed to make your reading of the book as fruitful as possible:

Revision Objectives

At the start of each chapter you will find a list of 'Revision Objectives'. These set out the key learning points of the chapter and are designed to focus your reading – enabling you to concentrate on what you really need to know. Look through these carefully before reading the chapter, consider what you already know and in which areas you need further revision.

Revision Summary

The 'Revision Objectives' are mirrored at the end of each chapter in the 'Revision Summary'. Again, this feature is designed to enable you to establish what you have learned. It can be used as a brief re-cap and is thus very useful for last minute revision.

Essential Notes

As you read through each chapter, you will see pertinent points highlighted as 'Essential Notes'. Each of our subject-specific authors has used this feature to highlight certain key learning notes you should remember.

Further Revision

The wide scope of this title makes it impossible for us to cover everything. We appreciate that you may feel the need to develop a deeper knowledge of a certain area, or indeed that you already have your future specialty in mind. The 'Further Revision' boxes include not only books, but also websites and journals that our specialist authors consider a vital source of specific information.

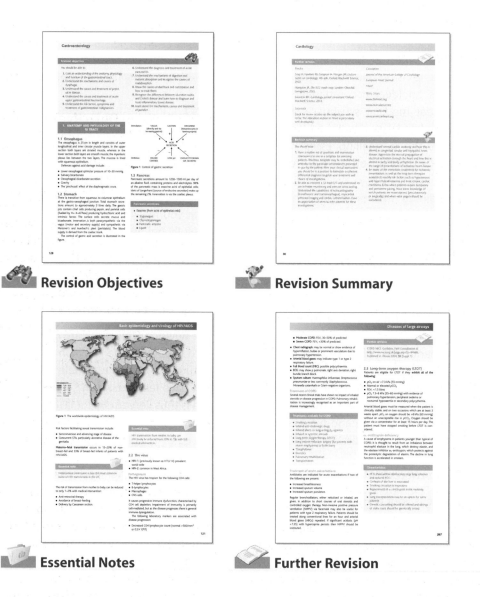

Revision Objectives

Revision Summary

Essential Notes

Further Revision

Notes on revision

Above all, it is important to be prepared. Leave yourself enough time to study and develop a true understanding of the subjects on which you are examined. Know where and when your examinations will be held and leave plenty of time to get there.

When you begin revising, you will soon discover what study techniques work best for you. Here are a few general tips to get you started:

Planning your revision

- Do not be too selective in your revision. It is dangerous to anticipate ('spot') specific questions and revise only those topics. Just because a particular topic appeared in an examination one year does not mean that it will not be examined in the following year.

- Aim to do equally well in all of your subjects. It is not a good tactic to attempt to do very well in some subjects and to neglect others.

- Make a realistic estimate of how much time you will be able to spend on concentrated revision. Make a timetable for your revision and try to keep to it. This will help you to be more organised in your revision. During revision of one subject you will worry less about how much or how little revision you have done in another subject. Also, if you keep to your revision timetable, you will be able to enjoy your relaxation time without feeling guilty that you are not revising.

- In planning your revision timetable, allow some spare time for unexpected problems; for example, illness, or relationship problems.

- Allow some time immediately before the examinations to practise answering questions from previous examinations. It is a fallacy to assume that if you know a subject well you will automatically be able to write well about it.

- *Do not let the construction and constant alteration of revision schedules become a substitute for revision itself!*

Revision

- At the beginning of your revision of a subject, scan through the section of your notes that you wish to revise to get an overview. Then split the subject area into smaller sections, and tackle these in turn.

- Read through your notes actively, thinking about what they mean. If you refer to text books at this stage, integrate the information from them into your notes.

- Make a set of skeleton notes using the main headings and sub-headings of the material. Use flow diagrams, annotated illustrations or lists of topics. For lists which that have to be learnt 'by heart', try making a mnemonic, that is, a word in which the letters, or sentence in which the first letters of the words, trigger your thoughts to items on the list. For example, Richard Of York Gave Battle In Vain, for the colours of the spectrum in their correct order, Red, Orange, Yellow, Green, Blue, Indigo, Violet.

- Using your skeleton notes alone, test yourself to see how much you can recall.

- Look at questions from past examination papers, and check how you would answer them. Do not write out answers in full, but do make a written plan of what you would include, and in what order. Remember that many examination questions will require the synthesis or comparison of material from more than one lecture, so to be fully prepared for an examination you should not learn lecture notes 'by heart', but you should understand and be prepared to apply the material which that you have been taught.

- Remember that during revision the general principles of private study apply. Familiar and reasonably comfortable surroundings aid concentration. There is an optimum time for concentrated study; too short a time interrupts your concentration, and after too long a time your ability to concentrate will decline.

- Immediately before the examinations, try to establish a routine with sufficient sleep and relaxation. There is little point in being full of facts but mentally or physically exhausted as you enter the examination.

The sections 'Planning your revision' and 'Revision' above are courtesy of the Study Skills sections of www.liverpool.ac.uk.

Notes on the exam

- Common things are common and these will be concentrated on in the MB exam. Think carefully if you find yourself answering a question by describing a rare disease – is there a more common condition you should be concentrating on?

- In general brevity is good – even in essays the examiner will have a mental tick list of important points and if these appear in your text you will generally do well.

- Read the newspapers – examiners do. They may light upon an item of topical medical news to discuss in an oral exam.

- When faced with an image that you do not recognise, describe it to yourself – many conditions in medicine have descriptive similes attached and describing the image may trigger the right memory.

- Knowledge learnt in one subject will overlap with other subjects, making the load of learning easier than it may first appear.

- In a multi-part question the subject (eg a disease) will usually be the same throughout.

- In oral examinations you dig your own holes – if you mention a rare and interesting condition that is relevant to the discussion then expect to be questioned about it.

Normal values for common biochemical and haematological tests

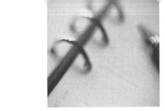

HAEMATOLOGY

Haemoglobin	
men:	13–18 g/dl
women:	11.5–16 g/dl
Mean cell volume MCV	76–96 fl
Platelets	$150–400 \times 10^9/l$
White cells (total)	$4–11 \times 10^9/l$
Differential WCC	
Neutrophils	$1.5–7 \times 10^9/l$
Lymphocytes	$1.5–4 \times 10^9/l$
Monocytes	$0–0.8 \times 10^9/l$
Eosinophils	$0.04–0.4 \times 10^9/l$
Basophils	$0–0.1 \times 10^9/l$
INR	0.9–1.2

Arterial blood gases (ABGs)

pH	7.35–7.45
PO_2	10–12 kPa
PCO_2	4.7–6 kPa
HCO_3^-	22–28 mmol/l
Base excess	±2 mmol/l

Urea and electrolytes (U&Es)

Sodium	135–145 mmol/l
Potassium	3.5–5 mmol/l
Creatinine	70–120 µmol/l
Urea	2.5–6.7 mmol/l
Albumin	35–50 g/l
Calcium	2.12–2.65 mmol/l
Phosphate	0.8–1.45 mmol/l

Normal values

Liver function tests (LFTs)

Bilirubin	3–17 µmol/l
Alanine aminotransferase (ALT)	3–35 u/l
Aspartate transaminase (AST)	3–35 u/l
Alkaline phosphatase (ALP)	30–150 u/l
Gamma glutamyl transferase (γGT)	11–51 iu/l

Other biochemical values

Amylase 0–180 units/dl
Glucose (fasting) 4–6 mmol/l
Glucose (random) <7 mmol/l
C-reactive protein (CRP) <10 mg/l
TSH 0.5–5.7 mu/l
T_4 (thyroxine) 70–140 nmol/l
T_3 (tri-iodothyronine) 1.2–3.0 nmol/l

CEREBROSPINAL FLUID

Opening pressure	50–180 mmH$_2$O
Total protein	0.15–0.45 g/l

Urine

Osmolality	350–1000 mosmol/kg
Albumin/creatinine ratio (untimed specimen):	
males	<2.5 mg/mmol
females	<3.5 mg/mmol
Total protein output	<200 mg/24 h

Cardiology

CONTENTS

Cardiology

Revision objectives

You should be able to

1. Develop a mental framework for clinical assessment of the cardiovascular system
2. Understand the principles, utility and limitations of major cardiac investigations
3. Relate disease processes to cardiac anatomy and physiology
4. Appreciate the relevance and application of therapeutic interventions on cardiac disease

---

1. HISTORY AND EXAMINATION

1.1 History

The cardinal presenting features of cardiac disease are

- Chest pain
- Breathlessness
- Palpitations
- Syncope and presyncope
- Peripheral oedema.

Chest pain is usually caused by ischaemia or inflammation (peri/myocarditis). Ischaemia is usually though not always due to coronary artery disease (CAD). Other causes of ischaemia include left ventricular hypertrophy (LVH), severe tachycardia and pulmonary thromboembolism (pain due to mixed pulmonary and myocardial ischaemia).

Cardiac breathlessness results from either failure of gas exchange (pulmonary oedema, pulmonary vascular insufficiency) or directly from the inability of the cardiac output to meet metabolic demands. Ischaemia, ventricular pressure or volume overload, tachy and bradycardia, pulmonary embolism and pulmonary hypertension may all present with dyspnoea.

> **Essential note**
>
> When taking a history from a cardiac patient ask specifically about chest pain, breathlessness, palpitations, syncope and ankle swelling

Palpitations are an awareness of the heartbeat, which is not infrequent in the normal population but may indicate an arrhythmia. All cardiac pathology predisposes to arrhythmias.

Syncope and presyncope are common features of tachy and bradycardias but also occur in left or right ventricular outflow tract obstruction as in aortic stenosis, hypertrophic cardiomyopathy and massive pulmonary embolism.

Peripheral oedema occurs in volume and pressure overload of the ventricles as well as in severe impairment of diastolic filling as seen in restrictive myocardial disease and constrictive pericardial disease.

1.2 Examination routine

A standard cardiovascular examination involves a variation on the following order:

- Introduction and position patient at 45°
- General inspection – scars, oxygen, IVIs, discomfort
- Hands – clubbing, vasculitis
- Pulses – rhythm, character, radioradial and radiofemoral delay
- Blood pressure
- Eyes and mouth – xanthelasma, corneal arcus, anaemia, cyanosis
- Jugular venous pressure
- Apex beat and RV impulse
- Auscultation – all areas with diaphragm, mitral area in left lateral position with bell, sitting forward in expiration at left sternal edge with diaphragm
- Auscultate lung bases
- Inspect and palpate for peripheral oedema.

> **Essential note**
>
> Examination follows the routine of inspection, palpation, auscultation, and works up from the hand, the arm to the face and neck before reaching the precordium

1.3 Jugular venous pulse (JVP)

This reflects the right atrial pressure (normal 3 cm above the clavicle with the subject at 45°). This should fall with inspiration, which increases venous return by a suction effect of the lungs, and with expansion of the pulmonary

---

Table 1

Normal waves in the JVP

a wave:	Due to atrial contraction – active push up SVC and into right ventricle (may cause an audible S4).
c wave:	An invisible flicker in the x descent due to closure of the tricuspid valve, before the start of ventricular systole.
x descent:	Downward movement of the heart causes atrial stretch and drop in pressure.
v wave:	Due to passive filling of blood into the atrium against a closed tricuspid valve.
y descent:	Opening of tricuspid valve with passive movement of blood from the right atrium to the right ventricle (causing an S3 when audible).

Pathological waves in the JVP

a waves:	Lost in atrial fibrillation, giant in tricuspid stenosis or in pulmonary hypertension with sinus rhythm (atrial septal defect will exaggerate the natural a and v waves in sinus rhythm).
giant V(S) waves:	Merging of the a and v into a large wave (with a rapid y descent) as pressure continues to increase due to ventricular systole in patients with tricuspid regurgitation.
steep x descent:	Occur in states where there is atrial filling due only to ventricular systole and downward movement of the base of the heart, ie compressed atrial states with tamponade or constrictive pericarditis.
rapid y descent:	Occurs in states where high flow occurs with tricuspid valve opening (eg tricuspid regurgitation (high atrial load) or constrictive pericarditis) – vacuum effect. A slow y descent indicates tricuspid stenosis.
cannon a waves:	Atrial contractions against a closed tricuspid valve due to a nodal rhythm, a ventricular tachycardia, ventricular-paced rhythm (regular), complete heart block or ventricular extrasystoles (irregular). They occur regularly but not consistently in type 1, second degree heart block.

---

beds. However, if the neck veins are distended by inspiration this implies that the right heart chambers cannot increase in size due to restriction by fluid or pericardium: Kussmaul's sign. Non-pulsatile JVP elevation occurs with superior vena cava (SVC) obstruction.

1.4 Arterial pulse associations

- **Collapsing**: aortic regurgitation, arterio-venous fistula, patent ductus arteriosus or other large extra-cardiac shunt
- **Slow rising**: aortic stenosis (delayed percussion wave)
- **Bisferiens**: a double shudder due to mixed aortic valve disease with significant regurgitation (tidal wave second impulse)
- **Jerky**: hypertrophic obstructive cardiomyopathy
- **Alternans**: severe left ventricular failure
- **Paradoxical (pulsus paradoxus)**: an excessive reduction in the pulse with inspiration (drop in systolic blood pressure (BP) >10 mmHg) occurs with left ventricular compression, tamponade, constrictive pericarditis or severe asthma, as venous return is compromised.

Causes of absent radial pulse

- Dissection of aorta with subclavian involvement
- Iatrogenic: post-catheterisation
- Peripheral arterial embolus
- Takayasu's arteritis
- Trauma

1.5 Cardiac apex

The normal apex beat (the most lateral and caudal point at which the cardiac impulse is palpable) is located in the mid clavicular line, fifth intercostal space.

An absent apical impulse

The apex may be impalpable in the following situations:

- Obesity/emphysema
- Right pneumonectomy with displacement
- Pericardial effusion or constriction
- Dextrocardia (palpable on right side of chest).

Apex associations

Palpation of the apex beat (reflecting counter clockwise ventricular movement striking the chest wall during isovolumic contractions) can detect the following pathological states:

- **Heaving**: left ventricular hypertrophy (and all its causes), sometimes associated with palpable fourth heart sound
- **Thrusting/hyperdynamic**: high left ventricular volume (eg in mitral regurgitation, aortic regurgitation (AR), patent ductus arteriosus (PDA), ventral septal defect (VSD))
- **Tapping**: palpable first heart sound in mitral stenosis
- **Displaced and diffuse/dyskinetic**: left ventricular impairment and dilatation (eg dilated cardiomyopathy, myocardial infarction)
- **Double impulse**: with dyskinesia is due to left ventricular aneurysm; without dyskinesia in hypertrophic cardiomyopathy (HCM)

- **Pericardial knock**: constrictive pericarditis
- **Parasternal heave**: due to right ventricular hypertrophy (eg atrial septal defect (ASD), pulmonary hypertension, chronic obstructive pulmonary disease, pulmonary stenosis)
- **Palpable third heart sound**: due to heart failure and severe mitral regurgitation.

1.6 Heart sounds

Third heart sound (S3)

Due to the passive filling of the ventricles on opening of the arteriovenous (AV) valves, audible in normal children and young adults. Pathological in cases of rapid left ventricular filling (eg mitral regurgitation, VSD, congestive cardiac failure (CCF) and constrictive pericarditis).

Table 2 Abnormalities of first heart sound (S1): closure of mitral and tricuspid valves

Loud	Soft	Split	Variable
Mobile mitral stenosis	Immobile mitral stenosis	RBBB	Atrial fibrillation
Hyperdynamic states	Hypodynamic states	LBBB	Complete heart block
Tachycardic states	Mitral regurgitation	VT	
Left to right shunts	Poor ventricular function	Inspiration	
Short PR interval	Long PR interval	Ebstein anomaly	

LBBB, left bundle branch block; RBBB, right bundle branch block; VT, ventricular tachycardia

---

Abnormalities of second heart sound (S2): closure of of aortic then pulmonary valves (<0.05 s apart)

Intensity		Splitting			
Loud:	Systemic hypertension (loud A2)	**Fixed:**	ASD	**Single S2:**	Severe PS/AS
	Pulmonary hypertension (loud P2)	**Widely split:**	RBBB		Hypertension
	Tachycardic states		Pulmonary stenosis		Large VSD
	ASD (loud P2)		Deep inspiration		Fallot's tetralogy
Soft or absent:	Severe aortic stenosis		Mitral regurgitation		Eisenmenger syndrome
					Pulmonary atresia
					Elderly
				Reversed split S2:	LBBB
					Right ventricular pacing
					PDA
					Aortic stenosis

Fourth heart sound (S4)

Due to the atrial contraction that fills a stiff left ventricle, such as in left ventricular hypertrophy, amyloid, HCM and left ventricular ischaemia. It is absent in atrial fibrillation.

Causes of valvular clicks

- **Aortic ejection**: aortic stenosis ± bicuspid aortic valve
- **Pulmonary ejection**: pulmonary stenosis
- **Mid-systolic**: mitral valve prolapse.

Opening snap (OS)

In mitral stenosis an opening snap may be present and occurs after S2 in early diastole. The closer it is to S2 the greater the severity of mitral stenosis. It is absent when the mitral cusps become immobile, due to calcification, as in very severe mitral stenosis.

---

2. CARDIAC INVESTIGATIONS

2.1 The ECG

- Interperate an ECG by identifying rate, rhythm and axis, then progress to assessing individual components of the electrogram. −30° to +90°: normal
- −30° to −90°: left axis
- +90° to +180°: right axis
- −90° to −180°: indeterminate.

Causes of common abnormalities in ECG

- **Causes of left axis deviation**

  - Left bundle branch block (LBBB)
  - Left anterior hemi block (LAHB)
  - Left ventricular hypertrophy (LVH)
  - Primum atrial septal defect (ASD)
  - Cardiomyopathies
  - Tricuspid atresia

- **Low voltage ECG**

  - Pulmonary emphysema
  - Pericardial effusion
  - Myxoedema
  - Severe obesity
  - Incorrect calibration
  - Cardiomyopathies
  - Global ischaemia
  - Amyloid

Causes of common abnormalities in ECG

- **Causes of right axis deviation**

  - Infancy
  - Right bundle branch block (RBBB)
  - Right ventricular hypertrophy (eg lung disease, pulmonary embolism, large secundum ASD, severe pulmonary stenosis, Fallot's)

- **Abnormalities of ECGs in athletes**

  - Sinus arrhythmia
  - Sinus bradycardia
  - 1° heart block
  - Wenckebach phenomenon
  - Junctional rhythm

Clinical diagnoses which may be made from the ECG of an asymptomatic patient

- Atrial fibrillation
- Complete heart block
- Hypertrophic cardiomyopathy (HCM)
- Atrial septal defects (with RBBB)
- Long QT syndromes
- Wolff–Parkinson–White syndrome (delta waves).

Short PR interval

This is rarely less than 0.12 s; the most common causes are those of pre-excitation involving accessory pathways or of tracts bypassing the slow region of the AV node; other causes do exist.

- **Pre-excitation**

  - Wolff–Parkinson–White (WPW) syndrome
  - Lown–Ganong–Levine syndrome (short PR syndrome)

- **Other**

  - Ventricular extrasystole falling after P wave
  - AV junctional rhythm (but P wave will usually be negative)
  - Low atrial rhythm
  - Coronary sinus escape rhythm

Causes of tall R waves in V1

It is easy to spot tall R waves in V1. This lead largely faces the posterior wall of the left ventricle and the mass of the right ventricle. As the overall vector is predominantly towards the bulkier LV in normal situations, the QRS is usually negative in V1. This balance is reversed in the following situations:

- Right ventricular hypertrophy
- RBBB
- Posterior infarction
- Dextrocardia
- Wolff–Parkinson–White (WPW) **type A** (ventricular conduction starts via a left posterior accessory pathway, ie towards V1)
- Hypertrophic cardiomyopathy (septal mass greater than posterior wall).

Bundle branch block and ST segment abnormalities

Complete bundle branch block is a failure or delay of impulse conduction to one ventricle from the AV node, requiring conduction via the other bundle, and the transmission within the ventricular myocardium; this results in abnormal prolongation of QRS duration (≥ 120 ms) and abnormalities of the normally iso-electric ST segment.

- **Causes of left bundle branch block (LBBB)**
  - Ischaemic heart disease (recent or old myocardial infarction (MI))
  - Left ventricular hypertrophy (LVH)
  - Aortic valve disease
  - Cardiomyopathy
  - Myocarditis
  - Post-valve replacement
  - Right ventricular pacemaker

- **Causes of right bundle branch block (RBBB)**
  - Normal in young
  - Right ventricular strain (eg pulmonary embolus)
  - Atrial septal defect
  - Ischaemic heart disease
  - Myocarditis
  - Idiopathic

- Causes of ST elevation
  - Early repolarisation
  - Acute MI
  - Pericarditis (saddle-shaped)
  - Ventricular aneurysm
  - Coronary artery spasm
  - During angioplasty

- Other ST-T wave changes (not elevation)
  - Ischaemia
  - Digoxin therapy
  - Hypertrophy
  - Post-tachycardia
  - Hyperventilation
  - Oesophageal irritation
  - Cardiac contusion
  - Mitral valve prolapse
  - Acute cerebral event (eg subarachnoid haemorrhage)
  - Electrolyte abnormalities

Q waves may be permanent (reflecting myocardial necrosis) or transient (suggesting failure of myocardial function, but not necrosis).

- Pathological Q waves
  - Transmural infarction
  - LBBB
  - Wolff–Parkinson–White syndrome
  - Hypertrophic cardiomyopathy
  - Idiopathic cardiomyopathy
  - Neoplastic infiltration
  - Myocarditis (may resolve)
  - Dextrocardia

- Transient Q waves
  - Coronary spasm
  - Hypoxia
  - Hyperkalaemia
  - Cardiac contusion
  - Hypothermia

Potassium and ECG changes

There is a reasonable correlation between plasma potassium and ECG changes.

- **Hyperkalaemia**

  - Tall T waves
  - Prolonged PR interval
  - Flattened/absent P waves.

- **Very severe hyperkalaemia**

  - Wide QRS
  - Sine wave pattern
  - Ventricular tachycardia/ventricular fibrillation/asystole.

- **Hypokalaemia**

  - Flat T waves, occasionally inverted
  - Prolonged PR interval
  - ST depression
  - Tall U waves.

ECG changes following coronary artery bypass surgery

- Osborne u waves (hypothermia)
- Saddle-shaped ST elevation (pericarditis)
- PR segment depression (pericarditis)
- Low voltage ECG in chest leads (pericardial effusion)
- Changing electrical alternans (alternating ECG axis – cardiac tamponade)
- $S_1Q_3T_3$ (pulmonary embolus)
- Atrial fibrillation
- Q waves
- ST segment and T wave changes.

Electrocardiographic techniques for prolonged monitoring

- **Holter monitoring**: the ECG is monitored in one or more leads for 24–72 h. The patient is encouraged to keep a diary in order to correlate symptoms with ECG changes.
- **External recorders**: the patient keeps a monitor with them for a period of days or weeks. At the onset of symptoms the monitor is placed to the chest and this records the ECG.
- **Wearable loop recorders**: the patient wears a monitor for several days or weeks. The device records the ECG constantly on a self-erasing loop. At the time of symptoms, the patient activates the recorder and a trace spanning some several seconds before a period of symptoms to several minutes afterwards is stored.
- **Implantable loop recorders**: a loop recorder is subcutaneously implanted in the pre-pectoral region. The recorder is activated by the patient or according to pre-programmed parameters. Again the ECG data from several seconds before symptoms to several minutes after are stored; data are uploaded by telemetry. The battery life of the implantable loop recorder is approximately 18 months.

2.2 Exercise stress testing

This is used in the investigation of coronary artery disease, exertionally induced arrhythmias, and in the assessment of cardiac workload and sinus node function. Exercise tests also give diagnostic and prognostic information post-infarction, and generate patient confidence in rehabilitation after myocardial infarction (MI).

The prerequisites for obtaining a diagnostic test are: an interpretable resting ECG and adequate effort tolerance.

The main contraindications to exercise testing include those conditions where fatal ischaemia or arrhythmias may be provoked, or those patients in whom cardiac function may be severely and acutely impaired by exertion.

Contraindications to exercise testing
- Severe aortic stenosis or HCM with marked outflow obstruction
- Acute myocarditis or pericarditis
- Pyrexial or 'flu'-like illness
- Severe left main stem disease
- Untreated congestive cardiac failure
- Unstable angina
- Dissecting aneurysm
- Adults with complete heart block
- Untreated severe hypertension

Interpretation of exercise test results

A positive result is indicated by the development of 2 mm or more of horizontal or downsloping ST segment depression.

A negative result is achieved if at least 6 minutes of exercise is achieved reaching at least 85% of the maximum predicted heart rate with a positive blood pressure response and no ECG changes.

Tests not conforming to either of these are classified as either non-diagnostic or equivocal.

2.3 Echocardiography

Echocardiography is the use of ultrasound to image the heart and derive functional information from the velocity of blood within the heart.

Conventional echocardiography includes 2D imaging and the use of Doppler to create colour flow maps and measure velocities. It is used in the diagnosis of:

- Pericardial effusion and tamponade
- Valvular disease (including large vegetations)
- Hypertrophic cardiomyopathy, dilated cardiomyopathy, LV mass and function
- Cardiac tumours and intracardiac thrombus
- Congenital heart disease (eg PDA; coarctation of the aorta).

Stress echo is used in the diagnosis of infarction and ischaemia.

Contrast echo is used in the diagnosis of atrial septal defects/ventricular septal defects.

Transoesophageal echo (TOE) provides much clearer pictures, particularly of posterior structures, and is therefore useful in the following:

- Diagnosis of aortic dissection
- Suspected atrial thrombus
- Assessment of vegetations or abscesses in endocarditis
- Prosthetic valve dysfunction or leakage
- Intra-operative assessment of left ventricular function
- Technically sub-optimal transthoracic echocardiogram.

2.4 Nuclear cardiology: myocardial perfusion imaging (MPI)

Perfusion tracers such as thallium or technetium can be used to gauge myocardial blood flow, both at rest and during stress (induced by drugs or exercise). Tracer uptake is detected using tomograms and displayed in a colour scale in standard views; stress and rest images are compared.

MPI may be used to:

- Detect infarction
- Investigate atypical chest pains
- Assess ventricular function
- Determine prognosis and detect myocardium that may be re-awakened from hibernation with an improved blood supply (eg after coronary bypass grafting).

2.5 Cardiac catheterisation

Cardiac catheterisation is the process of advancing catheters into the great vessels and heart chambers to measure pressures, oxygen saturations and to obtain angiograms.

Useful diagnostic information is obtained in:

- Coronary artery disease
- Valvular heart disease
- Cardiomyopathies
- Congenital heart disease.

In congenital and coronary artery disease there are also catheter-based therapeutic interventions (device closure of shunts and angioplasty).

Complications are uncommon (approximately 5%, including minor complications); these include contrast allergy, local haemorrhage from puncture sites with subsequent occurrence of thrombosis, false aneurysm or AV malformation. Vasovagal reactions are common. Occasionally a cerebrovascular accident (CVA) or myocardial infarction may be induced.

- Overall mortality rates are quoted at < 1/1000 cases.

2.6 24-hour ambulatory blood pressure monitoring

The limited availability and relative expense of ambulatory blood pressure monitoring prevents its use in all hypertensive patients. Specific areas of usefulness are in the following situations:

- Assessing for 'white coat' hypertension
- Borderline hypertensive cases that may not need treatment
- Evaluation of hypotensive symptoms
- Identifying episodic hypertension (eg in phaeochromocytoma)
- Assessing drug compliance and effects (particularly in resistant cases)
- Nocturnal blood pressure dipper status (non-dippers are at higher risk).

3. VALVULAR HEART DISEASE AND ENDOCARDITIS

3.1 Clinical assessment

Prior to auscultation of the precordium information regarding valvular heart disease is gained from the rate rhythm and character of the pulse, the blood pressure, the jugular venous pressure and palpable ventricular impulses (apex beat and right ventricular heave).

On examination murmurs are classified by their position in the cardiac cycle, their anatomical location and radiation and the effects that respiratory and other manoeuvres have on them.

The main positions for auscultation are:

- Mitral area, site of the apex beat, ie 5th intercostals space mid clavicular line in normals but displaced in cardiomegaly
- Aortic area, 2nd intercostal space right sternal edge
- Tricuspid area, 5th intercostal space left sternal edge
- Pulmonary area, 2nd intercostal space left sternal edge.

3.2 Mitral regurgitation

Often presenting with palpitations and breathlessness, characteristic examination findings are: atrial fibrillation, displaced apex beat, a pansystolic murmur loudest on expiration radiating into the axilla.

The full structure of the mitral valve includes the annulus, cusps, chordae and papillary musculature, and abnormalities of any of these may cause regurgitation.

The main causes of mitral regurgitation

- Annular dilatation (functional regurgitation)
- Mitral valve prolapse (floppy mitral valve)
- Myxomatous degeneration
- Ischaemic (eg papillary muscle dysfunction)
- Chronic rheumatic disease
- Other structural heart disease such as HCM and congenital heart defects
- Endocarditis, disorders of collagen such as Marfan's syndrome, connective tissue diseases.

Investigations

ECG – may show atrial fibrillation and high voltage QRS complexes

Chest radiograph (CXR) – LV and LA enlargement, prominent pulmonary vessels

Echo – dilated LA and LV, regurgitant jet on colour flow mapping and Doppler, in advanced disease right heart involvement (raised RV pressure, PR and TR)

Transoesophageal echocardiography (TOE) – demonstrates the anatomical reason for the regurgitation, eg leaflet prolapse, annular dilatation, papillary muscle rupture

Cardiac catheterisation – MR jet on LV injection, prominent V wave on PA wedge trace.

Indicators of severe mitral regurgitation

- Small volume pulse
- Left ventricular enlargement due to overload
- Presence of third heart sound
- Mid-diastolic flow murmur
- Praecordial thrill, signs of pulmonary hypertension or congestion (cardiac failure).

The presence of symptoms and increasing left ventricular dilatation are indicators for surgery in the chronic setting. Operative mortalities are 2–7% for valvular replacements in patients with mild to moderate symptoms.

Treatment options

Conservative – those with mild or moderate degrees of regurgitation and no evidence of distorted cardiac anatomy are followed up with regular clinical and echo assessment.

MV repair – if an operation is required, repairing a native valve offers excellent long-term results; the key investigation in determining whether a valve is repairable is the TOE.

Valve replacement – with either biological or mechanical prostheses should only be undertaken in highly symptomatic patients with unrepairable valves, as long-term outcome is poor due to disruption of left ventricular structures.

3.3 Mitral stenosis

Again presenting with palpitations and breathlessness with particularly marked exertional symptoms; two-thirds of patients presenting are women and in the UK almost all will be first-generation immigrants of South Asian origin. Haemoptysis and dysphagia also occur due to pulmonary hypertension and atriomegaly respectively.

Examination findings

- Low pulse pressure
- Soft first heart sound
- Long diastolic murmur
- Very early opening snap, ie closer to S2 (lost if valves immobile)
- In advanced disease right heart involvement is evidenced by right ventricular heave, loud P2, pulmonary regurgitation (Graham–Steell murmur), tricuspid regurgitation.

The causes of mitral stenosis are:

- Chronic rheumatic heart disease
- Congenital disease

- Carcinoid
- Systemic lupus erythematosus (SLE).

Stenosis may occur at the cusp, commisure or chordal level and, once atrial fibrillation develops, increases thrombo-embolism risk by 17 times. Anticoagulation with warfarin is therefore mandatory.

Investigations

- **ECG** – bifid high-voltage P waves or AF, RV strain pattern (high-voltage R waves V1–3 and right axis deviation)
- **CXR** – LA and RV enlargement, prominent pulmonary vessels, carinal angle > 90°
- **Echo** – enlarged LA and RV, calcified immobile mitral valve leaflets, reduced mitral valve orifice area, elevated RV pressure
- **Cardiac catheterisation** – gradient between LA (PA wedge pressure) and left ventricular end-diastolic pressure (LVEDP) > 15 mmHg either at rest or induced by exertion (straight leg raises).

Treatment options

- Percutaneous balloon mitral valvuloplasty. Only possible when leaflets are not excessively calcified or regurgitant
- Valve replacement.

Mitral regurgitation and stenosis commonly coexist; the dominant lesion is more likely to be regurgitation if the following are present:

- Third or fourth heart sounds
- Displaced and hyperdynamic apex (left ventricular enlargement)
- ECG shows left ventricular hypertrophy and left axis deviation.

3.4 Aortic stenosis (AS)

Patients often present with the classic triad of symptoms: angina, dyspnoea and syncope. Unfortunately sudden death is not an uncommon presentation.

Examination findings are of a crescendo decrescendo murmur in the aortic area radiating to the carotids. The apex may be thrusting and displaced due to hypertrophy and in advanced cases there may be pulmonary oedema.

Causes of AS

AS is conventionally divided into subvalvular, valvular and supravalvular.

Subvalvular includes HCM (discussed later) and sub aortic membranes (rare).

Valvular (true AS) results from either degeneration and calcification of a previously normal valve (incidence increases with age) or a congenitally abnormal valve (most commonly bicuspid), which degenerates prematurely often presenting in the sixth decade.

Supravalvular AS is rare.

Associations of AS

- **Sudden death**: may occur in AS or in subvalvular stenosis due to ventricular tachycardia. The vulnerability to ventricular tachycardia is due to LVH.
- **Complete heart block**: may be due to calcification involving the upper ventricular septal tissue housing the conducting tissue. This may also occur post-operatively (after valve replacement) due to trauma.
- **Calcified emboli**: causing transient ischaemic attacks (TIAs) may arise in severe calcific AS.

Investigations

ECG – LV strain pattern (high-voltage QRS complexes and left axis deviation with ST and T wave changes laterally)

CXR – may show LV enlargement and pulmonary oedema

Echo – calcified AV with restricted opening and increased velocity on Doppler

Cardiac catheter – tranduced LV to aortic pressure drop across valve – may not be possible (or advisable) to cross valve.

Treatment

The only treatment is valve replacement. This should be considered in anyone with symptomatic, rapidly progressive or severe disease.

Indicators of severe AS
<ul><li>Signs of left ventricular failure</li><li>Soft single S2 or paradoxically split A2</li><li>Presence of praecordial thrill</li><li>Slow rising pulse with narrow pulse pressure</li><li>Late peaking of long murmur</li><li>Valve area <0.5 cm² on echocardiography</li><li>Gradient >60 mmHg on catheter</li></ul>

Pitfalls in assessment of AS

In end-stage severe AS the ventricular function becomes impaired and this can result in an artificially reduced gradient and quiet or even inaudible murmur.

3.5 Aortic regurgitation

Aortic regurgitation presents predominantly with breath-lessness. Examination reveals a collapsing pulse, wide pulse pressure, a variety of eponymous pulse signs (*see* Box), a displaced dynamic apex and diastolic murmur beginning immediately after the second heart sound.

Causes of aortic regurgitation

- Congenitally abnormal valve – eg bicuspid AV
- Acquired valve abnormality – infection (endocarditis) or inflammation (rheumatic heart disease or connective tissue disease)
- Dilatation of the aortic root – hypertension, Marfan's, syphilis, type A aortic dissection

Eponymous signs associated with AR

- Quincke's sign – nail bed fluctuation of capillary flow
- Corrigan's pulse – (waterhammer); collapsing radial pulse
- Corrigan's sign – visible carotid pulsation
- De Musset's sign – head nodding with each systole
- Duroziez's sign – audible femoral bruits with diastolic flow (indicating moderate severity)
- Traube's sign – 'pistol shots' (systolic auscultatory finding of the femoral arteries)
- Austin Flint murmur – functional mitral diastolic flow murmur
- Müller's sign – pulsation of the uvula

Investigations

ECG – may show LV strain pattern

CXR – LV enlargement

Echo – AR is detected on colour flow and Doppler; the LV may be enlarged, as may the aortic root

Cardiac catheter – aortogram shows contrast passing retrogradely into the LV.

Indications for surgery

The principles for timing surgery in AR are similar to those in MR. Symptoms, severe disease and LV dilatation all indicate the need for valve replacement.

Acute severe AR will not be tolerated for long by a normal ventricle and therefore requires prompt surgery, except in the case of infection where delay for antibiotic therapy is preferable (if haemodynamic stability allows). At 10 years, 50% of patients with moderate chronic AR are alive, but once symptoms occur deterioration is rapid.

Valve replacement is the only definitive treatment option.

3.6 Other valvular lesions

Tricuspid regurgitation is characterised by giant V waves in the JVP and a pansystolic murmur louder at the lower left sternal edge and accentuated by inspiration.

Tricuspid stenosis is rare but causes gross peripheral oedema and a diastolic murmur.

Pulmonary stenosis causes an ejection systolic murmur which does not radiate to the carotids.

Pulmonary regurgitation causes an early diastolic murmur best heard in the pulmonary area.

3.7 Other causes of murmurs

- **Benign flow murmurs** are soft, short systolic murmurs heard along the left sternal edge to the pulmonary area, without any other cardiac auscultatory, ECG or chest X-ray abnormalities. Thirty per cent of children have an innocent flow murmur.
- **Hypertrophic cardiomyopathy** is associated with pansystolic and ejection systolic murmurs.
- **High output states** such as sepsis, pregnancy and exertion are all associated with flow murmurs.

Table 3 **Typical heart sounds and their diagnosis**

Heart sound	Most common lesion
Pan systolic murmur	Mitral regurgitation
Ejection systolic murmur	Aortic stenosis
Mid systolic click and late systolic murmur	Mitral valve prolapse
Opening snap and mid diastolic murmur	Mitral stenosis
Early diastolic murmur	Aortic regurgitation

3.8 Prosthetic valves

Valve prostheses may be metal or tissue (bioprosthetic). Mechanical valves are more durable but require full lifelong anticoagulation. All prostheses must be covered with antibiotic therapy for dental and surgical procedures; they have a residual transvalvular gradient across them.

Mechanical valves

- **Starr–Edwards**: ball and cage – ejection systolic murmur (ESM) in aortic area and an opening sound in mitral position are normal.

- **Bjork–Shiley**: single tilt disc – audible clicks without stethoscope.
- **St Judes/Carbomedics**: double tilt discs with clicks.

Tissue valves

- **Carpentier–Edwards**: porcine three-cusp valve – 3 months' anticoagulation needed until tissue endothelialisation. No need for long-term anticoagulation if patient is in sinus rhythm.
- **Homografts**: usually cadaveric and, again, need no long-term anticoagulation.

Anticoagulation in pregnancy

Warfarin may cause fetal haemorrhage and has a teratogenicity risk of 5–30%. This risk is dose-dependent and abnormalities include chondrodysplasia, mental impairment, optic atrophy and nasal hypoplasia. The risk of spontaneous abortion may be increased. At 36 weeks it is advised to switch to intravenous heparin for delivery. Breast-feeding is not a problem with warfarin. In all cases, consideration of the health of the mother should be paramount.

3.9 Infective endocarditis

- *Streptococcus viridans* (α haemolytic group) is still the most common organism, occurring in 50% of cases.
- Marantic (metastatic-related) and SLE-related (Libman–Sacks) endocarditis are causes of non-infective endocarditis.

See also Section 3.8 on Prosthetic valves.

Signs of infective endocarditis

As well as cardiac murmurs detected at auscultation, there are several other characteristic features of infective endocarditis:

- **Systemic signs of fever and arthropathy**
- **Hands and feet**: splinter haemorrhages, Osler nodes (painful), Janeway lesions (painless) and clubbing (late); needle track signs may occur in arm or groin
- **Retinopathy**: Roth spots
- **Hepatosplenomegaly**
- **Signs of arterial embolisation** (eg stroke or digital ischaemia).

Poor prognostic factors in endocarditis

- Prosthetic valve
- *Staphylococcus aureus* infection
- Culture-negative endocarditis
- Depletion of complement levels.

Indications for surgery

- Cardiac failure or haemodynamic compromise
- Extensive valve incompetence
- Large vegetations
- Septic emboli
- Abscess formation
- Fungal infection
- Antibiotic-resistant endocarditis
- Failure to respond to medical therapy

Antibiotic prophylaxis

This is indicated in the following:

Indications for antibiotic prophylaxis

Higher risk

- Prosthetic heart valves
- Previous infective endocarditis
- Cyanotic congenital heart disease
- PDA
- VSD
- AR/AS
- Mitral regurgitation (MR)
- Mitral stenosis (MS) and MR
- Coarctation

Intermediate risk

- Mitral valve prolapse with regurgitation
- Pure MS
- Tricuspid and pulmonary valve disease
- Asymmetrical septal hypertrophy
- Bicuspid aortic valve

- Antibiotic prophylaxis is indicated for all dental (including scaling of teeth), surgical, obstetric and gynaecological procedures, rigid bronchoscopy, urethral catheterisation (if urinary infection present) and vaginal delivery (if complicated by infection).
- Prophylaxis is not generally recommended for cardiac catheterisation or for upper GI endoscopy.
- Prophylaxis is not required for patients with isolated secundum ASD or mitral valve prolapse without regurgitation/murmur.

Infection of prosthetic valves

- Mortality is still as high as 60% depending on the organism.

- Within 6 months of implantation, it is usually due to colonisation by *Staphylococcus epidermidis*.
- Aortic root abscesses may cause PR interval lengthening.
- Valvular sounds may be muffled by vegetations; new murmurs may occur.
- Mild haemolysis may occur, and is detected by the presence of urobilinogen in the urine.
- Dehiscence is an ominous feature requiring urgent intervention.

4. CONGENITAL HEART DISEASE

Congenital heart disease is often divided into cyanotic and acyanotic disorders. Cyanotic heart disease is often associated with finger clubbing.

Causes of congenital acyanotic heart disease

- With shunts
  - VSD
  - ASD
  - PDA
  - Partial anomalous venous drainage
- Without shunts
  - Congenital aortic stenosis
  - Aortic coarctation

Causes of cyanotic heart disease

- With shunts
  - Fallot's tetralogy (VSD)
  - Severe Ebstein's anomaly (ASD)
  - Complete transposition of great vessels (ASD ± VSD/PDA)
- Without shunts
  - Tricuspid atresia
  - Severe pulmonary stenosis
  - Pulmonary atresia
  - Hypoplastic left heart

4.1 Atrial septal defect (ASD)

Atrial septal defects (ASDs) are the most common congenital defects found in adulthood. Rarely, they may present as stroke in young people, due to paradoxical embolus that originated in the venous system and reached the cerebral circulation via right to left shunting. Fixed splitting of the second heart sound is the hallmark of an uncorrected ASD. There may be a left parasternal heave and a pulmonary ejection systolic murmur due to increased blood flow. There are three main sub-types:

- **Secundum (70%)**: central fossa ovalis defects often associated with mitral valve prolapse (10–20% of cases). ECG shows incomplete or complete RBBB with *right* axis deviation. Note that the **patent foramen ovale** (slit-like deficiency in the fossa ovalis) occurs in 25% of the population, but this does not allow equalisation of atrial pressures, unlike ASD.
- **Primum (15%)**: sited above the atrio-ventricular valves, often associated with varying degrees of mitral and tricuspid regurgitation and occasionally a VSD, and thus usually picked up earlier in childhood. ECG shows RBBB, left axis deviation, 1° heart block. Associated with Down's, Klinefelter's and Noonan's syndromes.
- **Sinus venosus (15%)**: defect in the upper septum, often associated with anomalous pulmonary venous drainage directly into the right atrium.

Investigations should include chest X-ray, echo and cardiac catheterisation.

Operative closure is recommended if pulmonary to systolic flow ratios are above 1.5:1 to prevent development of pulmonary hypertension. Closure of secundum defects may be performed via cardiac catheterisation.

4.2 Ventricular septal defect (VSD)

Ventricular septal defects (VSD) are the most common isolated congenital defect (2/1000 births; around 30% of all congenital defects); spontaneous closure occurs in 30–50% of cases (usually muscular or membranous types). It is commonly associated with Down's syndrome.

- Irreversible pulmonary changes may occur from 1 year of age, with vascular hypertrophy and pulmonary arteriolar thrombosis, leading to Eisenmenger's syndrome.
- Parasternal thrill and pansystolic murmur are present. The murmur may be ejection systolic in very small or very large defects. With large defects the aortic component of the second sound is obscured, or even a single/palpable S2 is heard; a mitral diastolic murmur may occur. The apex beat is typically hyperdynamic.

There is a high risk of subacute bacterial endocarditis (SBE) with defects of any size and thus antibiotic prophylaxis is necessary.

Eisenmenger's complex describes the development of

reactive pulmonary hypertension. The thrill and left sternal edge (LSE) murmur abate and signs are of pulmonary hypertension ± regurgitation and right ventricular failure. Surgery should occur earlier to avoid this situation.

4.3 Patent ductus arteriosus (PDA)

Patent ductus arteriosus (PDA) is common in premature babies, particularly female infants born at high altitude; also if maternal rubella occurs in the first trimester. The connection occurs between the pulmonary trunk and the descending aorta, usually just distal to the origin of the left subclavian artery. PDA often occurs with other abnormalities.

Key features of PDA

- A characteristic left subclavicular thrill
- Enlarged left heart and apical heave
- Continuous 'machinery' murmur
- Wide pulse pressure and bounding pulse

4.4 Coarctation of the aorta

Coarctation may present in infancy with heart failure, or in adulthood (third decade) with hypertension, exertional breathlessness or leg weakness. This 'shelf-like' obstruction of the aortic arch, usually distal to the left subclavian artery, is 2–5 times more common in males and is responsible for about 7% of congenital heart defects.

Treatment is by surgical resection, preferably with end-to-end aortic anastomosis, or by balloon angioplasty for recurrence after surgery (which occurs in 5–10% of cases). Complications may occur despite resection/repair and these include hypertension, heart failure, Berry aneurysm rupture, premature coronary artery disease and aortic dissection (in the third or fourth decade of life).

4.5 Eisenmenger's syndrome

Reversal of left to right shunt, due to massive irreversible pulmonary hypertension (usually due to congenital cardiovascular malformations), leads to Eisenmenger's syndrome. This is significant as the pulmonary hypertension drastically alters the surgery required, from shunt closure to heart–lung transplantation.

4.6 Tetralogy of Fallot

The most common cause of cyanotic congenital heart disease (10%) usually presenting after age 6 months (as the condition may worsen after birth).

Key features of tetralogy of Fallot

- Pulmonary stenosis (causes the systolic murmur)
- Right ventricular hypertrophy
- VSD
- Overriding of aorta

5. ARRHYTHMIAS AND PACING

The normal heart beat is sinus rhythm with a rate between 60 and 100 bpm. Slower and faster rates are normal if there is adequate physiological explanation but apart from this any other activation sequence or rate is an arrhythmia.

Arrhythmias are subdivided into brady and tachy arrhythmias. Tachyarrhythmias are further subdivided anatomically into atrial and ventricular, by ECG into broad and narrow complex or by aetiology into re entry and automatic.

Atrial fibrillation remains the most common cardiac arrhythmia, with incidence increasing with age (Framingham data indicate a prevalence of 76/1000 males and 63/1000 females aged 85–94 years). It may be associated with brady or tachy rhythms or indeed remain within the range of 60–100 bpm.

Essential note

The risk of CVA in atrial fibrillation is reduced by more than two-thirds by formal anticoagulation with warfarin but absolute risk is low in under 50s with structurally normal hearts

Use of the term 'supraventricular tachycardia' (SVT) is best avoided as it is imprecise, particularly as radiofrequency ablation is changing the face of treatment in this condition. Ventricular tachycardia and fibrillation are life-threatening conditions, but implantable defibrillators and catheter or surgical ablation can now be used in addition to conventional pharmacological therapy.

5.1 Brady arrhythmias

Atrioventricular block

Complete heart block (CHB)

Untreated acquired CHB is associated with mortality that may exceed 50% at 1 year, particularly in patients aged over 80 years and in those with non-rheumatic structural heart disease.

- CHB is the most common reason for permanent pacing.
- It occurs mostly with right coronary artery occlusion, when related to an infarction, as the AV nodal branch is usually one of the distal branches of the right coronary artery.
- CHB rarely (3–7% of patients) requires permanent pacing when it occurs after acute infarction.
- In patients with an anterior infarct, CHB is a poor prognostic feature, indicating extensive ischaemia.

Mobitz type II AV block
A fixed proportion of atrial impulses are conducted to the ventricle resulting in 2:1, 3:1 or 4:1 block. It is also an indication for permanent pacing.

Mobitz type I (Wenkeback) AV block
The AV interval increases with each beat until a ventricular impulse is dropped. Not usually an indication for pacing.

First degree AV block
A PR interval >200 ms, not an indication for pacing unless associated with syncope and other conduction disturbance.

Narrow complex tachycardias
All of the rhythms listed in this section can also present with broad complexes

AV nodal re-entry tachycardia (AVNRT): also known as junctional tachycardia and often referred to as SVT, and involves a re-entry circuit in or around the AV node.

AV re-entry tachycardia (AVRT): this involves an abnormal connection between the atria and ventricles some distance from the AV node (eg Wolff–Parkinson–White syndrome).

Atrial flutter: the atrial rate is usually between 250 and 350 beats/min and is often seen with a ventricular response of 150 (2:1 block) beats/min. The block may vary between a 1:1 ratio to 1:4 or even 1:5. Isolated atrial flutter (without atrial fibrillation) is uncommon and has a lower association with thromboembolism; however, at the present time anticoagulation is often recommended with prolonged flutter.

The ventricular response may be slowed by increasing the vagal block of the AV node (eg carotid sinus massage) or by adenosine which 'uncovers' the flutter waves on ECG.

Atrial fibrillation (AF): this arrhythmia is due to multiple wavelet propagation in different directions. AF may be paroxysmal, persistent (but 'cardiovertable') or permanent, and in all three states is a risk factor for strokes. Treatment is aimed at ventricular rate control, cardioversion, recurrence prevention and anticoagulation.

Common associations with AF

- Ischaemic heart disease (IHD)
- Mitral valve disease
- Hypertension
- Thyroid disease
- Acute alcohol excess/chronic alcoholic cardiomyopathy
- Any structural heart disease

The overall risk of systemic emboli in AF is 5–7% annually (higher with rheumatic valve disease); this falls to 1.6% with anticoagulation.

5.2 Ventricular arrhythmias and long QT syndromes

Ventricular tachycardia (monomorphic)
Ventricular tachycardia (VT) has a poor prognosis when left ventricular function is impaired. After the exclusion of reversible causes such patients may need implantable defibrillators and anti-arrhythmic therapy.

- Ventricular rate is usually 120–200 beats/min.
- Patients should be DC cardioverted when there is haemodynamic compromise; overdrive pacing may also terminate VT.
- Amiodarone, beta blockers, flecainide and lignocaine may be therapeutic adjuncts or prophylactic agents; magnesium may also be useful.

Associations of ventricular tachycardia

- Myocardial ischaemia
- Hypokalaemia or severe hyperkalaemia
- Long QT syndrome (see below)
- Digoxin toxicity (VT may arise from either ventricle, especially with associated hypokalaemia)
- Cardiomyopathies
- Congenital abnormalities of the right ventricular outflow tract (VT with LBBB and right axis deviation pattern)

Features favouring ventricular tachycardia (VT) in broad complex tachycardia
It is often difficult to distinguish VT from SVT with aberration (disordered ventricular propagation of a supraventricular impulse); VT remains the most common cause of a broad complex tachycardia, especially with a previous history of myocardial infarction (MI). The following ECG observations favour VT:

- Capture beats: intermittent SA node complexes transmitted to ventricle
- Fusion beats: combination QRS from SA node and VT focus meeting and fusing
- Right bundle branch block (RBBB) with left axis deviation (LAD)
- Very wide QRS >140 ms
- Altered QRS compared to sinus rhythm
- V leads concordance with all QRS vectors, positive or negative
- Dissociated P waves: marching through the VT
- History of ischaemic heart disease: very good predictor
- Variable S1
- HR <170 beats/min with no effect of carotid sinus massage.

Essential note

In structurally abnormal hearts broad complex tachycardias should be assumed to be ventricular tachycardia until proven otherwise

Ventricular tachycardia (polymorphic) – torsades des pointes

Anti-arrhythmic agents (particularly class III) may predispose to torsades as the arrhythmia is often initiated during bradycardia. The VT is polymorphic (QRS complexes of different amplitudes twist around the isoelectric line), with QT prolongation when patient is in sinus rhythm.

- Intravenous magnesium and potassium may control the arrhythmia, whereas isoprenaline and temporary pacing may prevent bradycardia and hence the predisposition to VT
- May be due to QT prolongation of any cause (see later).

Long QT states

Abnormally prolonged QT (>460 ms) intervals may be familial or acquired, and are associated with syncope and sudden death, due to ventricular tachycardia (especially torsades des pointes). Mortality in the untreated symptomatic patient with congenital abnormality is high but some patients may reach the age of 50–60 years despite repeated attacks. Causes and associations are shown below.

Causes and associations of prolonged QT intervals

- Familial

    - Jervell–Lange–Neilsen syndrome
    - Romano Ward syndrome

- Ischaemic heart disease
- Metabolic

    - Hypocalcaemia
    - Hypothyroidism
    - Hypothermia
    - Hypokalaemia

- Rheumatic carditis
- Mitral valve prolapse
- Drugs

Cardiac causes of electro-mechanical dissociation (EMD)

When faced with a cardiac arrest situation it is important to appreciate the list of causes of electro-mechanical dissociation (EMD).

- Hypoxia
- Hypovolaemia
- Hypokalaemia/hyperkalaemia
- Hypothermia
- Tension pneumothorax
- Tamponade
- Toxic/therapeutic disturbance
- Thromboembolic/mechanical obstruction.

5.3 Pacing and ablation procedures

Temporary pacing

The ECG will show LBBB morphology (unless there is septal perforation when it is RBBB). Pacing may be ventricular (right ventricle apex) or atrio-ventricular (atrial appendage and right ventricle apex) for optimised cardiac output.

Complications include:

- Crossing the tricuspid valve during insertion causes ventricular ectopics, as does irritating the outflow tract.
- Atrial or right ventricular perforation and pericardial effusion.
- **Pneumothorax**: internal jugular route is preferable to subclavian as it minimises this risk and also allows control after inadvertent arterial punctures.

Permanent pacing

More complex permanent pacing systems include rate-responsive models which use piezocrystal movement sensors or physiological triggers (respiratory rate or QT interval) to increase heart rates. Although more expensive they avoid causing pacemaker syndrome and they act more physiologically for optimal left ventricular function.

Indications for temporary pacing

- Asystole
- Haemodynamically compromised bradycardia
- Prophylaxis of myocardial infarction complicated by second-degree or complete heart block
- Prior to high-risk cardiac interventions or pacemaker replacement
- Prevention of some tachyarrhythmias (eg torsades)
- Overdrive termination of various arrhythmias (eg atrial flutter, VT)

Indications for permanent pacing

- Chronic atrio-ventricular block
- Sick sinus syndrome with symptoms (including chronotropic incompetence – the inability to appropriately increase the heart rate with activity)
- Chronotropic incompetence
- Post-AV nodal ablation for arrhythmias
- Neurocardiogenic syncope
- Hypertrophic cardiomyopathy
- Dilated cardiomyopathy (may pace more than two chambers)
- Long QT syndrome
- Prevention of atrial fibrillation
- Post-cardiac transplantation

Pacing in heart failure

There are several synonymous terms for pacing in patients with cardiac failure. These include cardiac resynchronisation therapy, biventricular pacing or multisite pacing. The indications for pacing in heart failure are all of the following:

- NYHA III-IV heart failure
- QRS duration >130 ms
- Left ventricular ejection fraction <35% with dilated ventricle and patient on optimal medical therapy (diuretics, angiotensin-converting enzyme (ACE) inhibitors and beta blockers).

The atria and right ventricle are paced in the usual fashion and in addition to this a pacing electrode is placed in a tributary of the coronary sinus on the lateral aspect of the left ventricle. The two ventricles are paced simultaneously or near simultaneously with a short atrio-ventricular delay. The aim is to optimise AV delay and reduce inter- and intraventricular asynchrony. This therapy is known to improve exercise capacity, quality of life and to reduce hospital admissions.

Implantable cardioverter defibrillators (ICD)

ICD are devices that are able to detect life-threatening tachyarrhythmias and to terminate them by overdrive pacing or a counter shock. They are implanted in a similar manner to permanent pacemakers. Current evidence supports their use in both secondary prevention of cardiac arrest and also as targeted primary prevention (eg individuals with left ventricular impairment and those with familial syndromes predisposing to sudden cardiac death).

Radiofrequency ablation

Radiofrequency ablation is heat-mediated (65°C) protein membrane disruption causing cell lysis without the risk of coagulum forming on the electrode tip. Using cardiac catheterisation (with electrodes in right- or left-sided chambers) it interrupts electrical pathways in cardiac structures. Excellent results are obtained with accessory pathways, the His–Purkinje system or for AV nodal ablation. It is technically more difficult in atrial flutter (where a line of block across the atrium is required) and in VT (ventricular myocardium is much thicker than atrial). Ablation for atrial fibrillation is a rapidly developing technique. This involves isolating the pulmonary veins by ablation therapy, and it currently has a modest success rate of around a 60% cure. Complete heart block and pericardial effusions are rare complications of radiofrequency ablation.

6. ISCHAEMIC HEART DISEASE

Cardiovascular disease remains the largest cause of death in the UK, accounting for almost 250 000 deaths (77 000 from myocardial infarction) in 1994 (compared to 140 000 deaths from malignant disease). Ischaemic heart disease may present with an acute ischaemic event, heart failure or with arrhythmia.

Essential note

The major cardiovascular risk factors are smoking, diabetes, hypertension, dyslipidaemia and family history

Risk factors for coronary artery disease (CAD)

- **Primary**

  - Hypercholesterolaemia (LDL)
  - Hypertension
  - Smoking

- **Protective factors**

  - Exercise
  - Moderate amounts of alcohol
  - Low cholesterol diet
  - Increased HDL:LDL

- **Secondary**

  - Reduced HDL cholesterol
  - Obesity
  - Insulin-dependent diabetes mellitus (IDDM)
  - Non-insulin-dependent diabetes (NIDDM)
  - Family history of CAD
  - Physical inactivity
  - Stress and personality type
  - Gout and hyperuricaemia
  - Race (Asians)
  - Low birth weight
  - Male sex
  - Chronic renal failure
  - Increasing age
  - Low social class
  - Increased homocystine levels and homocystinuria

Smoking and its relationship to cardiovascular disease

Smokers have an increased incidence of the following cardiovascular complications:

- Coronary artery disease
- Malignant hypertension
- Ischaemic stroke
- Morbidity from peripheral vascular disease
- Sudden death
- Subarachnoid haemorrhage
- Mortality due to aortic aneurysm
- Thromboembolism in patients taking oral contraceptives

Both active and passive smoking increase the risk of coronary atherosclerosis by a number of mechanisms. These include:

- Increased platelet adhesion/aggregation and whole blood viscosity
- Increased heart rate; increased catecholamine sensitivity/release
- Increased carboxyhaemoglobin level and, as a result, increased haematocrit
- Decreased HDL cholesterol and vascular compliance
- Decreased threshold for ventricular fibrillation.

6.1 Angina

Other than the usual forms of stable and unstable angina, those worthy of specific mention include:

- **Decubitus**: usually on lying down – due to an increase in LVEDP or associated with dreaming, cold sheets, or coronary spasm during REM sleep.
- **Variant (Prinzmetal)**: unpredictable, at rest, with transient ST elevation on ECG. Due to coronary spasm, with or without underlying arteriosclerotic lesions.
- **Syndrome X**: this refers to a heterogeneous group of patients who have ST segment depression on exercise test, but angiographically normal coronary arteries. The patients may have very small vessel disease and/or abnormal ventricular function. It is commonly described in middle-aged females and oestrogen deficiency has been suggested to be an aetiological factor.
- **Vincent angina**: nothing to do with cardiology; infection of pharyngeal and tonsillar space!

Causes of non-anginal chest pains

- Pericardial pain
- Aortic dissection
- Mediastinitis

  - Associated with trauma, pneumothorax or diving

- Pleural

  - Usually with breathlessness in pleurisy, pneumonia, pneumothorax or a large peripheral pulmonary embolus.

- Musculoskeletal
- Gastrointestinal

  - Including oesophageal, gastric, gallbladder, pancreatic

Causes of non-anginal chest pains

- Hyperventilation/anxiety
- Mitral valve prolapse

  - May be spontaneous, sharp, superficial, short-lived pain

Symptomatic assessment of angina

The Canadian cardiovascular assessment of chest pain is useful for grading the severity of angina:

- **Grade I**: angina only on strenuous or prolonged exertion
- **Grade II**: angina on climbing two flights of stairs
- **Grade III**: angina on walking one block on the level
- **Grade IV**: angina at rest (indication for urgent intervention).

6.2 Myocardial infarction

Myocardial infarction (MI) occurs with an annual incidence of 5/1000 in the UK. The mortality associated with MI remains high, with an overall mortality of 27% at 28 days post-MI. The difference between MI and angina is the permanent damage which occurs in MI.

Diagnosis of MI

Acute, evolving or recent MI

Either one of the following criteria satisfies the diagnosis for an acute, evolving or recent MI.

- Typical rise and gradual fall (troponin) or more rapid rise and fall (CK-MB) of biochemical markers of myocardial necrosis with at least one of the following:

  - Ischaemic symptoms
  - Development of pathologic Q waves on the ECG
  - ECG changes indicative of ischaemia (ST segment elevation or depression)
  - Coronary artery intervention (eg coronary angioplasty).

- Pathologic finding of an acute MI (eg at post-mortem).

Established MI

Any one of the following criteria satisfies the diagnosis of an established MI:

- Development of new pathologic Q waves on serial ECGs. The patient may or may not remember previous symptoms. Biochemical markers of myocardial necrosis may have normalised, depending on the length of time that has passed since the infarct developed.
- Pathologic finding of a healed or healing MI.

Distinction between STEMI (ST segment elevation MI) and NSTEMI

An acute MI should be classified as **STEMI** when there is :

- ST segment elevation (≥2 mm in two or more chest leads, or ≥1 mm in two or more limb leads)
- A chronic MI with Q wave formation
- Pathological or imaging evidence of a full thickness scar.

Other MI that do not meet these criteria should be classified as **NSTEMI**.

Cardiac enzymes

A number of markers of cardiac damage are now available. Table 4 is a guide to the timing of the initial rise, peak and return to normality.

Table 4				
Marker	Initial rise	Peak	Return to normal	Notes
Creatine phosphokinase	4–8 h	18 h	2–3 days	CPK-MB is main cardiac isoenzyme
Myoglobin	1–4 h	6–7 h	24 h	Low specificity from skeletal muscle damage
Troponin	3–12 h	24 h	3–10 days	Troponins I and T are the most sensitive and specific markers of myocardial damage available
Lactate dehydrogenase (LDH)	10 h	24–48 h	14 days	Cardiac muscle mainly contains LDH

Troponins I and T

Troponins I and T are the most sensitive and specific markers of myocardial damage available. Troponin assays (INT) have proved to be extremely helpful in the diagnostic and prognostic assessment of patients presenting with acute coronary syndromes. They are reliably positive from 12 hours after the onset of ischaemia. False-positive troponin elevations occur in renal impairment and in uncontrolled diabetes.

Complications after MI

- Anterior infarctions

  - Late VT/VF
  - Left ventricular aneurysm
  - Left ventricular thrombus. Prescribe warfarin if present to prevent systemic embolism
  - CHB (rare)
  - Ischaemic mitral regurgitation
  - Congestive cardiac failure
  - Cardiac rupture – usually at days 4–10 with EMD
  - VSD with septal rupture
  - Pericarditis and pericardial effusion (**Dressler's** syndrome with high ESR, fever, anaemia, pleural effusions and anti-cardiac muscle antibodies is seen occasionally)

- Inferior infarctions

  - Higher re-infarction rate
  - Inferior aneurysm – with mitral regurgitation (rare)
  - Pulmonary embolism (rare)
  - CHB and other degrees of heart block
  - Papillary muscle dysfunction and mitral regurgitation
  - Right ventricular infarcts need high filling pressures (particularly if posterior extension)

Post-MI rehabilitation

After myocardial infarction, a patient should take 2 months off work and 1 month's abstinence from sexual intercourse and driving (see next section). Cardiac rehabilitation is particularly important for patient confidence. Depression occurs in 30% of patients.

Fitness to drive

The DVLA provides extensive guidelines for coronary disease and interventions, but the essential points are:

- Ordinary drivers do not need to inform the DVLA of cardiac events unless a continuing disability results. Driving should be avoided for 1 month after MI, coronary artery bypass grafting (CABG) and unstable angina, and for 1 week after percutaneous coronary angioplasty (PCI) or pacemaker insertion.
- Vocational drivers (HGV, etc) must inform the DVLA. They should not recommence driving until 3 months post-MI or CABG, and they must be symptom free and able to complete the first three stages of a Bruce protocol safely (off treatment for 24 hours), without symptoms, signs or ECG changes.
- Implantation of cardiac defibrillators usually results in loss of licence, although this may be reconsidered if the patient remains shock free for at least 6 months.

6.3 Thrombolysis

Thrombolysis is beneficial up to 6 hours after pain onset but may be given for up to 12 hours in the context of continuing pain or deteriorating condition. Recanalisation after thrombolysis occurs in 70% (vs. 15% without thrombolysis) of patients and results in a higher, earlier CPK rise (but a lower total CPK release). Reperfusion arrhythmias are common within the first 2 hours after thrombolysis. Theoretically (but often impractical in the UK) primary angioplasty is better than thrombolysis for acute MI if performed within the first few hours.

Tissue plasminogen activator (TPA) and similar recombinant agents are five to seven times more expensive than streptokinase (SK) and should be used only in patients to whom SK has previously been administered, or where local guidelines permit.

Contraindications to thrombolysis

Although there are numerous relative contraindications where the risk/benefit considerations are individual to the patient (eg a large anterior infarct in a patient where access to primary PCI is unavailable), there are several absolute contraindications to thrombolysis.

Contraindications to thrombolysis

- Absolute

  - Active internal bleeding or uncontrollable external bleeding
  - Suspected aortic dissection
  - Recent head trauma (<2 weeks)
  - Intracranial neoplasms
  - History of proven haemorrhagic stroke or cerebral infarction <2 months earlier
    Uncontrolled blood pressure (>200/120 mmHg)
  - Pregnancy

- Relative
  - Traumatic prolonged cardio-pulmonary resuscitation
  - Bleeding disorders
  - Recent surgery
  - Probable intracardiac thrombus (eg AF with mitral stenosis)
  - Active diabetic haemorrhagic retinopathy
  - Anticoagulation or INR >1.8
  - Active untreated diabetic haemorrhagic retinopathy

Groups particularly benefiting from thrombolysis (determined by the GUSTO, ISIS 2 and ISIS 3 trials) include:

- Large anterior infarction
- Pronounced ST elevation
- Elderly (>75 years)

- Poor left ventricular function or LBBB, or systolic BP <100 mmHg
- Early administration: within 1 hour of pain onset.

6.4 Cardiac revascularisation

Angioplasty

Often referred to as **percutaneous coronary intervention** (PCI), this procedure has evolved from plain balloon angioplasty, through bare metal stenting to drug eluting stents. Adjunct drug therapies are predominantly antiplatelet drugs.

Indications for PCI include acute ischaemia, either as a primary treatment or following failed thrombolysis, and stable angina.

The immediate complications include infarction (which may require emergency bypass grafting) and bleeding. In-stent thrombosis may occur within the first 6 months of a bare metal stent insertion or at any stage after drug eluting stenting.

Later restenosis of the dilated vessel occurs at a rate of 30% after plain balloon angioplasty but is very rare in drug eluting stents.

Table 5 Summary of clinical trials in patients with acute MI

Agents used for acute MI	Mortality in treated group (%)	Mortality in control subjects (%)	Number treated to save 1 life	Trials involved
Aspirin	9.4 (at 5 weeks)	11.8	42	ISIS 2
Thrombolytics	10.7* (at 21 days)	13.0*	43*	GISSI 1*, ISIS 2, TIMI II, GUSTO
Beta-blockers	3.9 (at 7 days)	4.6	143	ISIS 1
ACE inhibitors	35.2* (after 39-month mean follow-up)	39.7*	22*	SAVE, SOLVD*, AIRE
Lipid-lowering therapy (patients with average cholesterol)	10.2 (after 5 years)	13.2	33	CARE (note endpoints included second non-fatal MI and cardiac deaths)
Heparin with aspirin and any form of thrombolysis	8.6	9.1	200	Meta-analysis of 68, 000 patients
Magnesium: contradictory data but no mortality reduction				LIMIT 1, 2, ISIS 4
Nitrates: no clear benefit				ISIS 4, GISSI 3
Warfarin: no proven benefit above aspirin after thrombolysis				

* Data from that particular trial.

Coronary artery bypass grafting (CABG)

Coronary artery bypass grafting (CABG) has clear benefits in specific groups of patients with chronic coronary artery disease (when compared to medical therapy alone). Analysis has previously been limited because randomised trials included small numbers and were performed several decades ago; patients studied were usually males aged <65 years. The population now receiving CABG has changed, but so has medical therapy.

- Prognostic benefits are shown for symptomatic, significant left main stem disease (Veteran's Study), symptomatic proximal three-vessel disease and in two-vessel disease which includes the proximal left anterior descending (LAD) artery (CASS data).
- Patients with moderately impaired left ventricular function have greater benefit, but those with poor left ventricular function have greater operative mortality. Overall mortality is <2%, rising to between 5% and 10% for a second procedure; 80% of patients gain symptom relief.
- Peri-operative graft occlusion is around 10% for vein grafts, which otherwise last 8–10 years. Arterial grafts (internal mammary, gastro-epiploic) have a higher patency rate but long-term data are awaited.
- A 'Dressler-like' syndrome may occur up to 6 months post-surgery.
- Minimally invasive CABG involves the redirection of internal mammary arteries to coronary vessels without the need for cardiac bypass and full stenotomy incisions. Recovery times following this procedure are extremely short.

7. OTHER MYOCARDIAL DISEASES

7.1 Cardiac failure

Cardiac failure can be defined as the pumping action of the heart being insufficient to meet the circulatory demands of the body (in the absence of mechanical obstructions). A broad echocardiographic definition is of an ejection fraction (EF) <40% (as in the SAVE trial, which enrolled patients for ACE inhibitors post-MI). Overall 5-year survival is 65% with EF <40%, compared to 95% in those with EF >50%. The most common cause of cardiac failure in the Western world is ischaemic heart disease but there are several other possible aetiologies including toxins, viral and autoimmune conditions.

The ejection fraction is, however, only a guide and is dependent on other pre-load and after-load factors.

- **Pre-load**: will affect left ventricular end-diastolic pressure
- **After-load**: will affect left ventricular systolic wall tension.

Other echocardiographic features of LV dysfunction include reduced fractional shortening, LV enlargement and paradoxical septal motion.

The New York Heart Association (NYHA) classification is a helpful indication of severity.

Table 6 **NYHA classification**

NYHA class	Symptoms	One-year mortality (%)
I	Asymptomatic with ordinary activity	5–10
II	Slight limitation of physical activities	15
III	Marked limitation of physical activities	30
IV	Dyspnoeic symptoms at rest	50–60

Basic treatment of heart failure

- ACE inhibitors and beta blockers favourably alter neurohormonal activation, improving symptoms and prognosis in chronic heart failure
- Loop diuretics, spironolactone and digoxin all improve symptomatic status
- Anticoagulation is considered in some cases.

Essential note

ACE inhibitors and beta blockers are of prognostic benefit in heart failure and should be titrated up to maximum tolerated dose

7.2 Hypertrophic cardiomyopathy (HCM)

Hypertrophic cardiomyopathy is a heterogeneous group of genetic conditions linked by their propensity to cause left ventricular myocardial hypertrophy. The major risk associated with HCM is of arrhythmic death but there are also characteristic haemodynamic impacts. Thickening of the septum may impinge on the LV outflow tract causing a gradient and turbulent flow which sucks the anterior MV leaflet into the outflow tract (systolic anterior motion – SAM) exacerbating the obstruction and causing MR.

Characteristic features of HCM

- Jerky pulse with large tidal wave as outflow obstruction is overcome
- Large 'a' waves in JVP
- Double apical impulse (palpable atrial systole, S4, in sinus rhythm)
- LSE systolic thrill (turbulence) with harsh ESM radiating to axilla
- Often accompanied by mitral regurgitation
- Often paradoxical splitting of second heart sound
- The ejection systolic murmur increases with Valsalva manoeuvre and decreases with squatting.

Important points to remember

- ESM *increases* with: glyceryl trinitrate (GTN), digoxin and standing, due to volume reduction in diastole; ESM *decreases* with: squatting, beta-blockers, Valsalva release, handgrip.
- **Sudden death** may be due to catecholamine-driven extreme outflow obstruction, ventricular fibrillation related to accessory pathway or myocardial abnormalities – transmitted AF, or massive MI. Sudden death may occur without hypertrophy. Annual mortality of 2.5% in adults and 6% in children.
- Poor prognostic features include young age of diagnosis, family history of sudden death and syncopal symptoms, but there is no correlation with the left ventricular outflow tract gradient.
- HCM may be mimicked by long-term hypertension (so called HCMoid physiology).
- Some variants of HCM in some individuals may cause no hypertrophy but still increase arrhythmic risk.

Echocardiographic features of HCM (none alone are diagnostic)

- Asymmetrical septal hypertrophy: septum >30% thicker than left ventricular posterior wall
- Left ventricular outflow tract gradient ± turbulence
- Premature closure of aortic cusps
- Almost complete obliteration of left ventricular cavity
- Systolic anterior motion of anterior mitral valve cusp probably due to venturi effect (see on M mode)
- Hypertrophy which may only be apical

7.3 Dilated cardiomyopathy (DCM)

Dilated cardiomyopathy (DCM) is a syndrome of global ventricular dysfunction and dilatation, usually with macroscopically normal coronary arteries (if causes of ischaemic cardiomyopathy are excluded). Aetiology is often undetermined and the condition is more common in males and Afro-Caribbeans. There is often LBBB or poor R wave progression on ECG and anticoagulation may be warranted as the incidence of AF and ventricular thrombus is high.

Causes of DCM

- Alcohol
- Undiagnosed hypertension
- Autoimmune disease
- Nutritional deficiency (eg thiamine and selenium)
- Muscular dystrophies
- Viral infections (eg Coxsackie and HIV)
- Peripartum
- Drugs (eg doxorubicin)
- Infiltration (eg haemochromatosis, sarcoidosis)
- Tachycardia-mediated cardiomyopathy (uncontrolled fast heart rates, eg atrial fibrillation)

7.4 Restrictive cardiomyopathy

This produces identical symptoms to constrictive pericarditis (*see* Section 8.1) but surgery is of little use in restrictive cardiomyopathy. The ventricles are excessively rigid and impede diastolic filling. AF may supervene and stagnation of blood leads to thrombus formation.

- Causes
  - Idiopathic
  - Connective tissue disease
  - Amyloid (see below)
  - Sarcoid
  - Metabolic and storage disorders
  - Endomyocardial fibrosis
  - Carcinoid
  - Malignancy or radiotherapy

Cardiac amyloidosis

Cardiac amyloidosis behaves like restrictive cardiomyopathy but it may also be accompanied by pericardial thickening (due to nodular deposition), pericardial effusion and, rarely, tamponade. It is important to avoid digoxin in amyloid cardiac disease because of the risk of heart block and asystole.

7.5 Myocarditis

Myocarditis may be due to many different aetiological factors (eg viral, bacterial, fungal, protozoal, autoimmune, allergic and drugs). It may be self-limiting, relapsing or progressive resulting in a DCM picture. It is usually idiopathic but may be viral, toxic or autoimmune.

Rheumatic fever

This follows a group A streptococcal infection; pancarditis usually occurs and valvular defects are long-term sequelae. The cardiac histological marker is the Aschoff nodule. Patients are treated with penicillin and salicylates or steroids.

Criteria for diagnosis include the need for evidence of preceding β-haemolytic streptococcal infection (raised anti-streptococcal antibody titres (ASOT), positive throat swab or history of scarlet fever), together with two major (or one major and two minor) Duckett–Jones criteria (see below).

Rheumatic fever (Duckett–Jones diagnostic criteria)

- Major criteria

  - Carditis
  - Polyarthritis
  - Chorea
  - Erythema marginatum
  - Subcutaneous nodules

- Minor criteria

  - Fever
  - Arthralgia
  - Previous rheumatic heart disease
  - High ESR and CRP
  - Prolonged PR interval on ECG

7.6 Cardiac tumours

Myxomas are the most common cardiac tumours, comprising 50% of most pathological series.

Atrial myxomas: by far the commonest primary cardiac malignancy, they present with similar features to infective endocarditis with added heart sounds and features of vasculitis, embolism and occasionally obstruction. Slow growing, they are presumably present for years before diagnosis but once the diagnosis is made they are treated as a surgical emergency. They may be multiple and local recurrence is not uncommon.

Other primary cardiac tumours: these include papillomas, fibromas, lipomas, angiosarcomas, rhabdomyosarcomas and mesotheliomas, which are all rare lesions.

Metastatic involvement: the pericardium not infrequently becomes seeded by tumour resulting in effusions. Less commonly the myocardium may be involved.

7.7 Alcohol and the heart

Acute alcoholic intoxication is the most common cause of paroxysmal atrial fibrillation amongst younger individuals. Chronic excessive intake over 10 years is responsible for a third of the cases of dilated cardiomyopathy (DCM) in Western populations; alcohol is also aetiologically related to hypertension, CVA, arrhythmias and sudden death. Atrial fibrillation may be the first presenting feature (usually between the ages of 30 and 35 years).

Pathological mechanisms

- Direct myocardial toxic effect of alcohol and its metabolites
- Toxic effect of additives (eg cobalt)
- Secondary effect of associated nutritional deficiencies (eg thiamine)
- Effect of hypertension

Treatment includes nutritional correction and – most importantly – complete abstinence from alcohol, without which 50% with significant LV dysfunction will die within 5 years. Abstinence may lead to a marked recovery of resting cardiac function.

Beneficial mechanisms of modest amounts of alcohol

- Favourable effects on lipids (50% of this benefit is due to raised HDL levels)
- Anti-thrombotic effects (perhaps by raising natural levels of tissue plasminogen activator (t-PA))
- Anti-platelet effects (changes in prostacyclin:thromboxane ratios)
- Increase in insulin sensitivity
- Antioxidant effects of red wine (flavonoids and polyphenols)

7.8 Cardiac transplantation

With over 2500 heart-only transplants being performed in the USA each year, most often for intractable coronary disease and cardiomyopathy (44%), survival rates have been estimated at 80% at 1 year, 75% at 3 years and 40–50% at 10 years. Myocarditis is an indication, but may recur in the donor heart.

The major complications encountered after transplantation include accelerated coronary atheroma, lymphoma, skin cancer (and other tumours) and chronic renal failure (CRF) (due to ciclosporin toxicity)

8. PERICARDIAL DISEASE

8.1 Constrictive pericarditis

Rare in clinical practice, it presents in a similar way to restrictive cardiomyopathy, ie with signs of right-sided heart failure (cachexia, hepatomegaly, raised JVP, ascites and oedema) due to restriction of diastolic filling of both ventricles. It is treated by pericardial resection.

Other specific features include:

- A diastolic pericardial knock occurs after the third heart sound, at the time of the y descent of the JVP, and this reflects the sudden reduction of ventricular filling – 'the ventricle slaps against the rigid pericardium'.
- Soft heart sounds and impalpable apex beat.
- Severe pulsus paradoxus rarely occurs and indicates the presence of a co-existent tense effusion.
- Thickened, bright pericardium on echocardiography.

Causes of constrictive pericarditis

- Tuberculosis (usually post-pericardial effusion)
- Mediastinal radiotherapy
- Pericardial malignancy
- Drugs (eg hydralazine, associated with a lupus-like syndrome)
- Post-viral (especially haemorrhagic) or bacterial pericarditis
- Trauma/post-cardiac surgery
- Connective tissue disease
- Recurrent pericarditis

Signs common to constrictive pericarditis and restrictive cardiomyopathy

- Raised JVP with prominent x + y descents
- Atrial fibrillation
- Non-pulsatile hepatomegaly
- Normal systolic function

Some key features distinguish constrictive pericarditis from restrictive cardiomyopathy:

- Absence of LVH in constrictive pericarditis
- Absent calcification on chest X-ray, prominent apical impulse and conduction abnormalities on ECG, which are features of restrictive cardiomyopathy.

However, a combination of investigations, including cardiac CT, MRI and cardiac biopsy, may be necessary to differentiate between the two conditions.

8.2 Pericardial effusion

A slowly developing effusion of 2 litres can be accommodated by pericardial stretching and without raising the intrapericardial pressure. The classical symptoms of chest discomfort, dysphagia, hoarseness or dyspnoea (due to compression) may be absent. A large effusion can lead to muffled heart sounds, loss of apical impulse, occasional pericardial rub, small ECG complexes and eventually electromechanical dissociation.

Other key features are:

- **Pulsus alternans**: variable left ventricular output and right ventricular filling
- **Pulsus paradoxus**: exaggerated inspiratory fall in systolic BP
- **Electrical alternans on ECG**: 'swinging QRS axis'
- **Globular cardiac enlargement on chest X-ray**.

Causes of pericardial effusion

- All causes as listed for constrictive pericarditis
- Aortic dissection
- Iatrogenic due to pacing or cardiac catheterisation
- Ischaemic heart disease with ventricular rupture
- Anticoagulation associated with acute pericarditis

8.3 Cardiac tamponade

In contrast, if a small amount of intrapericardial fluid (eg <200 ml) accumulates rapidly, it can significantly limit ventricular filling, reduce cardiac output and elevate intracardiac pressures (particularly right-sided initially). Thus the 'y' descent due to right ventricular filling with tricuspid valve opening is lost as right ventricular pressures are high, and the 'x' descent of right atrium filling due to right ventricular contraction is prominent. The right atrium collapses in diastole as a result of impaired filling and high intrapericardial pressures. In early diastole even the right ventricle may collapse.

In hypotension with an elevated venous pressure consider cardiac tamponade as a diagnosis

Occasionally the stretched pericardium may compress the lingular lobe of the left lung, causing bronchial breathing at the left base (Ewart's sign). The QRS axis of the ECG may also be altered (electrical alternans).

Common signs of cardiac tamponade

- Elevated jugular venous pressure
- Kussmaul's sign
- Tachypnoea
- Systolic hypotension
- Pulsus paradoxus
- Tachycardia
- Diminished heart sounds
- Impalpable apex beat

Treatment is by urgent drainage – usually under echocardiographic control. Surgical 'pericardial' windows may be necessary for chronic (eg malignant) effusions.

9. DISORDERS OF MAJOR VESSELS

9.1 Pulmonary hypertension

Pulmonary hypertension is an important condition to recognise because prolonged episodes become irreversible due to thickening of the pulmonary arteries and arterioles (causing increased pulmonary vascular resistance) and hypertrophy of the right ventricle. This then results in a progressive condition which may only be curable by heart–lung bypass.

Pulmonary hypertension may be primary, or secondary to other conditions where early intervention may reverse the process.

Secondary causes of pulmonary hypertension

- Chronic pulmonary thromboembolism
- Chronic lung disease (eg COPD, pulmonary fibrosis)
- Mitral valve disease
- Heart failure of any cause
- Left to right shunt (eg ASD, VSD)

Primary pulmonary hypertension (PPH)

Primary pulmonary hypertension is a rare disease with an incidence of 2 per million per year; it is a disease of children and young adults, with a ratio of females:males of 2:1. PPH constitutes less than 1% of all cases of pulmonary hypertension and is characterised by a mean pulmonary artery pressure of >25 mmHg at rest, in the absence of another demonstrable cause. One in ten cases is familial. PPH is associated with connective tissue disease, vasculitis, HIV infection and also the use of appetite suppressants (eg fenfluramine). The pulmonary arteries become dilated and abnormally thickened; there is dilatation of the proximal pulmonary vessels with thick-walled, obstructed 'pruned' peripheral vessels. As a consequence of the high pulmonary pressure the right ventricle undergoes marked hypertrophy.

Treatment of primary pulmonary hypertension

- Advise avoidance of strenuous exercise and recommend contraception, as pregnancy is harmful.
- Anticoagulation to avoid thrombus formation in situ in the pulmonary arteries and also pulmonary embolism.
- Prostacyclin (PGI_2), a potent pulmonary and systemic vasodilator, is used, particularly to bridge patients to transplantation. The drug has an extremely short half-life and has to be given by continuous intravenous infusion, usually through a tunnelled central venous catheter. It is also very expensive.
- Calcium channel antagonists have been used to lower pulmonary (and systemic) pressure.
- Diuretics are helpful in the management of right heart failure.
- Continuous ambulatory inhaled nitric oxide is being developed, and this would provide good pulmonary vasodilatation, but without systemic effect.
- Sildenafil is a promising treatment.

The chief therapeutic option is transplantation, as other treatments are of limited benefit, or are difficult to administer.

9.2 Venous thrombosis and pulmonary embolism (PE)

The true incidence of pulmonary embolism (PE) is unknown but PE probably accounts for 1% of all admissions. Predisposing factors are discussed in Chapter 8, Haematology.

One or more predisposing risk factors are found in 80–90% of cases. The oral contraceptive increases the risk of deep vein thrombosis (DVT)/PE two to four times. However, thromboembolism is rare in women taking oestrogens without other risk factors.

Pulmonary embolism may present with subtle signs and a high index of suspicion is required. When complicated by hypotension thrombolysis is indicated

Clinical features

Nearly all patients have one or more of the following symptoms: dyspnoea, tachypnoea or pleuritic chest pain. With a large pulmonary embolus patients may present with collapse. Hypoxaemia may be present with moderate or large pulmonary emboli.

Investigations

- Chest X-ray
  - May be normal; pleural-based wedge-shaped defects described classically are rare and areas of oligaemia may be difficult to detect
- D-dimer
  - Will be raised in PE but the test is non-specific
- Helical CT scanning
  - Will demonstrate pulmonary emboli in the large pulmonary arteries but may not show small peripheral emboli
- ECG
  - May show sinus tachycardia and, in massive PE, features of acute right heart strain; non-specific S-T segment and T-wave changes occur
- Arterial blood gases
  - Shows a low or normal pCO_2 and may show a degree of hypoxaemia
- Ventilation/perfusion (V/Q) scanning
  - Shows one or more areas of ventilation perfusion mismatching (see below)
- Pulmonary angiography
  - Previously the 'gold standard', but this is being replaced by high resolution CT

In each case a clinical assessment of the probability of PE should be made. As demonstrated in the PIOPED study:

- Cases of high clinical probability combined with a high probability V/Q scan are virtually diagnostic of PE.
- Similarly, cases of low clinical suspicion combined with low probability or normal V/Q scans make the diagnosis of PE very unlikely.
- All other combinations of clinical probability and V/Q scan result should be investigated further.
- Patients who present with collapse need urgent echocardiography, helical CT scan or pulmonary angiogram to demonstrate pulmonary embolus.

Management

In all cases of moderate or high clinical probability of PE, anticoagulation with heparin should be started immediately after baseline coagulation studies have been taken. If unfractionated heparin is used, an initial loading dose of 5000–10 000 units should be given intravenously followed by a continuous infusion of 1300 IU/hour (adjusted according to the results of the activated partial thromboplastin time (APTT) which should be 1.5–2.5 times the control). Low molecular weight heparin, given as a once-daily subcutaneous injection, has recently been licensed for the treatment of PE; no monitoring is required. Patients should be treated with heparin for at least 5 days; during that time warfarin is introduced and the heparin is discontinued once the INR is two to three times the control.

- Warfarin is continued for 3–6 months in most cases; for PE occurring post-operatively, 6 weeks' anticoagulation is adequate. In recurrent PE, anticoagulation should be for longer periods (eg 1 year) and consideration should be given to life-long treatment.
- In cases of collapse due to massive PE, thrombolysis with streptokinase or recombinant t-PA given by peripheral vein should be considered. This should be avoided when the embolic material is an infected vegetation (eg iv drug abusers).
- Occasionally, pulmonary embolectomy is used for those with massive PE where thrombolysis is unsuccessful or contraindicated.
- Inferior vena caval filters should be considered in patients where anticoagulation is contraindicated or in those who continue to embolise despite anticoagulation.

9.3 Systemic hypertension

Hypertension is an important condition because it is asymptomatic until serious complications occur, is an important risk factor for vascular disease, and is easily screened for and treated.

A UK population survey in 1994 showed that 19.5% of a sample adult population would be classified as having hypertension using criteria of systolic blood pressure (SBP) >160 mmHg or diastolic blood pressure (DBP) >95 mmHg and/or receiving treatment for hypertension. Guidelines for treatment continually adapt to new clinical evidence, but the British Hypertension Society (BHS) would recommend the following:

- All adults should have their blood pressure measured every 5 years until the age of 80 years.
- Patients who have high normal blood pressure (SBP 135–139 mmHg or DBP 85–89 mmHg) should be monitored annually.
- Non-pharmacological measures (lifestyle) should be initiated in all hypertensive patients and those with borderline blood pressures. These measures include cessation of smoking; appropriate dieting for obesity; reduced cholesterol intake and improvement in exercise.
- Treatment is also indicated for all patients with sustained SBP >160 mmHg and/or DBP >100 mmHg.
- Treatment is also indicated for patients with sustained SBP >140–159 mmHg and/or DBP 90–99 mmHg if there is evidence of target organ damage, established cardiovascular disease, diabetes or if the patient would have an estimated 10-year coronary heart disease risk >15%.

Major antihypertensive classes

- Diuretics (loop, thiazide, potassium sparing)
- Beta blockers
- ACE inhibitors
- Angiotensin receptor blockers
- Calcium antagonists
- Alpha blockers.

> **Essential note**
>
> Risk factors such as hypertension and dyslipidaemia should be treated aggressively in higher risk cases such as secondary prevention and diabetics

> **Algorithm for blood pressure treatment endorsed by British Heart Foundation**
>
> - Stage 1: ACE inhibitor or beta blocker (for <55 years and non-black)
>   Calcium channel blocker or diuretic (black or >55 years)
> - Stage 2: ACE inhibitor or beta blocker plus calcium channel blocker or diuretic

> **Algorithm for blood pressure treatment endorsed by British Heart Foundation**
>
> - Stage 3: ACE inhibitor or beta blocker plus calcium channel blocker plus diuretic
> - Stage 4: Add alpha blocker or additional diuretic (eg spironolactone)
>
> Note: use of cardio-selective beta blockers may increase prognostic benefit.

> **Essential note**
>
> Patients with end organ disease will often not follow this algorithm as ACE inhibitors and beta blockers will both be indicated as they are known to have prognostic benefit in both coronary disease and heart failure

Recommended targets for blood pressure control

Blood pressure treatment targets have changed with evidence from recent large trials. Current recommendations are:

- Patients without diabetes mellitus <140/85 mmHg
- Patients with diabetes mellitus <140/80 mmHg
- Diabetic nephropathy <125/75 mmHg
- Chronic renal disease with persistent proteinuria (>1 g/24 hours) <125/75 mmHg.

Stepped antihypertensive therapy is probably outmoded as 50% of patients will be uncontrolled by monotherapy, and therapeutic gains with two- to three-agent low-dose therapy far outweigh the incidence of side-effects.

Other considerations in hypertension management

- Investigation of **phaeochromocytomas**: recommend three 24-hour urinary catecholamine metabolites (and off all drugs)
- Hypertension **increases the risk** (Framingham data) of: stroke ($\times$7); cardiac failure ($\times$4); coronary artery disease ($\times$3); peripheral vascular disease ($\times$2)
- Potassium salt should be substituted for sodium salt where possible
- **Drugs to avoid in pregnancy**: diuretics, ACE inhibitors, angiotensin II receptor blockers
- **Drugs with well-identified risks preferred in pregnancy**: beta-blockers (especially labetalol), methyldopa and hydralazine

- Young black men have a poor response to ACE inhibitors, thiazides and beta-blockers as they are salt conservers by background, and so are resistant to renin manipulation and are particularly likely to develop the side-effect of impotence.

9.4 Aortic dissection

Aortic dissection refers to the process of a tear in the intima of the aorta allowing blood to force open a false passage between the endothelium and adventitia. Two-thirds of tears occur in the ascending aorta with about one-fifth occurring in the descending aorta. Mortality is highest in the first few hours if the dissection is untreated. Ascending dissection should be included in the differential diagnosis for MI as the vulnerable right coronary ostium may be involved (giving rise to an inferior infarct pattern). This is particularly important when considering thrombolysis; aortic regurgitation provides supportive evidence of the diagnosis.

Ascending aorta dissections (often referred to as type A) are treated surgically due to the risk of the head and neck vessels becoming involved and also of retrograde extension into the aortic root.

Descending aorta dissections (type B) are treated conservatively if possible and only subjected to surgery in the event of continuing pain or major vessel involvement.

The major risks of surgery are death and paraplegia.

Associations with aortic dissection

- Systemic hypertension (present in 80%)
- Marfan's syndrome
- Cystic medial degeneration (rare in the absence of Marfan's syndrome)
- Noonan's, Turner's syndromes
- Trauma
- Aortic coarctation
- Congenital bicuspid aortic valve (present in 10–15% and dissection is therefore associated with aortic stenosis)
- Giant cell arteritis
- Pregnancy (particularly in patients with Marfan's syndrome)
- Cocaine abuse

Involvement of ascending aorta may cause

- Aortic regurgitation
- Inferior myocardial infarction
- Pericardial effusion (including cardiac tamponade)
- Carotid dissection
- Absent or decreased subclavian pulse.

Medical therapy to be considered for

- Old, stable dissections (>2 weeks)
- Uncomplicated dissection of descending aorta
- Isolated arch dissections.

Investigations for aortic dissection

- TOE, aortic MRI or contrast-enhanced spiral CT scans all have a high diagnostic sensitivity, but CT rarely identifies the site of tear or the presence of aortic regurgitation or coronary involvement.
- MRI is of the highest quality but is contraindicated in patients with pacemakers, certain vascular clips and metal valve prostheses.
- TOE is probably the most widely used investigation as it is available in the acute situation and has high sensitivity and specificity.
- Aortography is no longer the gold standard and coronary angiography is applicable only when deciding on the need for concomitant CABG.

APPENDIX I Normal cardiac physiological values

ECG

- PR interval 0.12–0.20 s
- QRS duration >0.10 s
- QTc (males) 380 ms, (females) 420 ms
- QRS axis −30° to + 90°.

Indices of cardiac function

- Cardiac index = cardiac output/body surface area (BSA) = 2.5–4.0 $l \cdot min^{-1} \cdot m^{-2}$
- Stroke volume index = stroke volume/BSA = 40–70 $ml \cdot m^{-2}$

Systemic vascular resistance (SVR) =

$$\frac{80 \times (Ao - RA)}{(Cardiac\ output)} = 770\text{--}1500\ dyn \cdot s \cdot cm^{-5},$$

where Ao is the mean aortic pressure and RA is the mean right atrial pressure.

- Ejection fraction = proportion of blood ejected from left ventricle = 50–70%.

Cardiology

Further revision

Books

Gray H, Dawkins KD, Simpson IA, Morgan JM. *Lecture notes on cardiology*. 4th edn. Oxford: Blackwell Science, 2002.

Hampton JR. *The ECG made easy*. London: Churchill Livingstone, 2003.

Swanton RH. *Cardiology pocket consultant*. Oxford: Blackwell Science, 2003.

Journals

(Look for review articles on the subject you wish to revise. The education section in *Heart* is particularly well developed.)

Circulation

Journal of the American College of Cardiology

European Heart Journal

Heart

Web Sites

www.theheart.org

www.incirculation.net

www.escardio.org

www.americanheart.org

Revision summary

You should now:

1. Have a routine set of questions and examination manoeuvres to use as a template for assessing patients. This basic template may be embellished and amended to the particular circumstances presented to you by the patient. After your clinical assessment you should be in a position to formulate a coherent differential diagnosis to guide your treatment and choice of investigations.

2. Be able to interpret a 12-lead ECG and understand its use in Holter monitoring and exercise stress testing. Understand the capabilities of echocardiography (transthoracic and transoesophageal), myocardial perfusion imaging and cardiac catheterisation. Have an appreciation of when to refer patients for these investigations.

3. Understand normal cardiac anatomy and how this is altered in congenital, vavular and myopathic heart disease. Appreciate the normal propagation of electrical activation through the heart and how this is altered in tachy and brady arrhythmias. Be aware of the range of presentations of ischaemic heart disease.

4. Be aware of the immediate treatments for ischaemic presentations as well as the long-term therapies available to modify risk factors such as hypertension and hypercholesterolaemia and treat chronic cardiac conditions. Know which patients require temporary and permanent pacing. Have some knowledge of which patients are revascularised (percutaneously or surgically) and when valve sugery should be considered.

Clinical pharmacology and toxicology

Chapter 2

CONTENTS

Revision objectives

You should:

1. Appreciate that genetic variation can alter drug effects
2. Recognise important drug interactions, including drugs that alter liver enzyme activity
3. Be aware of conditions that may significantly alter the response to certain drugs

4. Be able to identify drugs used to treat common medical conditions, and be able to give named examples
5. Recognise common drug-induced adverse effects
6. Understand the principles of managing patients after drug overdose

Clinical pharmacology and toxicology

1.1 Genetic polymorphisms of drug metabolism

Genetic variations can influence how drugs are metabolised. For example, around 50% of the UK population possess the slow acetylator phenotype, which can cause higher drug concentrations and greater adverse effects in these people:

- Drug-induced lupus
- Isoniazid-induced peripheral neuropathy.

Drug-induced lupus

Unlike autoimmune systemic lupus erythematosus (SLE), drug-induced lupus is equally prevalent in men and women. Laboratory findings include antibodies to histones and single-stranded DNA. Clinical features include:

- Arthralgia
- Butterfly rash
- Pleurisy.

Renal involvement (except with hydralazine) or neuropsychiatric manifestations are unusual.

Some causes of drug-induced lupus (*metabolised significantly by acetylation, hence lupus more common in slow acetylators)	
• Beta-blockers	• Phenytoin
• Chlorpromazine	• Procainamide*
• Hydralazine*	• Sulfasalazine*
• Isoniazid*	• Sulphonamides*
• Penicillin	

Poor metabolisers of other drugs

- **s-Mephenytoin**: 3–5% of the UK population have low s-mephenytoin hydroxylase activity, and metabolise this anti-epileptic agent slowly: higher drug concentrations may cause greater adverse effects
- **Codeine**: 7% of the UK population have low Cyp2D6 enzyme activity and cannot convert codeine to morphine; codeine is less effective in these people.

Rapid acetylators

Rapid acetylators may be exposed to lower drug concentrations (treatment less effective) and suffer adverse effects of high drug metabolite concentrations: eg isoniazid-induced hepatitis.

1.2 Liver enzyme induction

Certain drugs can induce the activity of liver enzymes. This can take a number of days to occur because of the time taken to synthesise more enzyme. Enzyme induction can cause more rapid metabolism of other drugs, thereby decreasing their effectiveness:

Drugs metabolised more rapidly in the setting of enzyme induction
• Hydrocortisone
• Oral contraceptive pill
• Phenytoin
• Warfarin

Drugs capable of causing enzyme induction can be remembered by the mnemonic **PC BRAS**:

(**P**henytoin, **C**arbamazepine, **B**arbiturates, **R**ifampicin, **A**lcohol (chronic excess), **S**ulphonylureas)

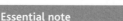

Essential note
Enzyme inducers increase hepatic metabolism so that other drugs may be less effective

1.3 Liver enzyme inhibition

A number of drugs can inhibit hepatic enzyme activity, often immediately. Other drugs are metabolised less extensively, so their plasma concentrations increase and adverse effects are more likely. Enzyme inhibition can increase the effects of the drugs listed in the following box:

Drugs metabolised more slowly in the setting of enzyme inhibition
• Carbamazepine
• Ciclosporin
• Phenytoin
• Theophyllines
• Warfarin

Drugs that are liver enzyme inhibitors may be recalled by the mnemonic **AODEVICES**:

(**A**llopurinol, **O**meprazole, **D**isulfiram, **E**rythromycin, **V**alproate, **I**soniazid, **C**imetidine (and ciprofloxacin), acute **E**thanol intoxication, **S**ulphonamides)

Enzyme inhibitors slow down hepatic metabolism and can increase the effects of other drugs

1.4 Failure of the combined oral contraceptive pill

Conditions that impair absorption of the oral contraceptive pill can cause treatment failure:

- Diarrhoea due to rapid gastrointestinal transit
- Broad-spectrum antibiotics, eg amoxicillin, eradicate gut flora that normally deconjugate bile and contribute to enterohepatic cycling of the oestrogen component.

In addition, oestrogen is metabolised more rapidly in the presence of enzyme inducers (see Section 1.2), leading to lower circulating concentrations and pill failure.

2. PRESCRIBING IN PARTICULAR CLINICAL STATES

European Law has recently required the use of Recommended International Non-proprietary Names (rINN) for medicines, which have replaced a number of older names used in the UK. rINN names are listed in the *British National Formulary* (BNF)

eg frusemide → furosemide
bendrofluazide → bendroflumethiazide

2.1 Drugs and breast-feeding

Infants <1 month are at greatest risk from drugs excreted in breast milk due to immature drug metabolism and excretion. Drugs that are contraindicated in breast-feeding mothers due to risks to the infant are:

- **Amiodarone**: thyroid anomalies
- **Cytotoxics and chloramphenicol**: blood dyscrasia.

Other drugs associated with adverse effects in the infants of breast-feeding mothers are:

- **Aspirin**: increased risk of bleeding and Reyes syndrome
- **Gold**: haematological reactions and renal impairment
- **Indometacin**: has been reported to cause seizures

- **Iodides**: thyroid disturbance
- **Lithium**: involuntary movements
- **Oestrogens**: feminisation of male infants.

2.2 Pregnancy and drug therapy

During the first 16 weeks of pregnancy, drugs may have teratogenic effects on the fetus leading to malformations. Particular associations are:

- **Lithium**: cardiac abnormalities
- **Phenytoin**: facial fusion abnormalities such as cleft lip and palate
- **Sodium valproate** and **retinoids**: neural tube defects
- **Warfarin**: abnormalities of long bones and cartilage.

Later in pregnancy some drugs may cross the placenta and harm the fetus:

- **Carbimazole**: neonatal goitre (can obstruct labour)
- **Gentamicin**: nerve deafness in the newborn.

2.3 Prescribing in liver failure

Accumulation of high drug or metabolite concentrations normally cleared by the liver can cause depressed CNS function. Patients with liver failure are more sensitive to the sedative effects of a number of drugs, which can provoke hepatic encephalopathy, eg opiates and benzodiazepines. Thiazides and loop diuretics can precipitate hypokalaemia and encephalopathy. Liver disease can have an important impact on drug effects:

- Drugs excreted in the bile, eg rifampicin, accumulate in obstructive jaundice
- Hypoalbuminaemia increases the proportion of free (active) drug versus protein-bound drug: higher risk of adverse effects
- Reduced clotting factor synthesis increases the effect of warfarin and increases bleeding risk
- Corticosteroids and non-steroidal anti-inflammatory drugs exacerbate salt and water retention in patients with advanced liver disease and can worsen ascites and oedema.

2.4 Prescribing in renal failure

Water-soluble drugs eliminated mainly by the kidneys will accumulate in patients with reduced glomerular filtration rate (GFR) and cause toxic effects, for example:

- **ACE inhibitors**: hyperkalaemia and worsened renal function
- **Digoxin**: cardiac arrhythmias, heart block
- **Erythromycin**: encephalopathy
- **Lithium**: cardiac arrhythmias and seizures

- **Penicillins** and **cephalosporins** (high dose): lead to encephalopathy.

Nephrotoxic drugs may cause an acute deterioration in patients with chronic renal impairment. If treatment is considered essential (eg gentamicin or vancomycin for severe infection) then therapeutic drug monitoring should be used.

Essential note

Drug clearance can be reduced in patients with renal failure: lower doses should be prescribed to avoid the risks of toxicity, eg digoxin

Some nephrotoxic drugs

- ACE inhibitors and angiotensin II receptor antagonists
- Aminoglycoside antibiotics (eg gentamicin)
- Amphotericin
- Ciclosporin
- Non-steroidal anti-inflammatory drugs

Other drugs may cause specific nephrotoxic effects, eg gold-induced proteinuria or nephrotic syndrome (*see* Chapter 12, Nephrology).

3. INDIVIDUAL DRUGS AND THOSE USED IN SPECIFIC CLINICAL CONDITIONS

3.1 Cardiology

Abciximab

This antibody irreversibly binds GpIIb/IIIa glycoprotein receptors, preventing platelet activation and aggregation. It is administered intravenously and used to prevent thrombosis and restenosis after coronary angioplasty, and appears effective in treatment of certain patients with unstable angina.

Adenosine

Adenosine binds to specific receptors and delays atrioventricular node conduction, and terminates supraventricular tachycardia (SVT). The effect of intravenous bolus administration can help distinguish between SVT and ventricular tachycardia. Normally, it has a short half-life of 8–10 s, but

this is prolonged by dipyridamole, which interferes with its metabolism.

Side-effects of adenosine

- Anxiety
- Bronchospasm (avoid in asthmatic patients)
- Chest tightening
- Facial flushing

Amiodarone

Amiodarone has a number of anti-arrhythmic actions, including prolongation of the refractory period (QT interval). It is used to treat SVT and ventricular arrhythmias, including cardioversion of atrial fibrillation to sinus rhythm. It can prevent life-threatening arrhythmia in some patients with recurrent VT or hypertrophic cardiomyopathy.

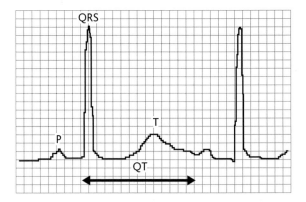

Figure 1 Amiodarone-induced prolongation of the QT interval

- It has a wide volume of distribution and long half-life (26–127 days)
- Effects occur within a few hours of intravenous administration, and up to several weeks after starting oral treatment
- High protein binding increases the risk of toxicity from digoxin and warfarin.

Essential note

Drugs that increase the QT interval are associated with a higher risk of arrhythmia

Side-effects of amiodarone

- Arrhythmias (torsades de pointes)
- Fibrosis (pulmonary and retroperitoneal)
- Hepatitis
- Hyperthyroidism/hypothyroidism
- Peripheral neuropathy
- Photosensitivity
- Reversible corneal microdeposits
- Slate grey skin discoloration.

Angiotensin converting enzyme (ACE) inhibitors

ACE inhibitors (eg lisinopril, enalapril) reduce mortality in patients after myocardial infarction or with heart failure. They are contraindicated in bilateral renal artery stenosis and should be used with caution in severe renal impairment.

Side-effects of ACE inhibitors

- Dry cough (due to accumulation of bradykinin): more common in women, who have a more sensitive cough reflex
- Hyperkalaemia
- Hypersensitivity (can cause angio-neurotic oedema)
- Renal failure (especially if reduced renal blood flow)

Angiotensin receptor blockers

Angiotensin II receptor antagonists (eg losartan, valsartan) prevent angiotensin-II-mediated vasoconstriction, and prolong survival in patients with hypertension and heart failure. Therapeutic and adverse effects are similar to ACE inhibitors, except that they do not cause cough.

Calcium channel blockers

These block calcium channel entry in vascular smooth muscle and neuronal tissue, and there are two broad groups: dihydropyridines (eg nifedipine, amlodipine, felodipine), which predominantly cause vascular relaxation and reduced peripheral resistance, and non-dihydropyridines (verapamil and diltiazem), which have predominantly cardiac effects resulting in bradycardia and delayed atrioventricular nodal conduction.

Adverse effects of calcium channel blockers

- Gingival hyperplasia
- Headache
- Hepatitis
- Hot flushes

Adverse effects of calcium channel blockers

- Peripheral oedema (especially dihydropyridine group)
- Bradycardia and AV block (especially verapamil or diltiazem)

Digoxin

Digoxin is derived from the purple foxglove, and delays atrioventricular node conduction, and reduces ventricular rate in patients with atrial fibrillation. It is a positive inotrope, and is used to treat patients with co-existent heart failure and atrial fibrillation, or severe heart failure even if in sinus rhythm.

- 85% is eliminated unchanged in urine, and accumulates in renal impairment
- Can cause gynaecomastia in chronic use
- Narrow therapeutic window, above which toxic effects are common.

Digoxin toxicity

- Amiodarone can cause digoxin toxicity due to protein-binding interaction: the dose of digoxin should normally be reduced by 50%.
- Arrhythmia: any can occur and the most common is heart block.
- Calcium channel blockers (eg nifedipine, verapamil) interfere with renal tubular clearance of digoxin and increase the risk of toxicity.
- Hypokalaemia, hypomagnesaemia and hypercalcaemia predispose to toxicity.
- 'Reversed tick' ST changes in the inferior and lateral ECG leads are a common feature of digoxin treatment, not necessarily indicative of toxicity.

Features of digoxin toxicity

- Anorexia
- Arrhythmias (eg atrial fibrillation, heart block)
- Diarrhoea
- Nausea/vomiting
- Yellow vision (xanthopsia)

HMG CoA reductase inhibitors

Statins (eg simvastatin, atorvastatin) inhibit the rate-limiting enzyme in cholesterol synthesis, which is predominantly active during fasting, and treatment is often given at bedtime. Low density lipoprotein (LDL) receptors are up-regulated, so that LDL cholesterol falls by around 30%, and high-density lipoprotein (HDL) increases. Statins have some triglyceride-lowering effect, particularly in high doses.

- Hepatitis, myositis and rhabdomyolysis can occur, especially with high doses or when given to patients with renal impairment. Treatment should normally be discontinued if symptoms are severe, or if creatinine kinase (CK) is elevated to more than 5 times the upper limit of normal, or if alanine transaminase is elevated to more than 3 times the upper limit of normal.
- Reduced morbidity and mortality in patients with established atherosclerotic disease.
- Treatment is escalated to target cholesterol <5.0 mmol/l and LDL cholesterol <3.0 mmol/l.

Essential note

Hepatitis and cholestatic jaundice are both recognised adverse effects of a number of different drugs

Nicorandil

A K⁺ channel opener that causes coronary artery dilatation and a nitrate-like action that causes systemic venous relaxation. It is used to treat angina, and can cause headache, flushing and dizziness and, in large doses, hypotension and reflex tachycardia.

Thiazide diuretics

Thiazides (eg bendroflumethiazide) lower blood pressure due to a direct vascular effect, independent of their diuretic effects. Maximum blood pressure reduction is achieved using low doses (eg bendroflumethiazide 2.5 mg daily). They are associated with a number of dose-dependent metabolic effects:

Adverse effects of thiazide diuretics

- Hyponatraemia, hypokalaemia, hypomagnesaemia and hypochloraemic alkalosis
- Hyperuricaemia due to reduced tubular clearance of urate; can predispose to gout
- Increased glucose and triglyceride concentrations thought due to increased insulin resistance
- Postural hypotension, photosensitivity, thrombocytopenia and impotence (mechanisms unclear)

Clopidogrel

Clopidogrel inhibits ADP-mediated platelet aggregation. It appears at least as effective as aspirin in secondary prevention of ischaemic heart disease and stroke, and the combination of aspirin and clopidogrel appears to confer additional benefits in high-risk patients. It should be considered for patients who do not tolerate aspirin due to gastrointestinal bleeding.

3.2 Endocrinology

Carbimazole

Carbimazole blocks peroxidase-mediated thyroid hormone synthesis, and can take up to 6 weeks to lower circulating concentrations. Hormone concentrations can increase transiently after commencing therapy, and a beta-blocker (eg propranolol) can suppress symptoms such as tachycardia and anxiety.

- Agranulocytosis can occur; patients should seek medical help if they develop a sore throat.
- Carbimazole crosses the placenta and can cause fetal hypothyroidism and goitre.

Hormone replacement therapy

Around 60–75% of menopausal women experience vasomotor symptoms. These can be reduced by hormone replacement therapy (HRT), which is taken by 10–15% of post-menopausal women in the UK.

- Women aged 70 or more have reduced bone mass: around half will have an osteoporosis-related fracture.
- HRT reduces osteoporosis-related fractures by up to 50%.
- HRT does not appear to significantly reduce cardiovascular risk effect.
- See also Chapter 4, Endocrinology, section 4.4.

Some oral treatments for diabetes

- Nateglinide and repaglinide: These agents have a short duration of action and stimulate insulin release prior to meals. They can be given alongside metformin in type 2 diabetes. They are associated with gastrointestinal adverse effects and hypersensitivity reactions
- Acarbose: Acarbose inhibits intestinal alpha-glucosidase. It delays absorption of starch and sucrose, and reduces post-prandial hyperglycaemia. It is used as an adjunct to metformin or sulphonylureas to improve blood glucose lowering. Excess flatus is a common adverse effect
- Thiazolidinediones (eg rosiglitazone and pioglitazone): These reduce peripheral insulin resistance, and can be added to metformin or sulphonylureas to delay the need for insulin in patients with type 2 diabetes. Hepatic impairment is an important adverse effect.

3.3 Gastroenterology

Mesalazine and olsalazine

Mesalazine and olsalazine differ from sulfasalazine by being 5-amino salicylic acid (5-ASA) molecules that have a local action in the colon. They suppress local inflammation in ulcerative colitis.

- Adverse effects are nausea, abdominal pain, headache and sometimes worsening of colitis
- Rare side-effects include pancreatitis, blood dyscrasias and interstitial nephritis.

Sulfasalazine

Sulfasalazine comprises 5-ASA (active part) and a sulfonamide carrier to deliver active drug to the colon. It is used to treat colitis and rheumatoid arthritis. Adverse effects include:

- Gastrointestinal symptoms: common (due to sulfonamide component)
- Oligospermia and male infertility (usually reversible)
- Orange discoloration of body fluids
- Slow acetylators are at greater risk of toxicity due to higher sulfonamide concentrations
- Rare side-effects are Stevens–Johnson syndrome, agranulocytosis and nephrotic syndrome.

Orlistat

Orlistat inhibits pancreatic lipase and is used in patients with a BMI >30 kg/m^2 and where they have already lost >2.5 kg in weight over a four-week period. It causes liquid, oily stools and may reduces absorption of fat-soluble vitamins.

3.4 Neurology

Treatment of Parkinson's disease

Treatments generally aim to enhance dopaminergic neurotransmission:

- **Selegiline** inhibits monoamine oxidase type B (MAO-B), thereby increasing dopamine. It is used to reduce end-of-dose akinesia.
- **Amantadine** potentiates dopamine by preventing re-uptake into pre-synaptic terminals.
- **Levodopa** (L-dopa) is converted to dopamine within the nigro-striatal pathway by catechol-*o*-methyl transferase. After prolonged treatment, many patients develop on–off symptoms and end-of-dose akinesia. This is managed by switching to controlled-release preparations and splitting the total daily dose over more frequent administrations.

- **Dopamine receptor agonists** include bromocriptine, cabergoline, lisuride, pergolide, pramipexole and ropinirole. They cause less dyskinesia than L-dopa, but more neuropsychiatric adverse effects. They can be associated with pulmonary and retroperitoneal fibrosis. **Apomorphine** is a powerful dopamine agonist given by parenteral administration. It is highly emetogenic (stimulates vomiting) and domperidone should be given before treatment is started.

Side-effects of L-dopa

- Cardiac arrhythmias
- Involuntary movements (dyskinesia) are common
- Nausea and vomiting
- Postural hypotension (important contributor to falls)
- Psychosis (depression or mania)
- Somnolescence

Treatment of epilepsy

Most anti-epileptic agents are believed to have effects on ion channel conductance or neurotransmitter availability.

- **Diazepam and lorazepam** stimulate the benzodiazepine receptor, thereby increasing affinity of GABA receptors for GABA (inhibitory CNS neurotransmitter), and increasing seizure threshold.
- **Carbamazepine** suppresses sodium channel conduction, and is used to treat epilepsy, mood disorder and neuralgia. Adverse effects include headache and diplopia, weight gain, generalised morbilliform rash and hepatic enzyme induction.
- **Gabapentin** stimulates the CNS receptor for GABA, an inhibitory neurotransmitter. It can cause drowsiness, particularly if taken with alcohol.
- **Lamotrigine** inhibits the action of glutamate, an excitatory neurotransmitter. Adverse effects include mood change, flu-like symptoms, rash and Stevens–Johnson syndrome.
- **Phenytoin** is used to treat and prevent generalised seizures. Mechanism of action believed to be sodium channel blockade. Adverse effects include hepatic enzyme inhibition, cerebellar toxicity and ataxia, gingival hyperplasia, hirsutism, macrocytosis, osteomalacia and hepatitis.
- **Sodium valproate** is used for absence attacks and temporal lobe epilepsy. It inhibits liver enzymes and, therefore, may potentiate the effects of other drugs,

including phenytoin. Adverse effects include cerebellar toxicity and ataxia, hepatitis, hepatic enzyme inhibition thrombocytopenia and weight gain.

- **Vigabatrin** irreversibly inhibits GABA transaminase, thereby increasing GABA and decreasing glutamate CNS concentrations. It is used to treat partial seizures with secondary generalisation, in patients who have not responded to other anti-epilectic drugs. Adverse effects include psychosis in 5%, and visual field defects (regular visual field assessment is required).

5-HT agonists (eg sumatriptan and rizatriptan)

These are effective for migraine if taken sufficiently early by either the oral or sublingual route. They promote vasoconstriction, and prevent headache in the vasodilator phase of migraine. They must not be given in hemiplegic migraine, or within 24 hours of ergotamine, as intense vasospasm may lead to permanent neurological damage. They may also cause angina due to coronary vasospasm.

3.5 Psychiatry

Chlorpromazine

Chlorpromazine acts at many CNS sites, resulting in blockade of dopamine, alpha-adrenergic, cholinergic and histamine receptors.

Adverse effects of chlorpromazine

- Agranulocytosis
- Contact dermatitis and purple pigmentation of the skin
- Drowsiness
- Dystonia (including oculogyric crisis)
- Neuroleptic malignant syndrome
- Photosensitivity
- Prolonged QT interval (and ventricular tachycardia in high doses)
- Tardive dyskinesia

Lithium

Lithium carbonate is used for prophylaxis and treatment of bipolar affective disorder. It has a narrow therapeutic range (0.6–1.2 mmol/l), and toxic effects are especially common >2.0 mmol/l.

- **Toxicity** is more likely in patients with renal impairment, hyponatraemia, or if taking diuretics, ACE inhibitors or non-steroidal anti-inflammatory drugs.
- **Long-term treatment** is associated with diabetes insipidus and hypothyroidism due to de-coupling of

ADH and thyroid stimulating hormone (TSH) receptors respectively from intracellular second messenger systems.

Toxic and side-effects of lithium

- (At 1–2 mmol/l)

  - Anorexia and vomiting
  - Ataxia and dysarthria
  - Blurred vision
  - Drowsiness
  - Muscle weakness
  - Tremor

- (Severe toxicity >2 mmol/l)

  - Circulatory failure
  - Coma
  - Hyper-reflexia
  - Seizures
  - Death

3.6 Rheumatology

Allopurinol

Inhibits xanthine oxidase, the rate-limiting enzyme in formation of uric acid in purine metabolism, thereby lowering serum concentrations by up to 35%. Initiation of treatment can occasionally provoke acute gout. Established tophi may regress with chronic allopurinol treatment. Allopurinol causes accumulation of 6-mercaptopurine, an active metabolite of azathioprine, and cyclophosphamide. Allopurinol should be avoided in patients receiving these treatments, otherwise potentially fatal bone marrow toxicity can occur.

Colchicine

Inhibits macrophage migration into gouty joints and has powerful anti-inflammatory effects, but its usefulness is limited by the frequent occurrence of diarrhoea. It has been said of colchicine that 'you run before you can walk'!

Penicillamine

Penicillamine is a disease-modifying agent in rheumatoid arthritis. It also chelates cysteine and copper in cystinuria and Wilson's disease, respectively. In the first 6 weeks of therapy reversible loss of taste may occur. Adverse effects include:

- Impaired taste sensation
- Neutropenia and thrombocytopenia: patients should seek medical advice if they develop sore throat or easy bruising

- Proteinuria due to membranous glomerulonephritis after chronic use
- Stevens–Johnson syndrome, myasthenia and drug-induced lupus have been reported.

Urate oxidase

Urate oxidase enzymatically degrades urate to allantoin, and causes a significant reduction in serum urate concentrations (up to around 98%). It is used to prevent renal impairment in tumour lysis syndrome.

3.7 Miscellaneous

A description of the mechanism of action, pharmacokinetics and characteristic adverse effects of commonly used antimicrobials is provided in Chapter 10, Infectious diseases and tropical medicine.

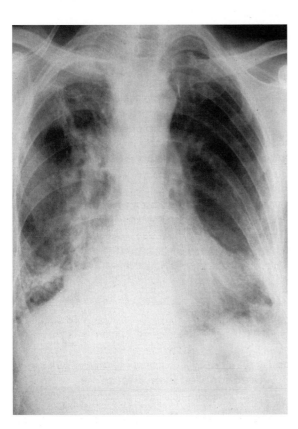

Figure 2 Plain chest radiograph showing pulmonary fibrosis affecting bilateral lung bases and right mid and upper zones.

Source *Wellcome Trust Medical Photographic Library*

Ciclosporin A

Ciclosporin A is an immune suppressant that prevents transplant rejection. It causes dose-dependent renal impairment and has a narrow therapeutic range; therefore, therapeutic drug monitoring is necessary. Other adverse effects include gingival hyperplasia, hypertrichosis, hyperkalaemia, fluid retention and, as with other immunosuppressants, an increased risk of lymphoma and soft tissue malignancy (*see also* Chapter 12, Nephrology).

Cytotoxics

Most cytotoxic agents have the potential to cause marrow suppression.

Side-effects of individual cytotoxic agents

- **Bleomycin**
  - Dose-dependent lung fibrosis; comparatively few myelotoxic effects
- **Cisplatin**
  - Ototoxicity, nephrotoxicity (interstitial nephritis), hypomagnesaemia and peripheral neuropathy
- **Cyclophosphamide**
  - Haemorrhagic cystitis in up to 10%, with subsequent bladder scarring and contracture. Risks are reduced by treatment with sodium 2-mercaptoethanesulfonate (MESNA)
- **Doxorubicin**
  - Cardiomyopathy is common with high cumulative dose exposure
- **Methotrexate**
  - May cause severe mucositis and myelosuppression, which is prevented by the use of folinic acid rescue. During chronic administration pneumonitis and liver fibrosis may occur, and retroperitoneal fibrosis is a rare complication (Fig 3)
- **Vincristine and vinblastine**
  - Cause a reversible peripheral neuropathy

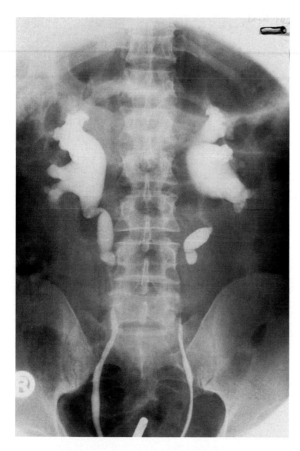

Figure 3 Bilateral ureteric obstruction and dilatation of the proximal ureters and renal calyces due to retroperitoneal fibrosis caused, for example, by methotrexate, methyldopa, amiodarone and pergolide.

Source *Wellcome Trust Medical Photographic Library*

4. SPECIFIC ADVERSE EFFECTS

4.1 Secondary amenorrhoea due to drugs
Dopamine inhibits prolactin release, therefore dopamine-blocking drugs such as chlorpromazine and metoclopramide cause hyperprolactinaemia and may cause amenorrhoea. Sodium valproate also may cause amenorrhoea.

4.2 Bronchospasm
Bronchospasm may be induced by **aspirin** and **non-steroidal anti-inflammatory drugs**, particularly in patients with late-onset asthma. The mechanism is not immunological but appears related to prostaglandin metabolism and is thus termed 'pseudoallergic'.

- **Adenosine** binds to bronchial smooth muscle receptors and causes bronchoconstriction; it should be avoided in patients with asthma.
- Even **cardioselective beta-blockers**, such as atenolol, may provoke bronchospasm.
- **Sodium chromoglicate** is a mast cell stabiliser; it is an inhaled, preventative agent in asthma. However, bronchospasm has occasionally been reported, because the dry powder can exert an irritant effect.
- *N*-Acetyl cysteine is used as an antidote in paracetamol overdose, and may cause bronchospasm and anaphylactoid reactions that usually resolve without specific treatment.

4.3 Dyskinesia and dystonia
A number of agents are recognised causes of movement disorders.

- **Dopamine agonists** used to treat Parkinson's disease may cause dyskinesia (L-dopa, bromocriptine, lysuride and pergolide).
- **Drugs with dopamine-antagonist properties** such as antipsychotics (eg chlorpromazine, haloperidol), or dopamine antagonist antiemetics (eg metoclopramide and domperidone) may also cause dyskinesias.
- **Serotonin-selective re-uptake inhibitors (SSRIs)**, eg fluoxetine and paroxetine, are associated with dystonias.

4.4 Gynaecomastia
Gynaecomastia can complicate treatment with drugs that have oestrogen-like or anti-androgen properties.

Recognised causes of gynaecomastia
- Cimetidine - Digoxin - Spironolactone - Diethylstilbestrol

4.5 Drug-induced liver disease
Drugs can cause dose-dependent or dose-independent liver impairment.

- Dose-dependent liver disease includes paracetamol-induced hepatitis, and steatosis caused by tetracyclines and ethanol.
- Dose-independent liver disease typically causes **hepatitis** or **cholestasis**.

Drug-induced hepatitis occurs with

- Amiodarone
- HMG CoA reductase inhibitors (eg simvastatin)
- Isoniazid metabolite
- Methyldopa (antibody-mediated)
- Nifedipine (can also cause cholestasis)
- Paracetamol
- Phenytoin
- Pyrazinamide
- Valproate

Causes of drug-induced cholestasis

- Chlorpromazine
- Co-amoxiclav (due to clavulanic acid)
- Erythromycin
- Nifedipine (can also cause hepatitis)
- Sulphonylureas

Androgens and oestrogens increase the risk of liver tumours. Methotrexate can cause fibrosis within the liver and at other sites (lung, retroperitoneal, etc).

4.6 Drug-induced myasthenia

- **Aminoglycosides**, certain **beta-blockers** (propranolol, oxprenolol), **phenytoin**, **lignocaine** and **quinidine** impair acetylcholine release, and can worsen or unmask myasthenia.
- **Penicillamine** causes formation of antibodies against the acetylcholine receptor, and myasthenia gravis-like syndrome, which normally resolves after treatment is stopped.
- **Lithium** may cause a myasthenia-like pattern of weakness.

4.7 Photosensitivity

A number of drugs increase the risks of ocular and dermal photosensitivity, and precautions should be taken to avoid potentially hazardous sunlight exposure.

Drugs causing photosensitivity

- Amiodarone
- Ciprofloxacin
- Griseofulvin
- Loop and thiazide diuretics
- Oral contraceptives
- Retinoids
- Sulphonylureas
- Tetracyclines

4.8 Drug-induced vasculitis

Drug-induced vasculitis can affect the skin or internal organs.

Some drugs causing vasculitis

- Allopurinol
- Captopril
- Cimetidine
- Hydralazine
- Leukotriene antagonists
- Penicillin
- Quinidine
- Sulphonamides

4.9 Acute pancreatitis

Acute pancreatitis is a recognised adverse effect of a number of drugs:

Drugs causing acute pancreatitis

- Anti-retrovirals (ritonavir, didanosine, zalcitabine, stavudine, lamivudine)
- Azathioprine
- Corticosteroids
- Fibrates
- HMG CoA reductase inhibitors
- Omega-3 fish oils
- Thiazide diuretics

4.10 Syndrome of inappropriate antidiuretic hormone (SIADH)

SIADH is characterised by hyponatraemia, concentrated urine and low plasma osmolality, in the absence of oedema, diuretic use or hypovolaemia.

Drugs causing SIADH

- Carbamazepine
- Chlorpropamide
- Cytotoxic agents
- Opiates
- Oxytocin
- Psychotropic agents

There are also many non-pharmacological causes, including malignancy, central nervous system disorders, suppurative pulmonary disease and porphyria (*see* Chapter 4, Endocrinology).

5. POISONING

5.1 Paracetamol overdose

This is the most common cause of self-poisoning in the UK. Early features are usually absent or minor (nausea and vomiting), but hepatic or renal failure are late complications. Typically, liver damage becomes apparent at 1–2 days after ingestion. Hepatotoxicity arises because excess toxic metabolites overwhelm the normal glutathione-linked mechanisms of detoxification, and these accumulate in the liver.

Essential note

Liver toxicity may take a number of days to develop after paracetamol overdose

- Hepatic transaminases and the INR, or prothrombin ratio, are the most useful indicators of liver damage. Hypoglycaemia is a feature of advanced liver damage.
- INR >3.0, raised serum creatinine or plasma pH <7.3 at 24 hours after overdose indicate poor prognosis.
- Patients taking enzyme inducers such as phenytoin are at increased risk of hepatic damage due to rapid formation of toxic metabolite.
- Renal failure tends to develop later, typically around 4–5 days after ingestion.
- *PARVOLEX* *N*-Acetyl cysteine improves prognosis in paracetamol poisoning, even after hepatic encephalopathy has developed. It is often administered continuously until the INR has stabilised or is returning to normal.

5.2 Tricyclic antidepressant overdose

Tricyclic antidepressants have anti-cholinergic effects (pupillary dilatation, confusion and tachycardia) and alpha-blocking effects (hypotension). Sympathomimetic over-activity results.

- Prolonged QRS interval on the ECG indicates increased risk of ventricular arrhythmia and seizures; intravenous bicarbonate is indicated in these situations.
- Treatment is supportive, with early consideration of activated charcoal and gastric lavage, and subsequent maintenance of fluid and electrolyte balance. Seizures should be controlled with lorazepam or diazepam.

5.3 Theophylline toxicity

Theophylline inhibits phosphodiesterase, raises intracellular cAMP and can cause tachycardia and arrhythmias in overdose. Arrhythmia is more likely in the presence of severe acidosis or hypokalaemia. Other features include severe vomiting, seizures and coma.

- Treatment with activated charcoal reduces absorption, which can be prolonged after theophylline overdose. Fluid and electrolyte status should be monitored.
- Haemodialysis or charcoal haemoperfusion is indicated for patients with severe toxicity.

5.4 Carbon monoxide poisoning

Carbon monoxide binds to haemoglobin with high affinity (>200 times that of oxygen), and decreases its oxygen-carrying ability. Normal carboxyhaemoglobin levels are <3% in non-smokers, around 5–6% in smokers. At 10–30%, exposed patients' features are usually mild, including headache and mild exertional dyspnoea.

Signs of marked CO toxicity (carboxyhaemoglobin 30–60%)

- Acute renal failure
- Agitation and confusion
- Cardiac ischaemia (clinical and/or ECG features)
- ECG changes and arrhythmias
- Hyperpyrexia
- Hypertonia and hyperreflexia
- Muscle necrosis
- Pink mucosae
- Vomiting

Treatment of severe toxicity:

- 100% oxygen should be administered by mask
- Hyperbaric oxygen (2.5 atmospheres pressure) will enhance elimination of CO, but the risks associated with transfer to a specialist centre require consideration.
- Neuropsychiatric changes may become apparent several weeks or more after CO poisoning, including intellectual deterioration and personality change.

5.5 Quinidine and quinine toxicity

Poisoning may result in severe dose-dependent features, that may be delayed:

- **Blindness** which can be irreversible
- **Blurred vision**
- **Cardiac arrhythmias** and prolonged QT interval
- **Hypotension**
- **Tinnitus**.

5.6 Iron poisoning

Clinical features of iron poisoning

- Abdominal pain
- Diarrhoea
- Haematemesis
- Lower gastrointestinal blood loss
- Nausea and vomiting

Severe poisoning

- Coma
- Delayed hepatocellular necrosis
- Hypotension
- Death

Gastric lavage should be considered if the patient presents within 1 hour of ingestion. Intravenous desferrioxamine chelates iron and improves clinical outcome in severe cases.

5.7 Salicylate overdose

Salicylate poisoning causes direct stimulation of the respiratory centre (respiratory alkalosis), and accumulation of organic acids (metabolic acidosis).

Early features of salicylate poisoning

- Hypokalaemia
- Respiratory centre stimulation in the CNS, and hence alkalosis
- Sweating
- Tinnitus

Later features of salicylate poisoning

- Acute renal failure
- Hypoglycaemia
- Hypoprothrombinaemia
- Metabolic acidosis
- Pulmonary oedema

Key aspects of management of salicylate poisoning involve:

- Activated charcoal.
- Correction of electrolyte and metabolic abnormalities.
- Intravenous fluids to ensure adequate hydration (forced diuresis is unsafe and not recommended).
- **Haemodialysis**: for very severe salicylism (blood salicylate >750 mg/l).

5.8 Ethylene glycol poisoning

Ethylene glycol (1,2-ethanediol) is a major component of antifreeze and other industrial fluids. In the first 12 hours, poisoning can give the appearance of alcohol intoxication with cerebellar symptoms and signs, but without the smell of alcohol. Breakdown of ethylene glycol to oxalate causes metabolic acidosis with raised anion gap due to exogenous organic acid, and a raised osmolar gap. Acute tubular necrosis develops after 2–3 days due to accumulation of glycolates and oxalates, and cardiac failure and pulmonary oedema can occur.

5.9 Haemodialysis for overdose or poisoning

Dialysis assists elimination of certain drugs or metabolites. It is generally **ineffective** for those with a large volume of distribution (eg amiodarone and paraquat) and those with high protein binding (eg digoxin and phenytoin). Repeated or continuous dialysis might be required for drugs that are widely distributed throughout the body, eg lithium.

Removal of drugs or toxins by haemodialysis/haemoperfusion

- Haemodialysis effective

  - Alcohol
  - Barbiturates
  - Ethylene glycol
  - Lithium
  - Methanol
  - Salicylate

- Charcoal haemoperfusion

  - Paracetamol metabolites
  - Theophylline

Further revision

Rang HP, Dale MM, Ritter JM, Moore P. *Pharmacology*, 5th Edn. London: Churchill Livingstone, 2005.

The *British National Formulary* contains valuable information about drug treatment of a wide range of diseases, with details of drugs licensed in the UK, including indications, dose, route and cost (requires on-line registration) at http://www.bnf.org.

Drugs and Therapeutics Bulletin provides reviews of specific drugs and therapeutic strategies for common diseases at http://www.dtb.org.uk/dtb/.

The British Pharmacology Society (BPS) website contains a core curriculum for undergraduate students, and provides access to computer-assisted learning modules, at
http://www.bps.ac.uk/education/resources.jsp.

The British Toxicology Society provides Continuing Professional Development with an online area dedicated to young toxicologists at www.thebts.com.

United Kingdom Medicines Information Pharmacists Group (UKMIPG) website at http://www.ukmi.nhs.uk.

In the UK, information on poisoning is provided by the National Poisons Information Services (NPIS) using TOXBASE®, an internet-based resource available to hospital departments and GP surgeries, and via telephone enquiries to NPIS centres. The NPIS is part of the Chemicals and Hazards division of the Health Protection Agency, and more information is available via their website http://www.hpa.org.uk/chemicals/poisoning.htm (accessed November 2005).

You should now understand that:

1. A number of important genetic variations can influence how people metabolise and respond to drugs, eg rapid and slow acetylators.

2. Certain drugs can enhance liver enzyme activity (enzyme inducers), which means that other drugs may be metabolised more rapidly. For example, phenytoin is an important enzyme inducer that makes the oral contraceptive pill less effective.

3. Certain drugs can reduce liver enzyme activity (enzyme inhibitors), so that other drugs are metabolised less extensively. For example, ciprofloxacin is an enzyme inhibitor that may increase the risk of theophylline toxicity.

4. For drugs normally cleared extensively by renal elimination, the dose and frequency of administration need to be reduced in patients with renal impairment (eg gentamicin).

5. Drugs that are extensively cleared by hepatic metabolism need to have their dose reduced in patients with liver disease (eg rifampicin).

6. Drugs can cause a wide range of adverse effects including rash, anaemia, pancreatitis, hepatitis, dyskinesia and gynaecomastia. Adverse effects can occur early (eg anaphylaxis) or late (eg fibrosis after methotrexate). They can be dose-dependent (eg renal failure due to ACE inhibitors) or idiosyncratic (eg neutropenia due to carbimazole). Management of overdose patients involves supportive care, monitoring of fluid and electrolyte balance and consideration of antidote treatment if available. Haemodialysis may be effective in enhancing clearance of certain drugs.

Dermatology

CONTENTS

Revision objectives

1. Understand how to approach the history and examination of a patient with a skin problem
2. Have an awareness of the common dermatological dermatoses and their appearances
3. Have an awareness of how infection can affect the skin
4. Understand how the skin can give clues to systemic diseases
5. Understand how drugs can affect the skin
6. Be aware of the different types of skin malignancy
7. Be aware of hair and nail disorders

1. STRUCTURE AND FUNCTION OF SKIN AND TERMINOLOGY OF SKIN LESIONS

1.1 Structure

The skin consists of three distinctive layers: the epidermis, dermis and the subcutis.

- **Epidermis:** this forms the outermost layer and is the largest organ in the body. The principal cell is the keratinocyte. The epidermis has four layers, which are the basal cell layer, stratum spinosum, stratum granulosum and the stratum corneum.
- **Dermis:** this lies beneath the epidermis and is a support structurally and nutritionally, and contributes 15–20% of total body weight. The principal cell is the fibroblast, which makes collagen (giving the skin its strength), elastin (providing elasticity) and proteoglycans. It also contains adnexal structures including hair follicles, sebaceous glands, apocrine glands and eccrine glands.
- **Dermo-epidermal junction:** separates the epidermis from the dermis. Anomalies of this can give rise to some of the blistering disorders.
- **Subcutis:** contains adipose tissue, loose connective tissue, blood vessels and nerves.

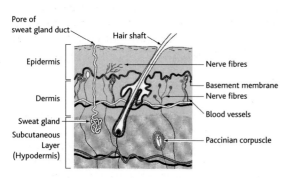

Figure 1 The anatomy of the skin
Source www.nurse-prescriber.co.uk

1.2 Function

The skin has numerous functions, all of which are designed to protect the rest of the body.

- **Barrier properties:** the skin acts as a two-way barrier, preventing the inward or outward passage of fluid and electrolytes.
- **Mechanical properties:** the skin is highly elastic and so can be stretched or compressed.
- **Immunological function:** the skin provides defence against foreign agents. In the epidermis, antigen presentation is carried out by Langerhans' cells.

- **Sensory function:** the skin perceives the sensations of touch, pressure, cold, warmth and pain.
- **Endocrine properties:** as a result of exposure to ultraviolet B radiation, vitamin D3 is synthesised from previtamin D3.
- **Temperature regulation:** the rich blood supply of the dermis plays an important role in thermoregulation.
- **Respiration:** the skin plays a minor role in gaseous exchange with the environment.

2. TAKING A HISTORY

2.1 History of presenting complaint

Find out exactly when and where on the body the eruption started and how it has evolved up to the present. Have the lesions been constant or do they come and go? Are there any associated symptoms such as itch? Was there an initiating event? Are there any factors that exacerbate or relieve the eruption?

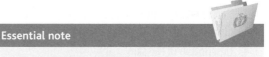

> **Essential note**
>
> A full detailed description is necessary and depends on a thorough examination of all the skin, preferably in good natural light

2.2 Past medical history

Elicit if there is a history of skin problems. Other medical disorders may well be relevant including symptoms of atopy.

2.3 Social history

Occupational history may be relevant especially in cases of irritant or contact dermatitis. Sun exposure is relevant both to photosensitive conditions and chronic sun damage leading to development of skin cancers. Alcohol intake should be noted.

2.4 Family history

This helps identify those conditions that have a strong hereditary component, eg psoriasis and atopic eczema. It may also indicate whether the eruption is contagious, eg scabies.

2.5 Drug history

As well as taking a full drug history, elicit whether any of the medications have been recently commenced and whether there is a history of true drug allergy. It is important to directly enquire whether the patient has used any over-the-counter drugs or creams.

3. EXAMINATION OF THE SKIN

All of the skin should be examined, preferably in good natural light.

- Look carefully at the skin eruption and consider the following points:

  - Distribution of the eruption:

    - Localised/widespread
    - Symmetrical/non-symmetrical
    - Are other sites affected?
    - Scalp/nails/mouth/genitalia

  - For each individual lesion:

    - Size
    - Shape
    - Colour
    - Border (well/ill defined)
    - Surface – smooth/shiny/irregular
    - Presence of other features, eg scale, crust, erosions.

- Palpate the skin to determine skin texture, consistency and whether the rash is raised or not.

4. DESCRIPTION OF THE SKIN

A full, detailed description is necessary and depends on a thorough examination. It is helpful to imagine you are describing the eruption to a person on the telephone.

Start with the distribution – exactly where on the body the rash or lesion is, and continue with each of the points above. The following terminology is used for individual lesions.

4.1 Terminology of skin lesions

Macule: a flat lesion due to a localised colour change; when >1 cm in diameter, this is termed a patch
Papule: a small solid elevation of skin <1 cm diameter
Plaque: a raised flat-topped lesion >1 cm diameter
Nodule: a raised lesion with a rounded surface >1 cm diameter
Bulla: a fluid-filled lesion (blister) >1 cm diameter
Vesicle: a fluid-filled skin lesion <1 cm diameter
Pustule: a pus-filled lesion
Wheal: a raised compressible area of dermal oedema
Scale: flakes arising from abnormal stratum corneum
Crust: dried serum, pus or blood.

5. SPECIFIC DERMATOSES AND INFECTIONS OF THE SKIN

5.1 Psoriasis

Psoriasis is a chronic, non-infectious, inflammatory disease of the skin characterised by well-demarcated erythematous plaques bearing silvery scales.

Essential note

Chronic plaque psoriasis is characterised by well-demarcated erythematous plaques with silvery scale

Psoriasis is a genetically determined, inflammatory and proliferative disorder of the skin, occurring in 1–2% of the UK population. Its aetiology is unknown but there is an association with HLA Cw6, B13 and B17 in skin disease and HLA B27 in psoriatic arthropathy. The disease is more common in the second and sixth decades, with females generally developing psoriasis at an earlier age than males.

Psoriasis tends to affect the extensor surfaces and demonstrates the Köbner phenomenon (trauma to the epidermis and dermis, such as a scratch or a surgical scar can precipitate psoriasis in the damaged skin). Other affected areas include the scalp, nails, genitalia and flexures.

Clinical presentation

- **Chronic plaque**: well-defined red, disc-like plaques covered by white scale, which classically affect elbows, knees and scalp.
- **Pustular (generalised pustular)**: sheets of small, sterile yellow pustules on a red background. This presentation may be accompanied by systemic symptoms and progression to erythroderma. (Erythroderma is involvement of 90% or greater of the skin surface by an inflammatory dermatosis.)
- **Pustular (palmo-plantar pustulosis)**: yellow/brown sterile pustules and erythema on palms or soles. Strongly associated with smoking. This is most often seen in middle-aged women.
- **Guttate**: an acute eruption of drop-like lesions often following a streptococcal sore throat.
- **Erythrodermic**: confluent areas affecting most of the skin surface.
- **Nail psoriasis**: onycholysis, pitting and subungal hyperkeratosis.

- **Flexural**: affects axillae, submammary areas and the natal cleft. Lesions are often smooth, red and glazed in appearance.

Associations with psoriasis

- **Arthropathy**: arthritis occurs in about 8% of patients with psoriasis. There are several different forms (*see* Chapter 16, Rheumatology) – distal inter-phalangeal joint disease, large single joint oligoarthritis, arthritis mutilans, sacro-iliitis and psoriatic spondylitis have all been described.
- **Gout**
- **Malabsorption**: Crohn's and ulcerative colitis are associated with psoriasis.

Factors that can exacerbate psoriasis

- **Trauma**: the Köbner phenomenon (see above)
- **Infection**: eg streptococci (guttate psoriasis as above) and HIV
- **Endocrine**: psoriasis generally tends to improve during pregnancy and deteriorate in the post-partum period
- **Drugs**: beta-blockers, lithium, antimalarials and the withdrawal of oral steroids can exacerbate psoriasis
- **Alcohol**
- **Stress**: severe physical or psychological stress.

Causes of the Köbner phenomenon

- Psoriasis
- Lichen planus
- Vitiligo
- Viral warts
- Molluscum contagiosum

Causes of erythroderma

- Psoriasis
- Eczema
- Mycosis fungoides
- Adverse drug reactions
- Underlying malignancy

Management of psoriasis

A careful explanation of the disease process and the likely necessity for long-term treatment should always be given. The type and severity of psoriasis influences the choice of treatment. However, it is usual to prescribe topical agents as the first-line treatment.

softening/soothing

- **Topical therapy**: emollients, tar preparations, dithranol, vitamin D analogues, topical steroids (for face, genitalia and flexures).

For widespread or severe disease further treatment options are **ultraviolet radiation**, **systemic treatment**, or newer **biological agents**.

Ultraviolet radiation

- PUVA (oral/topical psoralen and UVA)
- UVB narrowband (311–313 nm) is now replacing broadband UVB (290–320 nm).

Systemic treatment

The benefits must be weighed against side-effects of the drugs. Treatments include retinoids (vitamin A derivatives), methotrexate, ciclosporin, azathioprine, hydroxyurea, mycophenolate mofetil (MMF).

Biological agents

These are promising new treatments but as yet they are not licensed for use in psoriasis. Etanercept and efalizumab are presently under review by NICE.

5.2 Eczema (dermatitis)

Eczema is an inflammatory skin disorder with characteristic histology and clinical features, which include itching, redness, scaling and a papulovesicular rash. Eczema can be divided into two broad groups, exogenous or endogenous.

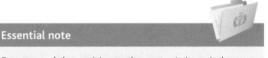

Essential note

Eczema and dermatitis are the same. It is an itchy, erythematous rash often with papules, vesicles and exudation

- Exogenous eczema – irritant dermatitis, allergic contact dermatitis
- Endogenous eczema – atopic dermatitis, seborrhoeic dermatitis, pompholyx.

Seborrhoeic dermatitis is a red, scaly rash caused by *Pityrosporum ovale*. The eruption occurs on the scalp, face and upper trunk and is more common in young adults and HIV patients.

Pompholyx is characterised by itchy vesicles occurring on the palms and soles.

Atopic dermatitis is a characteristic dermatitic eruption associated with a personal or family history of atopy. The age of onset is usually between two and six months, with males being more affected than females. The disease is chronic but tends to improve during childhood. The flexural sites are commonly affected and features include itching, exudative papules or vesicles, dryness and lichenification. There is an increased risk of bacterial (staphylococcal or streptococcal) and viral (Herpes simplex) infection.

Management of atopic eczema

Initial treatment consists of avoidance of irritants and of exacerbating factors. Thereafter:

- **Topical therapy**: regular emollients, topical steroids, tar bandages, wet wraps and antibiotic ointment (for minor infections). Topical tacrolimus and pimecrolimus are indicated as second-line treatments for moderate to severe atopic dermatitis in patients who have not been controlled on topical steroids or who have had adverse effects to topical steroids.
- **Ultraviolet radiation**: UVB or PUVA (*see* Section 5.1, Psoriasis).
- **Systemic treatment**: this can be with ciclosporin, azathioprine, antihistamines, as well as antibiotics for any infective episodes.

5.3 Lichen planus

This presents as an itchy, shiny, violaceous, flat-topped, polygonal, papular rash with white lines on the surface known as Wickham's striae. Other affected sites include mucous membranes, genitalia, palms, soles, scalp and nails. Lichen planus causes a white lace-like pattern on the buccal mucosa.

5.4 Erythema multiforme

This is usually a maculo-papular, targetoid rash, which can occur anywhere, including the palms, soles and oral mucosa. The most common cause is thought to be herpes simplex virus (HSV).

Stevens–Johnson syndrome – this is erythema multiforme that is more likely to affect mucosal surfaces; it is usually associated with drug reactions.

Causes of erythema multiforme

- Infections: HSV, mycoplasma, hepatitis B virus, orf, HIV
- Drug reactions: eg sulphonamides, penicillins
- Others: SLE, sarcoidosis, malignancy

5.5 Erythema nodosum

This is a hot, tender, nodular, erythematous eruption lasting three to six weeks, which is more common in the third decade and in females.

Causes of erythema nodosum

- **Bacterial infection**
  - Streptococcal throat infection
- **Mycoses**
- **Sarcoidosis**
- **Tuberculosis**
- **Malignancy**
- **Viral/chlamydial infection**
- **Other infections**
  - Salmonella gastroenteritis
  - Campylobacter colitis
- **Inflammatory bowel disease**
- **Drugs**
  - Penicillin
  - Tetracyclines
  - Oral contraceptive pill
  - Sulphonamides
  - Sulphonylureas

5.6 Acne and rosacea

Acne vulgaris

Acne vulgaris is a disease of the pilosebaceous units and is characterised by inflammatory papules and pustules and open and closed comedones (blackheads). There is an increased sebum rate. The peak age for acne is 18 years in both sexes.

Treatment

Topical treatments include benzoyl peroxide and tretinoin. Systemic treatments include oral tetracyclines or erythromycin, co-cyprindiol (Dianette®, an anti-androgenic oral contraceptive) and oral isotretinoin.

Rosacea

Rosacea is a disease of the middle-aged and elderly and is characterised by facial erythema, telangiectasia, papules and sterile pustules. There is no increase in sebum rate. Rhinophyma – hyperplasia of the sebaceous glands and connective tissue of the nose and eye involvement by blepharitis and conjunctivitis are complications. Treatment is with oral tetracycline or topical metronidazole.

6. BULLOUS ERUPTIONS

This is a rare group of disorders characterised by the formation of bullae. The development of blisters can be due to congenital, immunological or other causes. The level of split within the epidermis or within the dermo-epidermal junction determines the type of bullous disorder.

Causes of bullous eruptions

- Congenital

  - Epidermolysis bullosa

- Others

  - Staphylococcal scalded-skin syndrome
  - Toxic epidermal necrolysis
  - Friction/burns
  - Bullous impetigo
  - Herpes simplex/zoster
  - Acute eczema

- Immunological

  - Pemphigus
  - Bullous pemphigoid
  - Cicatricial pemphigoid
  - Pemphigoid gestationis
  - Dermatitis herpetiformis

Epidermolysis bullosa is the term used for a group of genetically determined disorders characterised by blistering of the skin, palms, soles and mucosae, especially the mouth and oesophagus.

Staphylococcal scalded skin syndrome is caused by a toxin released by some strains of s.aureus – often in only a minor infection. The toxin causes a split to occur in the epidermis and large areas of the epidermis can be loosened and shed. It responds well to systemic antibiotics.

Toxic epidermal necrolysis is a medical emergency and has a high mortality rate. It is due to a drug hypersensitivity or toxicity causing a split which is supepidermal. The eutine epidermis may become necrotic and comes off in sheets like a scald. Treatment is stopping the drug, intensive fluid balance and nursing care. The use of systemic steroids or IV immunoglobulin is controversial.

Pemphigus is a severe, often life threatening blistering disorder of the skin and mucous membranes. It is due to autoantibodies to the intercellular areas of the epidermis. The split is intraepidermal. Treatment is with systemic steroids or other immunosuppressive agents.

Bullous pemphigoid is more common than pemphigus. It is a disorder characterised by large tense blisters found on limbs, trunk and flexures in the elderly. Oral mucosal involvement is rare. It is due to autoantibodies to the basement membrane – the split is subepidermal causing intact blisters.

Cicatricial pemphigoid is a rare, chronic blistering disease of the mucous membranes and skin, which results in permanent scarring, particularly of the conjunctivae.

Dermatitis herpetiformis is an itchy, vesiculo-bullous eruption mainly occurring on the extensor areas. The majority of patients have asymptomatic gluten-sensitive enteropathy. Lesions contain IgA. IgA is found in the dermis.

7. SPECIFIC SKIN INFECTIONS

These can be sub-divided into bacterial, fungal and viral infections as well as infestations.

Specific infections of the skin

- Bacterial infections

  - Streptococcal: cellulitis, erysipelas, impetigo, necrotising fasciitis, rheumatic fever (erythema marginatum), scarlet fever
  - Staphylococcal: folliculitis, impetigo, staphylococcal scalded-skin syndrome, toxic-shock syndrome
  - Mycobacterial: TB (lupus vulgaris, scrofuloderma), fish tank granuloma, Buruli ulcer, leprosy
  - Spirochaetal: syphilis, Lyme disease (erythema chronicum migrans)

- Fungal

  - Dermatophytes: *Trichophyton rubrum, Trichophyton interdigitale, Epidermophyton floccosum* (tinea pedis, tinea corporis, tinea cruris, tinea unguium)
  - Yeasts: *Candida* (intertrigo, oral, genital or systemic)
  - *Pityrosporum orbiculare*: pityriasis versicolor

- Viral

  - Human papilloma virus: warts
  - Herpes virus: varicella (chickenpox), zoster (shingles), simplex I (face and lips), simplex II (genital)

Specific infections of the skin

- Viral

  - Pox virus: molluscum contagiosum, parapox virus (orf)
  - Parvovirus B19: erythema infectiosum (fifth disease)
  - RNA virus: measles, rubella
  - Coxsackie A16: hand, foot and mouth disease
  - HIV/AIDS: skin disease is common, affecting 75% of patients who can be at any stage of HIV disease (*see* Chapter 7, Genito-urinary medicine and AIDS)

- Infestations

  - *Sarcoptes scabiei*: scabies mite infestation
  - Lice infestation (pediculosis): head lice, pubic lice

8. THE SKIN IN SYSTEMIC DISEASES

8.1 Systemic sclerosis

This is a rare, multisystem, connective tissue disease of unknown aetiology, characterised by fibrosis of the skin and visceral organs and accompanied by the presence of relatively specific antinuclear antibodies. The incidence peaks in the fifth and sixth decades and females are more affected than males. Prognosis is poor.

Morphoea (localised scleroderma) consists of indurated plaques of sclerosis in the skin; systemic features are not found.

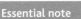

Essential note

Signs in the skin often give clues to systemic disease

Skin changes in systemic sclerosis

- Facial telangiectasia
- Restricted mouth opening
- Peri-oral puckering
- Smooth shiny pigmented indurated skin
- Raynaud's phenomenon with gangrene

Skin changes in systemic sclerosis

- Sclerodactyly
- Pulp atrophy
- Dilated nail fold capillaries
- Ragged cuticles
- Calcinosis cutis
- Livedo reticularis
- Leg ulcers

8.2 Rheumatoid arthritis

Specific skin changes in rheumatoid arthritis

- Rheumatoid nodules
- Nail fold infarcts
- Vasculitis with gangrene
- Pyoderma gangrenosum.

8.3 Dermatomyositis

Specific skin changes in dermatomyositis

- Heliotrope rash around eyes
- Gottron's papules: red plaques on extensor surfaces of finger joints
- Gottron's sign: erythema over knees and elbows
- Dilated nail fold capillaries and prominent, ragged cuticles
- Nail fold infarcts.

8.4 Lupus erythematosus

Discoid lupus erythematosus is associated with scaly erythematous plaques with follicular plugging, on sun-exposed sites. These tend to heal with scarring.

Systemic lupus erythematosus (SLE) is commonly associated with dermatological manifestations. These include malar rash, photosensitivity, vasculitis, Raynaud's phenomenon, alopecia and oropharyngeal ulceration.

8.5 Sarcoidosis

Skin lesions are found in approximately 25% of patients with systemic sarcoid and can occur in the absence of systemic disease.

- Erythema nodosum
- Scar sarcoid
- Lupus pernio
- Scarring alopecia.

8.6 Diabetes

Skin signs in diabetes mellitus

- Necrobiosis lipoidica
- Disseminated granuloma annulare
- Diabetic rubeosis
- Candidiasis and infection
- Neuropathic foot ulcers.

Diabetic rubeosis is an odd redness of the face, hands and feet thought to be due to diabetic microangiopathy.

9. GENERALISED PRURITUS

Pruritus is an important skin symptom and occurs in dermatological diseases such as atopic eczema. In the absence of localised skin disease or skin signs, patients should be fully investigated to exclude an underlying cause.

Causes of generalised pruritus

- Obstructive liver disease
- Haematological
  - Iron deficiency anaemia
  - Polycythaemia
- Endocrine
  - Hyperthyroidism
  - Hypothyroidism
  - Diabetes mellitus
- Chronic renal failure
- Malignancy
  - Internal malignancies
  - Lymphoma
- Drugs
  - Morphine
- Other
  - Pregnancy
  - Senility

10. CUTANEOUS MARKERS OF INTERNAL MALIGNANCY

Dermatological features can be seen in all types of malignant disease but some are more common in certain types of neoplasia. Some are:

- **Acanthosis nigricans**: gastrointestinal adenocarcinoma
- **Acanthosis palmaris (tripe palms)**: bronchial carcinoma
- **Generalised pruritus**: lymphoma
- **Dermatomyositis (in adults)**: bronchial, breast and ovarian tumours
- **Erythema gyratum repens**: bronchial carcinoma
- **Acquired hypertrichosis lanuginosa**: gastrointestinal and bronchial tumours
- **Necrolytic migratory erythema**: glucagonoma
- **Migratory thrombophlebitis**: pancreatic carcinoma
- **Acquired ichthyosis**: lymphoma
- **Clubbing**: bronchial carcinoma

Other causes of acanthosis nigricans

- Internal malignancy
- Insulin-resistant diabetes mellitus
- Familial
- Acromegaly
- Cushing's disease
- Obesity
- Oral contraceptive pill
- Nicotinic acid
- Hypothyroidism

11. DRUG ERUPTIONS

The incidence of drug eruptions is approximately 2%.

Essential note

Drug eruptions are common and have many different forms

The most common drug eruptions are:

- **Toxic erythema**: the commonest type of eruption. It is usually characterised by a morbilliform or maculopapular eruption which may become confluent. Causes include antibiotics (including sulphonamides), carbamazepine, allopurinol, gold, thiazides and anti-tuberculous drugs.
- **Fixed drug eruption**: this occurs in a localised site each time the drug is administered (see below).
- **Toxic epidermal necrolysis**: a life-threatening eruption due to extensive skin loss. This can be associated with allopurinol, sulphonamides, penicillin, carbamazepine, phenytoin, NSAIDs, gold, salicylates and barbiturates.
- **Urticaria**: (see below).
- **Photosensitivity** (*see* Chapter 2, Clinical pharmacology, toxicology and poisoning).
- **Lupus erythematosus-like syndrome**: a number of drugs have been implicated to cause this relatively rare disorder (*see* Chapter 2, Clinical pharmacology, toxicology and poisoning).
- **Vasculitis** (*see* Chapter 2, Clinical pharmacology, toxicology and poisoning).
- **Erythema multiforme**: this is associated with penicillins, sulphonamides, phenytoin, carbamazepine, ACE inhibitors, NSAIDs, gold, barbiturates, thiazides.
- **Contact dermatitis.**
- **Hyperpigmentation** (see above): associated with amiodarone, minocycline, bleomycin, chlorpromazine, antimalarials.

Urticaria is a transient, itchy, erythematous rash characterised by the presence of weals. It is thought to occur due to histamine release from mast cells, but other mediators such as prostaglandins and leukotrienes have also been implicated. 95% of cases are idiopathic. Drug causes include salicylates, ACE inhibitors and penicillins. **Angio-oedema** is similar to urticaria, but histologically there is greater swelling of the subcutaneous tissue and mucosal sites are often affected.

12. NAEVI AND SKIN TUMOURS

A naevus is a benign proliferation of cells of the skin. The most common type is where there is a proliferation of melanocytes – a melanocytic naevus. Other types of naevi include vascular naevi (eg port wine stain), the epidermal naevus and connective tissue naevi.

Melanocytic naevi can be classified according to where the naevus cells lie in the skin.

Epidermis

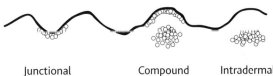

Junctional   Compound   Intradermal

Dermis

Figure 2 Types of melanocytic naevi

12.1 Benign tumours

Some common benign skin tumours

- **Seborrhoeic wart**: very common in middle aged/elderly. Flat with irregular/warty surface. Have the appearance of being 'stuck on'
- **Dermatofibroma**: a firm often pigmented dermal papule, often found on the lower legs
- **Lipoma**: a fatty mass in the subcutaneous tissue
- **Pyogenic granuloma**: a rapidly growing red lesion often in an area of trauma
- **Epidermoid cyst**: a firm skin-coloured keratin-filled cyst with a central punctum
- **Campbell de Morgan spot (cherry angioma)**: bright red papules, 1–4 mm, found on trunk

12.2 Malignant skin tumours

Malignant melanoma

This has an incidence of around 10 per 100 000 per year; and this is doubling every decade. The prognosis is related to tumour thickness. Early lesions are often curable by surgical excision. Any changing mole (bleeding, increase in size, itching, etc) should be viewed suspiciously.

The different types of melanoma are:

- **Superficial spreading**: this is the most common. An irregularly pigmented macule or plaque which may have an irregular edge and colour variation.
- **Nodular**: a pigmented nodule, often rapidly growing and aggressive.
- **Lentigo maligna melanoma**: occurs in the elderly in a long-standing lentigo maligna (a slowly expanding, irregularly pigmented macule).
- **Acral lentiginous melanoma**: occurs on the palms, soles and nail beds. This is the commonest type of melanoma in Chinese and Japanese people.

Basal cell carcinoma

This is the commonest skin cancer and are seen most commonly on the face of elderly or middle-aged patients. They only very rarely metastasise. Predisposing factors for basal cell carcinoma are:

- Prolonged sun exposure (most common)
- Radiation treatment
- Chronic scarring
- Ingestion of arsenic (tonics)
- Basal cell naevus syndrome (Gorlin's syndrome).

Basal cell carcinomas are classified as:

- Nodular/cystic
- Superficial
- Morphoeic
- Pigmented.

Essential note

Skin cancers are the most common malignancies seen in the UK

Squamous cell carcinoma

These lesions may metastasise and therefore early diagnosis and treatment is important. There are several predisposing factors for squamous cell carcinoma:

- **Pre-malignant conditions**: these include Bowen's disease, actinic keratosis (solar keratosis – a red scaly plaque in sun-damaged skin) and actinic cheilitis (actinic keratosis of the lip)
- **Actinic damage**: squamous carcinomas can also develop in just sun-damaged skin (in the absence of actinic keratosis)
- **X-irradiation**
- **Chronic scarring or inflammation**
- **Smoking (particularly lesions of the lip)**
- **Arsenic ingestion**
- **Organic hydrocarbons**
- **Immunosuppression**
- **Human papilloma virus.**

Other skin tumours

Keratoacanthoma

- A rapidly growing tumour arising in sun-exposed skin
- This is normally thought of as benign but histologically it is similar to squamous cell carcinoma

Cutaneous T-cell lymphoma (mycosis fungoides)

- A lymphoma that evolves in the skin, usually over a protracted course of many years
- The clinical pattern may be varied

13. HAIR AND NAILS

13.1 Alopecia

Loss of hair is called alopecia and can be scarring or non-scarring.

- **Scarring alopecia** is loss of hair with destruction of the hair follicles. This condition can result from: burns/irradiation, infection or inflammatory causes such as lichen planus or lupus erythematosus.
- **Non-scarring alopecia** is when the hair follicles are preserved. A good example of this is the 'exclamation mark' hair seen in the patchy hair loss of alopecia areata. Other causes include androgenetic (male/female pattern hair loss) and diffuse alopecia, which may be due to hypothyroidism, iron deficiency and drugs such as cytotoxics.

13.2 Disorders of nails

Nails are derived from keratin. This is a protein complex, which gives the nail its hard property. The nail can be affected in a variety of skin and systemic disorders.

Causes of nail changes associated with skin disorders

- **Psoriasis**: nail changes include onycholysis, nail pitting, hyperkeratosis, pustule and occasional loss of nail.
- **Fungal**: signs include discoloration, onycholysis and thickening of the nail.
- **Bacterial**: usually due to staphylococcal infections. *Pseudomonas* infections give a green discoloration to the nail.

- **Lichen planus**: nail changes occur in 10% of cases, with thinning of the nail plate and longitudinal linear depressions. Occasionally there is destruction of the nail (pterygium),
- **Alopecia areata**: pitting, thickening and ridging of the nail (sandpaper nail) is seen.

Causes of nail changes associated with systemic disease

- **Koilonychia**: the nails are thin, brittle and concave. There is an association with iron deficiency anaemia.
- **Yellow nail syndrome**: the nails are yellow and excessively curved. The syndrome is associated with recurrent pleural effusions, chronic bronchitis, bronchiectasis, nephrotic syndrome and hypothyroidism.

- **Beau's lines**: these are transverse depressions in the nail due to temporary arrest in growth. They usually occur after a period of illness or infection.
- **Half and half nails**: the proximal nail bed is white and distal, pink or brown. They are associated with chronic renal failure and rheumatoid arthritis.

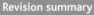

Further revision

Buxton P K. *ABC of dermatology*. 3rd edn. London: BMJ Publishing Group, 1998.

Revision summary

1. Be able to take a full history relevant to dermatology. Should be able to undertake a full detailed examination of the skin and a full description of the findings. Know the terminology of skin lesions.
2. Have an understanding of the different types of psoriasis and eczema and their management. Know which factors can exacerbate psoriasis.
3. Know the causes of erythema nodosum.
4. Should understand the clinical presentations of bacterial, fungal and viral infections.
5. Be aware of the skin changes that can occur in connective tissue diseases, rheumatoid arthritis and diabetes. Know the various causes of pruritus and cutaneous markers for internal malignancy.
6. Be aware of the different types of drug eruptions in the skin and the likely drug precipitants.
7. Understand the types of melanoma, basal cell carcinoma and squamous cell carcinoma and factors that predispose to their development.
8. Have an awareness of the types of alopecia and nail changes that can occur with skin disorders and systemic diseases.

Endocrinology

CONTENTS

Endocrinology

Revision objectives

You should:

1. Be aware of the different types of hormones and their modes of action
2. Be aware of hormonal changes related to disease states and the appropriate investigations
3. Be aware of the structure and role of the pituitary gland, and associated diseases
4. Be aware of the clinical features, investigation and treatment of abnormal thyroid gland function
5. Be aware of the clinical features, investigations and treatment of abnormal adrenal gland function
6. Be aware of the different types of diabetes mellitus and their treatment

1. HORMONE ACTION

The way a hormone acts in cells and much of its physiology can be predicted by knowing the type of hormone concerned. There are three main types of hormone:

- Amine
- Steroid
- Peptide.

Thyroxine is an exception to this as shown below.

1.1 Types of hormone

- **Amine**: catecholamines, serotonin, **thyroxine**
- **Steroid**: cortisol, aldosterone, androgens, oestrogens and progestogens and **vitamin D**
- **Peptide**: everything else! (made up of a series of amino-acids).

Thyroxine is chemically an amine but it acts like a steroid. Vitamin D has the structure of a steroid hormone and it acts like one.

Essential note

There are three main types of hormone: amine, steroid and peptide

Amines/peptides

- Short half-life (minutes)
- Secretion may be pulsatile
- Act on a cell surface receptor
- Often act via a second messenger

Steroids

- Longer biological half-life (hours)
- Act on an intracellular receptor
- Act on DNA to alter gene expression

This information can be used to predict hormone action. For example, aldosterone is a steroid hormone so it must have a biological half-life of several hours, bind to an intracellular receptor and affect gene transcription. Glucagon is not a steroid or an amine so it must be a polypeptide hormone which has a short circulation half-life, acts via a cell-surface receptor and probably utilises a second messenger (cAMP in fact).

1.2 Hormones that act at the cell surface

Peptide and amine hormones act at the cell surface via specific membrane receptors. The signal is transmitted intracellularly by one of three mechanisms:

- Via cAMP
- Via a rise in intracellular Ca^{2+} levels
- Via receptor tyrosine kinases.

If in doubt, assume the action of a peptide or amine hormone (excluding thyroxine) is via cAMP unless it is insulin or has the word 'growth' in its name, in which case it is likely to act via a receptor tyrosine kinase.

Essential note

Peptide and amine hormones act via cell surface receptors

Via cAMP	Via Ca²⁺	Via receptor tyrosine kinases
Adrenaline (β receptors)	GnRH	Insulin
All pituitary hormones except GH, PRL	TRH	GH, PRL
Glucagon	Adrenaline (α receptors)	'Growth factors': IGF-1, EGF
Somatostatin		

cAMP = cyclic adenosine monophosphate; GnRH = gonadotrophin releasing hormone; GH = growth hormone; PRL = prolactin; TRH = thyrotrophin releasing hormone; IGF-1 = insulin-like growth factor 1; EGF = epidermal growth factor.

1.3 Hormones that act intracellularly

Steroids and vitamin D are sufficiently lipid soluble that they do not need cell surface receptors but can diffuse directly through the cell membrane. They then bind to receptors in the cytoplasm which results in shedding of heat shock proteins that protect the empty receptor. The hormone–receptor complex migrates into the nucleus where the complex alters the transcription of a large number of genes.

Essential note

Steroids diffuse through the cell membrane to act intracellularly

2. SPECIFIC HORMONE PHYSIOLOGY

2.1 Hormones from the hypothalamus and pituitary

There are certain facts about hormone physiology which are particularly relevant to medicine.

Figure 1 summarises the hormones released from the hypothalamus and pituitary.

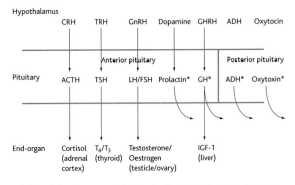

Figure 1 Hormones released from the hypothalamus and pituitary

* These pituitary hormones act directly rather than by releasing another hormone. GH acts directly and by releasing IGF-1 from the liver

Essential note

The anterior pituitary secretes growth hormone, prolactin, follicle-stimulating hormone, luteinising hormone, thyroid-stimulating hormone, ACTH and endorphins. The posterior pituitary secretes oxytocin and ADH

2.2 Hormone changes in illness

During illness/stress, the body closes all unnecessary systems down 'from the top', eg the thyroid axis closes down by a fall in thyrotrophin releasing hormone (TRH), thyroid-stimulating hormone (TSH) and L-thyroxine/tri-iodo-thyronine (T_4/T_3). It is orchestrated by the hypothalamus, not by the end organs. Hormones involved in the stress response may rise.

Hormones which fall	May rise (stress hormones)
TSH, T_4/T_3*	GH (though IGF-1 falls)
LH, FSH	ACTH, glucocorticoids
Testosterone, oestrogen	Adrenaline
Insulin (starvation)	Glucagon (starvation)
	Prolactin

Continued over

Continued

TSH = Thyroid-stimulating hormone; GH = growth hormone; IGF-1 = insulin-like growth factor 1; LH = luteinising hormone; FSH = follicle-stimulating hormone; ACTH = adrenocorticotrophic hormone; T_3 = L-thyronine; T_4 = L-thyroxine.

*In this case conversion of T_4 to T_3 is inhibited so T_3 falls more than T_4

2.3 Leptin, adipokines and other hormones involved with appetite and weight

Leptin was identified as a product of the *ob* gene in 1994; *ob/ob* mice make no leptin owing to a homozygous *ob* gene mutation and are grossly obese.

- Leptin is a polypeptide hormone, released from fat cells, that acts on specific receptors in the hypothalamus to reduce appetite.
- Circulating leptin levels are directly proportional to fat mass, and hence they tell the brain how fat an individual is.
- Leptin appears to have stimulatory effects on metabolic rate and levels fall in starvation (appropriate change for weight homeostasis).
- Adequate leptin levels are required for the onset of puberty.
- Persistently obese individuals appear relatively resistant to leptin.
- Hereditary leptin deficiency (very rare) results in grossly obese children due to a voracious appetite.

Several other hormones have recently been shown to affect appetite and weight:

- **Ghrelin**: this was first identified as a growth hormone releasing hormone. It is released from the stomach when subjects are fasting and triggers hunger. Ghrelin levels fall after gastric by-pass surgery which may help weight loss (by reducing appetite).
- **Peptide YY** (a member of the neuropeptide Y family): released from the small and large bowel. Levels rise after meals and reduce appetite. This may be the main regulator of day-to-day appetite.
- **Glucagon-like-peptide-1** (GLP-1): released from the intestine after meals and powerfully stimulates insulin secretion and possibly reduces appetite as well.
- In the hypothalamus itself, **neuropeptide Y (NPY)** and **Agouti-related protein (AgRP)** increase appetite while **α-MSH** (a melanocortin) reduces appetite.

In addition to leptin a number of other hormones have recently been identified as being released from fat cells. These 'adipokines' include **adiponectin**, which reduces insulin resistance, and **resistin** and **acylation stimulating protein (ASP)**, which both increase insulin resistance. Their exact role in the association between obesity and type 2 diabetes (insulin resistance) remains to be confirmed.

2.4 Investigations in endocrinology

The plasma level of almost all hormones varies throughout the day (because of pulsatile secretion, environmental stress or circadian rhythms) and is influenced by the prevailing values of the substrates they control. This makes it hard to define a 'normal range'. For example, insulin values depend on the glucose level, and GH levels depend on whether a pulse of GH has just been released or the blood sample is taken in the trough between pulses.

Dynamic testing is therefore frequently used, ie suppression or stimulation tests. The principle is, 'If you think a hormone level may be high, suppress it; if you think it may be low, stimulate it'.

- **Suppression tests** are used to test for hormone EXCESS – eg dexamethasone suppression for Cushing's syndrome, glucose tolerance for GH in acromegaly.
- **Stimulation tests** are used to test for hormone DEFICIENCY – eg synacthen tests for hypoadrenalism, insulin-induced hypoglycaemia for GH deficiency and/or hypoadrenalism.

Essential note

Suppression tests are used when suspicious of high hormone levels; stimulation tests when suspicious of low levels

2.5 Growth hormone

This is secreted in pulses lasting 30–45 minutes separated by periods when secretion is undetectable. The majority of GH pulses occur at night ('children grow at night'). In response to GH pulses, the liver makes insulin-like growth factor-1 (IGF-1, previously called somatomedin C), the plasma level of which is constant and which mediates almost all the actions of GH, ie GH does not act directly. The effective levels of IGF-1 are influenced by changes in the level of its six binding proteins (IGF-BP I–G).

2.6 Prolactin (galactorrhoea gynaecomastia)

Prolactin causes galactorrhoea (milk from the breast) but not gynaecomastia (oestrogen does this). Raised prolactin levels are essentially the only cause of galactorrhoea, although occasionally prolactin levels in the normal range can cause milk production in a sensitised breast. Raised prolactin levels also 'shut down' the gonadal axis 'from the top' (hypothalamic level) resulting in low GnRH, LH and oestrogen/testosterone levels. Surprisingly, prolactin is a stress hormone and levels rise after an epileptic fit.

Prolactin release from the pituitary is under **negative** control by dopamine from the hypothalamus. Levels therefore rise after hypothalamic or pituitary stalk damage (eg large pituitary tumours pressing on the stalk as the dopamine cannot reach the rest of the pituitary) or with dopamine-blocking drugs (typically anti-emetics, eg metoclopramide, prochlorperazine or major tranquillisers, eg haloperidol). Dopamine agonists (bromocriptine, cabergoline) are used to lower prolactin and treat prolactin-secreting pituitary tumours very effectively. Oestrogens (the pill, pregnancy) and nipple stimulation raise prolactin.

Essential note

Aide memoire: 'Female psychiatric patients may complain of galactorrhoea – doctors may not believe them but the patients are right and it is due to the doctor's treatment!'

Gynaecomastia (breast enlargement)

This is due to a decreased androgen:oestrogen ratio in men. Gynaecomastia is unrelated to galactorrhoea (which is always due to prolactin). Breast enlargement is not necessary to make milk.

Causes of gynaecomastia:

- Pubertal (normal)
- Obesity – not true gynaecomastia
- Hypogonadism (eg Klinefelter's, testicular failure)
- Cirrhosis, alcohol
- Hyperthyroidism
- Drugs: including spironolactone, digoxin, oestrogens, cimetidine, anabolic steroids, marijuana
- Tumours, including adrenal or testicular making oestrogen; lung, pancreatic, gastric – make hCG; hepatomas converting androgens to oestrogens.

2.7 Adrenal steroids

These are made in the adrenal cortex, released into the blood stream and act intracellularly in cells to alter the transcription of DNA to mRNA (see Section 1, Hormone action). In humans, cortisol (also known as hydrocortisone) is the key glucocorticoid and aldosterone is the key mineralocorticoid. Release of cortisol is controlled by adrenocorticotrophic hormone (ACTH) from the pituitary which is itself controlled by cortocotrophin releasing hormone (CRH) release from the hypothalamus (see Figure 1). Surprisingly, the mineralocorticoid (aldosterone) and glucocorticoid receptors have an equal affinity for cortisol. However, the cellular enzyme **11-beta hydroxysteroid dehydrogenase** 'protects' the mineralocorticoid receptor by chemically modifying any cortisol that comes near the receptor to an inactive form while having no effect on aldosterone itself. Inactivating mutations of this enzyme or inhibition of it by liquorice causes 'apparent mineralocorticoid excess' since cortisol (which circulates at much higher concentrations than aldosterone) is able to stimulate the mineralocorticoid receptor. Prednisolone and dexamethasone are synthetic glucocorticoids; fludrocortisone is a synthetic mineralocorticoid.

Essential note

Cortisol is the key glucocorticoid and aldosterone the key mineralocorticoid

2.8 Thyroid hormone metabolism

More than 95% of thyroid hormones are bound to plasma proteins in the circulation, predominantly thyroid binding globulin (TBG) and thyroid binding prealbumin (TBPA). T_4 (L-thyroxine, four iodine atoms per molecule) has a half-life of seven days (so if a patient is in a confused state it is possible to administer his/her total weekly dose of thyroxine once a week). It is converted partly in the thyroid and partly in the circulation to T_3 (tri-iodo-thyronine, three iodine atoms per molecule), which is the active form and has a half-life of one day.

There are three deiodinase enzymes that act on thyroid hormones (termed D_1–D_3). D_1 and D_2 promote the generation of active hormone (T_3) by converting T_4 to T_3, and they can also convert reverse T_3 (rT_3, inactive) to T_2 (see Figure 2). D_3 opposes this by promoting conversion of T_4 to rT_3 and destroying T_3 by conversion to T_2. The D_1 and D_2 enzymes are inhibited by illness, propranolol, propylthiouracil, amiodarone and ipodate (formerly used as X-ray contrast medium for study of gall bladder disease). This reduces the

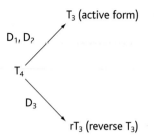

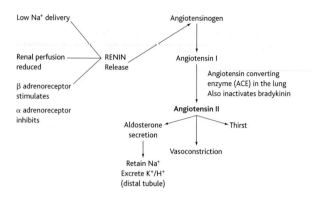

Figure 2 Metabolism of thyroid hormones. D_1–D_3 – different deiodinase enzymes that act on thyroid hormone

level of active hormone, T_3, with little change or a rise in T_4. rT_3 levels rise (T_4 spontaneously converts to rT_3 if the mono-deiodinase is not available) but rT_3 is *not* detected in routine laboratory tests of T_3 levels.

2.9 Renin–angiotensin–aldosterone

Aldosterone secretion is controlled almost completely by the renin–angiotensin system, not by ACTH. The initial letters of the zones of the adrenal cortex from outside inwards spell 'GFR', like glomerular filtration rate: glomerularis, fasciculata, reticularis. Aldosterone is the 'outsider hormone' and is made on the 'outside' (zona glomerulosa).

Renin is released from the JGA (juxtaglomerular apparatus) of the kidney in response to low Na^+ delivery or reduced renal perfusion. Renin is an enzyme which converts angiotensinogen to angiotensin I (10 amino acids). ACE (angiotensin converting enzyme) in the lung converts angiotensin I to angiotensin II which is the active form. ACE also breaks down bradykinin: ACE inhibitors (eg captopril) are believed to cause cough by causing a build up of bradykinin in the lung. The renin–angiotensin system (Figure 3) is designed to restore circulating volume. It is therefore activated by hypovolaemia (*See* above and Neurology, chapter 13) and its end product, angiotensin II, has three actions which restore volume:

- Releasing aldosterone from the adrenal (retains Na^+, excretes K^+ in the distal tubule)
- Vasoconstriction (powerful)
- Induction of thirst (powerful).

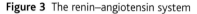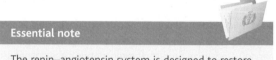

Figure 3 The renin–angiotensin system

Essential note

The renin–angiotensin system is designed to restore circulating volume

2.10 Calcium, PTH and vitamin D

(*See also* Chapter 11, Metabolic Diseases.)

Plasma calcium is tightly regulated by parathyroid hormone (PTH) and vitamin D acting on the kidney (PTH), bone (PTH) and the gut (vitamin D).

PTH controls Ca^{2+} levels minute to minute by mobilising Ca^{2+} from bone and inhibiting Ca^{2+} excretion from the kidney. Vitamin D has a more long-term role, predominantly by promoting Ca^{2+} absorption from the gut. Its actions on the kidney and bone are of lesser importance. Calcium levels are sensed by a specific calcium-sensing receptor on the parathyroid glands.

Precursor vitamin D, obtained from the diet or synthesised by the action of sunlight on the skin, requires activation by two steps:

- 25-hydroxylation in the liver
- 1-hydroxylation in the kidney.

Calcitonin (from the C-cells of the thyroid) behaves almost exactly as a counter-hormone to PTH (secreted by high Ca^{2+}, acts to lower serum Ca^{2+} by inhibiting Ca^{2+} release from bone) but its physiological importance is in doubt (thyroidectomy does not affect Ca^{2+} levels).

Essential note

Calcium homeostasis is controlled by PTH (calcium-raising) and vitamin D (calcium absorption enhancing)

2.11 Natriuretic peptides

There are three natriuretic peptides, A-type, B-type and C-type natriuretic peptides (ANP, BNP and CNP). BNP is similar to ANP, and is produced from the heart especially in heart failure and promotes diuresis and vascular dilatation. Serum levels are more stable than ANP, and BNP is proving to be a useful test of heart failure. CNP is produced by the vascular endothelium rather than by cardiac myocytes.

3. THE PITUITARY GLAND

3.1 Anatomy

The anatomical relations of the pituitary are important as enlarging pituitary tumours may press on surrounding structures. The commonest feature is visual field change (bitemporal hemianopia).

- **Above**: optic chiasm (causing bitemporal hemianopia if compressed), pituitary stalk, hypothalamus, temporal lobes.
- **Below**: sphenoid sinus (in front and below to allow transphenoidal surgery), nasopharynx.
- **Lateral**: cavernous sinus, internal carotid arteries, III, IV, V_1, V_2 and VI cranial nerves.

Expanding pituitary tumours may also compromise remaining anterior pituitary function but very rarely affect posterior pituitary hormones.

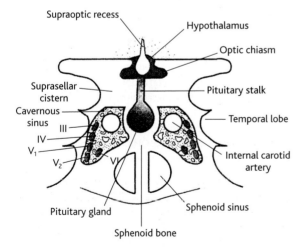

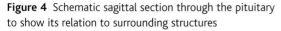

Figure 4 Schematic sagittal section through the pituitary to show its relation to surrounding structures

---

> **Essential note**
>
> If the pituitary enlarges it may cause changes in visual fields (bitemporal hemianopia) by pressing on the optic chiasm

3.2 Pituitary tumours

A microadenoma is a pituitary tumour less than 1 cm in size. The size and frequency of pituitary tumours are related.

Pituitary tumours	
Large – non-secreting (typically 'chromophobe', may be LH/FSH positive)	50% of all tumours
Large – prolactinomas in men	25% of all tumours
Medium – acromegaly (GH secreting, typically 'acidophil', 70% are >1 cm)	12% of all tumours
Small – Cushing's disease (ACTH secreting, often undetectable on CT/MRI, typically basophil)	5–10% of all tumours
Small – TSH-secreting	1% – very rare

The commonest tumours are small, non-functioning micro-adenomas which have been reported to occur in up to 20% of people at post-mortem. Note that **prolactinomas** in women are usually picked up at the microadenoma size due to their effects upon menstrual disturbance.

Craniopharyngiomas are benign tumours that arise from remnants of Rathke's pouch. Two-thirds arise in the hypothalamus itself (suprasellar), one-third in the pituitary. Although they represent an embryonic remnant, they not infrequently present for the first time in adulthood.

3.3 Diabetes insipidus

Anti-diuretic hormone (ADH, also called vasopressin or arginine-vasopressin, AVP) is synthesised in the hypothalamus and transported to the posterior pituitary, along with oxytocin, for storage and release. Diabetes insipidus (DI) is caused either by a failure to secrete vasopressin from the posterior pituitary (**central or cranial DI**, eg congenital or caused by craniopharyngiomas in the hypothalamus, or damage to the hypothalamus at pituitary surgery) or resistance to **the action of vasopressin in the kidney** (nephrogenic DI – X-linked congenital inactivity of the ADH receptor). To cause **cranial DI**, the hypothalamic nuclei (supraoptic and paraventricular) need to be damaged – it is not sufficient simply to compress the posterior pituitary as vasopressin can be secreted directly from the hypothalamus itself. Pituitary tumours therefore rarely cause DI. A 'water deprivation test' is sometimes required to diagnose diabetes insipidus.

Causes of polydipsia/polyuria

There are six causes of excess thirst (polydipisa) and increased urine output (polyuria):

Causes of polydipsia/polyuria

- Diabetes mellitus (commonest)
- Diabetes insipidus
- High calcium
- Low potassium
- Renal disease
- Psychogenic excess water drinking

3.4 Acromegaly

Acromegaly is the condition that results from excessive secretion of growth hormone in adulthood. In childhood, growth hormone excess causes gigantism.

Common features of acromegaly

- Hands and feet enlarge (rings no longer fit, shoe size increases)
- Coarse facial features, broad nose, prominent supraorbital ridges, enlarged prominent jaw
- Splaying of teeth and underbite of lower jaw
- Sleep apnoea
- Diabetes
- Hypertension
- Twofold increase in death from cardiovascular disease
- Left ventricular hypertrophy
- Arthropathy – often pseudogout
- Carpal tunnel syndrome
- Increase in malignancies, especially colonic polyps

Acromegaly is diagnosed by failure of GH to suppress to less than 2 mU/l at any time in a standard 75 g glucose tolerance test (GTT). This may produce a double diagnosis as the GTT may diagnose acromegaly-induced diabetes at the same time. The IGF-1 level is usually also raised.

First-line treatment is **transphenoidal surgery** to the pituitary tumour (or transcranial surgery if there is a large suprasellar extension of the tumour). The cure rate (40–70%) depends on the initial tumour size. Alternative therapies are **octreotide** (long-acting analogue of somatostatin), **pituitary radiotherapy** (may take years to take effect and result in hypopituitarism), **pegvisomant** (GH antagonist derived from the GH receptor) or **bromocriptine** (effective in less than 20% of cases). After successful treatment of acromegaly (GH <5 mU/l, IGF-1 in the normal range), most physical features do **not** regress. Features of active disease are increased sweating and oedema of hands and feet which can regress after therapy.

3.5 Hypopituitarism and growth hormone deficiency in adults

Hypopituitarism

- Hypopituitarism refers to failure of secretion of one or more pituitary hormones. Pan-hypopituitarism (failure of all anterior pituitary hormones) can be caused by enlarging pituitary tumours, cranial irradiation (including specific pituitary radiotherapy), pituitary apoplexy and Sheehan's syndrome (infarction following post-partum haemorrhage). Important features include the following:
- Patients present with a soft, smooth 'baby' skin, 'crows' feet' lines around the eyes and possibly features of other specific hormone loss (eg hypotension associated with hypoadrenalism, hypothyroidism).
- Only replacement therapy with steroids and thyroxine is essential for life.
- In suspected hypopituitarism, the steroids should be given first and certainly before thyroid replacement therapy. This is because correction of hypothyroidism will accelerate cortisol metabolism and would precipitate a hypo-adrenal crisis (if thyroxine is given before exogenous steroids).
- If the pituitary is damaged, GH production is lost early so that most patients are growth hormone deficient (see below).
- Despite conventional hormone replacement therapy (thyroxine, glucocorticoid and sex steroids), mortality rates are increased in hypopituitarism owing to either an increase in cardiovascular events or malignancy. The potential for GH therapy to reverse this trend is currently under research.

GH is required for growth in children. It was thought to have little function in adults but recently the following have been ascribed to **adult GH deficiency**:

- Reduced muscle, increased fat

- Low mood (some patients improve markedly with GH therapy)
- Raised lipids
- Reduced left ventricular function
- Osteoporosis
- Impaired endothelial function.

Treatment of adult GH deficiency with daily GH injections is now recommended in patients whose quality of life is shown to improve significantly after a three-month trial of GH therapy.

4. THE THYROID GLAND

4.1 Thyroid function tests

TSH is the most sensitive measure of thyroid status in patients with an intact pituitary. It is usually the first test done by laboratories but can be misleadingly normal in pituitary disease (see below). T_4 and T_3 are over 95% protein bound, predominantly to thyroxine binding globulin (TBG). Raised oestrogen levels (eg the pill and pregnancy) alter TBG levels and hence total but not free hormone levels. Nowadays, many laboratories report free not total T_4 and T_3 levels.

Primary hypothyroidism (myxoedema – underactivity of the thyroid gland) results in a **raised TSH** and low T_4 (more so than T_3).

Rarely hypothyroidism is due to pituitary failure (secondary hypothyroidism) – T_4 is low but TSH is not raised in this situation.

Primary hyperthyroidism (thyrotoxicosis – overactivity of the thyroid gland) results in a **low TSH** and raised T_3 (more so than T_4).

Hyperthyroidism due to a pituitary tumour producing TSH (secondary hyperthyroidism) is extremely rare.

4.2 Clinical features of hyperthyroidism and hypothyroidism

The common features of hyperthyroidism and hypothyroidism are shown in Table 1.

Table 1 Features of hyper and hypothyroidism

Features	Hyperthyroidism	Hypothyroidism
General	Weight loss	Weight gain
Skin	Feel hot, sweating	Dry skin, thin eye brows
	Hair loss	Hair loss, feel cold
Neuro	Tremor, agitation	Slowed up, coma
CVS	Tachycardia	Bradycardia
	Atrial fibrillation	Raised cholesterol
	Cardiac failure, angina	
GI	Diarrhoea	Constipation
Gynae	Amenorrhoea	Menorrhagia, reduced fertility
Bone	Osteoporosis Hypercalcaemia	
Eyes	Eye signs (see Section 4.4)	Periorbital oedema
Muscle	Proximal myopathy	Cramps

Amenorrhoea is predictable in hyperthyroidism because of associated weight loss. In hypothyroidism, everything slows down except the periods! In the GI tract, the symptoms of hyperthyroidism are almost indistinguishable from those of anxiety. The diarrhoea is actually more like the increased bowel frequency before an examination.

4.3 Causes and treatment of abnormal thyroid function

The three common causes of **hyperthyroidism** are:

- Graves' disease (65%)
- Toxic multinodular goitre (20%)
- Toxic (hot) nodule (5%).

Graves' disease is an autoimmune disease caused by a stimulating anti-TSH receptor antibody. Anti-thyroid peroxidase (anti-TPO) and anti-thyroglobulin (anti-Tg) antibodies are frequently present and the thyroid may be diffusely enlarged with a bruit. It can occur at any age and is six times more common in women than men. It is associated with thyroid eye disease (see Section 4.4). After 18 months of treatment with anti-thyroid drugs, 50% of cases go into remission. Toxic multinodular goitre and toxic nodules are due to benign adenomas of the thyroid and are rare under the age of 40. Autoantibodies are absent and the hot nodules can be demonstrated on a radionucleotide thyroid scan. Hyperthyroidism in these conditions does not go into remission after drug treatment and radioiodine or surgery is needed for a permanent cure. Not all multinodular goitres overproduce thyroid hormone. Severe hyperthyroidism with confusion is termed 'thyroid storm' and is a medical emergency.

The three main treatments of primary hyperthyroidism are:

- Antithyroid drugs (carbimazole, propylthiouracil)
- Radioiodine
- Surgery (thyroidectomy).

All three are effective. A rare but important side-effect of carbimazole or propylthiouracil is agranulocytosis (often presenting with mouth ulcers) and requires **immediate** drug cessation. Radioiodine (^{131}I) can take up to six months to work and frequently results in hypothyroidism. Thyroidectomy has a (low) risk of recurrent laryngeal nerve damage (causing hoarseness) and parathyroid gland damage (causing hypocalcaemia).

The common causes of **primary hypothyroidism** are:

- Chronic autoimmune thyroiditis (Hashimoto's disease) – very common – anti-TPO and anti-Tg antibodies usually present.
- Post-thyroidectomy
- Post-radioiodine

Worldwide, iodine deficiency is the commonest cause of hypothyroidism but this is rare in the UK. Other rare causes of hypothyroidism include congenital hypothyroidism and defects in thyroid hormone biosynthesis (Pendred's syndrome). Transient hypothyroidism can also follow hyperthyroidism in post-viral (De Quervain's), post-partum or lymphocytic thyroiditis.

Treatment of hypothyroidism is with **thyroxine (T_4)** which is well absorbed orally and has a long half life (approximately seven days).

4.4 Eye signs in thyroid disease

The eye signs in thyroid disease are shown below (*see also* Chapter 14, Ophthalmology). Retro-orbital inflammation and swelling of the extra-ocular muscles is an autoimmune process and is only seen in Graves' disease. The target of the antibody or T-cell reaction causing this inflammation is not known for certain and eye disease activity can occur in the absence of thyrotoxicosis.

Graves' disease only	Thyrotoxicosis from any cause
Soft tissue signs: periorbital oedema, conjunctival injection, chemosis	Lid retraction
	Lid lag
Proptosis/exophthalmos	
Diplopia/ophthalmoplegia	
Optic nerve compression causing visual failure	

4.5 Thyroid cancer and nodules

Only 5–10% of thyroid nodules are malignant (the rest are benign adenomas). Thyroid cancer virtually never causes hyperthyroidism so 'hot nodules' can usually be presumed to be benign. In order of increasing malignancy and decreasing frequency the thyroid epithelial cancers are:

- Papillary
- Follicular
- Anaplastic.

Lymphomas occur in Hashimoto's disease. Medullary thyroid cancer is from the C-cells (calcitonin), not from the thyroid epithelium. Serum calcitonin is a tumour marker for this cancer, which often occurs in families, sometimes as part of the multiple-endocrine neoplasia type 2 syndrome (*see* Section 6).

5. ADRENAL DISEASE

5.1 Cushing's syndrome

Clinical features: Cushing's syndrome refers to the sustained overproduction of cortisol (hypercortisolism) which causes:

- Centripetal obesity with moon face
- 'Buffalo hump'
- Hirsutism
- Recurrent infections
- Osteoporosis
- Oligomenorrhoea
- Hypokalaemia
- Striae
- Acne
- Proximal muscle weakness
- Hyperglycaemia
- Psychiatric disturbances
- Hypertension

If untreated, death is usually due to infection. Other than due to steroid treatment, Cushing's syndrome is rare. In the first instance, it needs to be distinguished from simple obesity. Once Cushing's syndrome is confirmed, the cause needs to be identified.

Causes of Cushing's syndrome

- Pituitary tumour (Cushing's disease)
- Ectopic production of ACTH – either from cancer (eg small cell cancer of lung) or from a benign tumour, eg bronchial adenoma (often very small)
- Adrenal tumour – may be malignant
- [Treatment with exogenous steroids].

Diagnosis of Cushing's syndrome

Diagnosis is made in two phases:

- **Tests to confirm overproduction of cortisol (Cushing's syndrome):** overnight dexamethasone or low-dose dexamethasone suppression test; 24 hour urinary free cortisol; persistently raised midnight serum cortisol.
- **Tests to determine the cause of the excess cortisol production:** ACTH level (very low in adrenal tumour). High-dose dexamethasone suppression tests; MRI or CT of the pituitary (though tumour may be too small to see); CT of adrenals (for adrenal tumour).

Treatment of Cushing's syndrome

Surgical removal of source – pituitary, adrenal or ectopic source.

Essential note

Cushing's syndrome may be due to an adrenal tumour, excess ACTH from the pituitary or ectopic secretion of ACTH from a lung tumour.

5.2 Primary hyperaldosteronism and Conn's syndrome

Excess production of aldosterone (primary hyperaldosteronism) is a rare cause of secondary hypertension and is associated with hypokalaemia (80% of cases) and metabolic alkalosis. It accounts for approximately 3% of all cases of hypertension. In the majority of cases, the cause is benign adrenal tumour (Conn's syndrome). Proving the endocrine diagnosis can be complex but the first test is the non-recumbent serum renin:aldosterone ratio which will show a low renin and high aldosterone. CT of the adrenals may show a unilateral tumour. Treatment comprises unilateral adrenalectomy to remove the lesion or aldosterone blockade with spironolactone or amiloride if this is not possible.

5.3 Hypoadrenalism

In the UK, spontaneous primary hypoadrenalism (adrenal gland failure) is most commonly due to autoimmune destruction of the adrenal glands (Addison's disease – adrenal autoantibodies present in 70% of cases). Vitiligo is present in 10–20% of cases. Other causes include TB, HIV or haemorrhage into the adrenal glands and anterior pituitary disease (secondary hypoadrenalism). Hypoadrenalism after withdrawal of long-standing steroid therapy is similar to secondary hypoadrenalism.

The clinical features of a hypoadrenalism/hypoadrenal crisis are shown below. They are important to recognise, because if the diagnosis is missed the patient may die. The skin pigmentation means that the patient may look deceptively well ('tanned'), although examination of the arm pits or pubic area will show 'tanning' in non-sun-exposed area.

Clinical features of hypoadrenalism (Addisonian crisis)

- Weight loss
- Increased skin pigmentation (including in non-sun-exposed areas)
- Abdominal pain (in some cases)
- Hypotension/collapse with low BP
- Hypoglycaemia
- Hyperkalaemia

Hypoadrenalism is confirmed using a short synacthen test – the cortisol level fails to rise adequately after an im or iv injection of synthetic ACTH (Synacthen®). Treatment is with hydrocortisone (glucocorticoid) and fludrocortisone (mineralocorticoid). In a hypoadrenal crisis, intravenous saline and correction of hypoglycaemia are also required.

Note that patients on long-term steroid replacement for hypoadrenalism need to increase their doses (by two or three times) during acute illness.

6. PHAEOCHROMOCYTOMA AND MULTIPLE-ENDOCRINE NEOPLASIA (MEN) SYNDROMES

Phaeochromocytomas are rare tumours of the adrenal medulla or ganglia of the sympathetic nervous system that secrete adrenaline or noradrenaline and can induce a fatal hypertensive crisis. They are the 'tumour of 10%':

- 10% are outside the adrenal glands – paragangliomas (including organ of Zuckerkandl)

- 10% are multiple (eg bilateral)
- 10% are malignant
- 10% are familial.

Diagnosis of phaeochromocytoma is by measurement of urinary catecholamines (this has now replaced measurement of urinary catecholamine metabolites – 3-methoxy-4-hydroxymandelic acid (VMAs)). As is the case with most endocrine tumours, the histology is not a reliable guide to the malignant potential in phaeochromocytomas. The diagnosis of malignant phaeochromocytoma can only be made if metastases are present.

Familial phaeochromocytomas occur in

- Multiple endocrine neoplasia type II (see below)
- Von Hippel–Lindau syndrome (retinal and cerebral haemangioblastomas and renal cystic carcinomas)
- Spontaneously in some families (not associated with a syndrome)
- von Recklinghausen's disease (neurofibromatosis) – 1–2%

Important features of phaeochromocytomas

- Hypotension or postural hypotension may occur particularly if adrenaline is produced
- The triad of headache, sweating and palpitations with a hypertnsive crisis is said to be >90% predictive
- Hypertension – 70% have persistent rather than episodic raised blood pressure
- Treatment is surgical removal
- Pre-operatively it is essential that the patient is treated with alpha adrenergic blockade (eg phenoxybenzamine) first and then beta blockade (eg atenolol) to avoid a hypertensive crisis during the operation.

Multiple endocrine neoplasia (MEN) syndromes are syndromes with multiple benign or malignant endocrine neoplasms. They should not be confused with polyglandular autoimmune syndromes which relate to autoimmune endocrine diseases.

Table 2 Classification of multiple endocrine neoplasia

	MEN-1	MEN-2A	MEN-2B
Genetics			
	menin gene	ret gene	ret gene
	Chromosome 11	Chromosome 10	Chromosome 10
Tumours			
	Parathyroid	Parathyroid	Parathyroid
	Pituitary*	Phaeochromo	Phaeochromo
	Pancreas*	Medullary thyroid cancer	Medullary thyroid cancer
			Marfanoid
			Mucosal neuromas

* Gastrinomas and insulinomas are the most common pancreatic tumours in MEN-1. Of the pituitary tumours, prolactinomas are the most common, followed by acromegaly and Cushing's disease.

Medullary thyroid cancer (MTC) is always malignant, secretes calcitonin and is preceded by C-cell hyperplasia. Prophylactic thyroidectomy in patients with confirmed MEN-2 should be performed to prevent this most serious manifestation.

7. DIABETES MELLITUS

Diabetes may be defined as chronic hyperglycaemia at levels sufficient to cause microvascular complications:

- 85% of cases are due to insulin resistance of unknown origin (type 2, maturity-onset, non-insulin dependent)
- 10% of cases are due to autoimmune destruction of the pancreatic islets causing insulin deficiency (type 1, juvenile-onset, insulin-dependent)
- Around 5% of cases are due to miscellaneous secondary causes (see Section 7.3).

Common presenting features are polydipisa, polyuria, blurred vision, and oral or genital Candida infection (thrush). In the case of type 1 diabetes, weight loss and possibly vomiting, if ketosis has developed, may occur.

Diabetes mellitus is a clinical syndrome characterised by chronic hyperglycaemia and takes two main forms. Type 1: failed insulin production, treatment with insulin. Type 2: insulin resistance, treatment with lifestyle modification and medication (commencing orally, but insulin may eventually be necessary)

7.1 Risk factors and clinical features of type 1 and type 2 diabetes mellitus

The following table summarises the differences between type 1 and type 2 diabetes mellitus. Note that type 2 diabetes mellitus is more common in non-Caucasian races and that, despite being 'late-onset', is more strongly inherited than the juvenile-onset form.

In addition to insulin resistance, there is relative failure of the beta cells in type 2 diabetes: they are unable to maintain the very high insulin levels required.

Maturity-onset diabetes of the young (MODY) is the term used to describe type 2 diabetes occurring in patients under the age of 25 with a strong family history. Single gene defects with an autosomal dominant mode of inheritance have been found in the majority of cases, eg in the hepatic transcription factor HNF-1α (MODY 1) or glucokinase (MODY 2). At least five separate MODY genes resulting in inheritance of type 2 diabetes have now been defined.

Table 3 Summary of type 1 and type 2 diabetes mellitus

	Type 1	Type 2
Genetics	Both parents affected: 10–20% risk for child	Both parents affected: 70–100% risk for child
	Identical twins: 50% concordance	Identical twins: up to 90% concordance
	Caucasians	Asian, Black, Pima Indians, other indigenous peoples
	Increased risk: HLA DR3/4, DQ8, CTLA-4	No HLA association
Autoantibodies	60–90% Islet cell Ab (ICA) positive at diagnosis	No association with antibodies
Other risk factors		Impaired glucose tolerance, obesity
		Gestational diabetes (50% diabetic in 10 years)
Incidence	Approx 1/10 000 per year	Approx 1–2/1000 per year
Prevalence	Approx 1/1000	Approx 3/100
	Age <40	Age>40 (except MODY – see above) often asymptomatic
Clinical features (at diagnosis and pathology)	Weight loss	Overweight
	Ketosis prone	Ketone negative
	Insulin-deficient	Insulin-resistant
	Autoimmune aetiology (associated with other autoimmune disorders)	Acanthosis nigricans _hyperpigmentation of skin_
		Associated with 'metabolic syndrome': hypertension, IHD, hyperinsulinaemia, glucose intolerance

7.2 Diagnostic criteria for diabetes

Many people are on the 'borderline' of type 2 diabetes and the exact criteria for diagnosing diabetes remains controversial. The following criteria may be used:

- In the presence of typical symptoms (see Section 7.1 above) – a single fasting blood of >7.0 mmol/l or a random blood glucose >11.1 mmol/l.
- If no symptoms are present, these results must be repeated on two separate occasions for confirmation.
- If in doubt, a glucose tolerance test can be performed (75 g of glucose and blood sugar measured 2 h later) and a 2-h value of >11.1 mmol/l confirms the diagnosis.

Borderline glucose tolerance that is abnormal but as yet cannot be diagnosed as diabetes can be defined as:

- A fasting glucose level of between 5.6 and 7.0 mmol/l ('impaired fasting glucose')
- A blood glucose 2 h after a 75-g oral glucose load that is >8.1 mmol/l, but <11 mmol/l ('impaired glucose tolerance').

In impaired glucose tolerance (IGT) glucose levels are insufficient to cause microvascular complications (see Section 7.6) but there is still an increased macrovascular risk (see Section 7.6). Twenty per cent or more of individuals with IGT will progress to type 2 diabetes within 10 years.

7.3 Secondary diabetes

A variety of conditions can lead secondarily to chronic hyperglycaemia fulfilling the criteria of diabetes either by reducing insulin secretion (type 1-like) or by increasing insulin resistance (type 2-like). A pigmented rash in the axillae, neck and groin (acanthosis nigricans) is seen in many conditions associated with insulin resistance.

Causes of secondary diabetes

- Insulin deficiency

  - Pancreatitis
  - Haemochromatosis
  - Pancreatic cancer/surgery
  - Cystic fibrosis
  - Somatostatin

Causes of secondary diabetes

- Insulin resistance

  - Polycystic ovarian syndrome
  - Cushing's, steroid use
  - Acromegaly
  - Glucagonoma
  - Phaeochromocytoma
  - Insulin-receptor or signalling defect
  - Anti-insulin receptor antibodies
  - Partial lipodystrophy

7.4 Treatment of diabetes mellitus

Type 1 diabetes must be treated with insulin, typically two to four subcutaneous injections daily. In type 2 diabetes, lifestyle modification (weight loss, increased exercise, low sugar high fibre diet) and tablet treatment are also used to lower glucose levels. A gradual decline in insulin reserve leads to an increasing requirement for medication over time and around 30% of type 2 diabetes patients ultimately require insulin therapy to achieve satisfactory glycaemic targets. **Weight loss** (diet and exercise, orlistat and other weight loss drugs), **antihypertensive agents** and drugs to **reduce cardiovascular risk** (aspirin, statins and other lipid-lowering drugs) are also equally important in the management of diabetes mellitus.

Drugs used in treatment of type 2 diabetes mellitus

Drug	Action/comments
Sulphonylureas	Increase insulin secretion
Biguanides (eg metformin)	Reduce insulin resistance (less hepatic glucose production)
	Do not cause hypoglycaemia but risk of lactic acidosis
Alpha-glucosidase inhibitor (acarbose)	Slows carbohydrate absorption, not complicated by hypoglycaemia
Glitazones (eg rosiglitazone and pioglitazone). Troglitazone has been withdrawn in the UK because of cases of liver failure	Activate intracellular peroxisome proliferator activated receptors (PPAR-gamma) so reducing insulin resistance

Drugs used in treatment of type 2 diabetes mellitus	
Drug	Action/comments
Insulin	Often used in combination with other drugs (eg metformin). Leads to weight gain

Insulin analogues: these have now been introduced for the treatment of both type 1 and type 2 diabetes mellitus. Examples are lispro (a lysine to proline substitution) and insulin-aspart (an asparagine substitution) both of which are designed to replace soluble (regular) insulin. They have an ultra-fast absorption and elimination so reducing late hypoglycaemia. Newer intermediate-acting insulin analogues have also been developed with a smoother 24-h profile ('peakless') and these include insulin glargine (which is soluble in the vial at pH 4 but precipitates under the skin at pH 7) and insulin detemir (whose action is prolonged by binding to albumin and dissolving in fat due to a fatty acid side-chain). These analogues also reduce the likelihood of hypoglycaemia.

7.5 Glycated haemoglobin (HbA1, HbA1c)

Red cell haemoglobin is non-enzymically glycated at a low rate according to the prevailing level of glucose. The percentage of glycated haemoglobin provides an accurate estimate of mean glucose levels over the preceding six weeks and correlates well with the risk of microvascular complications. HbA1c is a more specific fraction of glycosylated haemoglobin than HbA1 and values are 1–2% lower. Optimal control equates to an HbA1c of 7% in most assays.

7.6 Microvascular and macrovascular complications of diabetes

Long-term diabetic complications are due to vascular damage. Damage to the microvasculature and its consequences (see below) correlate well with levels of glycaemic control and can be delayed or prevented by maintaining near-normal glucose levels. Microvascular complications take a minimum of five years to develop even with poor glycaemic control. However, they may be apparently present 'at diagnosis' in type 2 diabetes as hyperglycaemia has often been present for many years prior to diagnosis. Neuropathy (70–90%) and retinopathy (90%) occur in virtually all patients if control is not perfect and diabetes is present for long enough. Thirty to forty per cent of patients will develop diabetic nephropathy, usually within 20 years of onset of the diabetes (see Chapter 12, Nephrology).

The incidence of microvascular complications was reduced by around 50% in the 'Diabetes Control and Complications Trial' (DCCT) by tight glycaemic control.

In contrast, macrovascular disease (see below), which is responsible for most of the increased mortality in diabetes, does not appear to be related to the level of glycaemic control. However, the increased risk of macrovascular disease in diabetes is at least partly explained by a combination of higher blood pressure, lower HDL and higher triglyceride levels, although absolute cholesterol levels are not raised. Macrovascular complications are markedly reduced by hypertension treatment (which also reduces microvascular complications) and treatment of dyslipidaemia. Proteinuria is a strong risk factor for ischaemic heart disease in diabetes, presumably as it is a marker for endothelial dysfunction.

Essential note
The increased mortality of diabetics is predominantly related to macrovascular disease

Micro- and macrovascular complications of diabetes	
Microvascular	Macrovascular
Retinopathy (90%)*	Ischaemic heart disease (accounts for up to 70% of deaths in diabetes)
Neuropathy (70–90%)*	Peripheral vascular disease

Micro- and macrovascular complications of diabetes	
Microvascular	Macrovascular
Nephropathy (30–40%)*	CVA, hypertension
HbA1c dependent	HbA1c independent
	(Also present in impaired glucose tolerance)

* Approximate percentages of diabetics who will have this complication to some degree during their lifetime (data from retrospective studies)

7.7 Autonomic neuropathy

Autonomic complications of diabetes mellitus occur in very long-standing disease and include the following:

Manifestations of diabetic autonomic neuropathy

- Postural hypotension
- Gustatory sweating
- Cardiac arrhythmia ('dead-in-bed')
- Gastroparesis
- Generalised sweating
- Diarrhoea
- Reduced appreciation of cardiac pain
- Sexual impotence

8. HYPOGLYCAEMIA

8.1 Hypoglycaemia in diabetes mellitus

Hypoglycaemia can occur in diabetic patients taking either insulin or sulphonylurea drugs. Autonomic symptoms (sweating, tremor) appear when the blood glucose is <3.5 mmol/l and cerebral function becomes progressively impaired at glucose levels <2.5 mmol/l. In patients on insulin, failure of the normal counter-regulatory responses (sympathetic nervous system activation, adrenaline and glucagon release) may develop in long-standing insulin-treated diabetes, particularly in the presence of frequent hypoglycaemic episodes. This results in **hypoglycaemia unawareness**. The patient has no warning of impending neurological impairment and cannot take appropriate action (eg glucose ingestion). More frequent hypoglycaemic episodes result, exacerbating the problem – 'hypos beget hypos'. Hypoglycaemia awareness can be restored by relaxing control to allow a prolonged (3-month) hypoglycaemia-free period. There is no proof that hypoglycaemia unawareness is more common with human as compared with animal insulin.

8.2 Hypoglycaemia unrelated to diabetes

True hypoglycaemic episodes unrelated to diabetes therapy are rare. A blood sugar of 2.5 mmol/l or less should be documented, associated with appropriate symptoms which resolve after treatment (eg food) – 'Whipples' triad'. A supervised 72-h fast can be used to precipitate and document an episode, particularly to diagnose an insulinoma.

Causes can be classified as follows:

Causes of hypoglycaemia

- **Fasting**

  - Insulinoma*
  - Tumour (IGF-2)
  - Hypoadrenalism
  - Alcohol
  - Severe liver failure
  - Factitious (insulin or sulphonylurea)*
  - Drugs (pentamidine, quinidine)
  - Anti-insulin antibodies (delayed post-prandial release of insulins)*

- **Post-prandial**

  - Post-gastrectomy ('rebound hypoglycaemia')
  - Idiopathic (rare)

* Associated with detectable insulin levels and low β-hydroxybutyrate levels at the time of hypoglycaemia

Further information

The American Endocrine Society at http://www.endo-society.org/

The Society for Endocrinology at http://www.endocinology.org

British Thyroid Association at http://www.british-thyroid-association.org/

British Society for Paediatric Endocrinology and Diabetes at http://www.bsped.org.uk/

The Pituitary Society at http://www.pituitarysociety.org//

Diabetes UK at http://www.diabetes.org.uk/

American Diabetes Association at http://www.diabetes.org.

Brook CGD, Marshall NJ. *Essential endocrinology.* 2001. Oxford: Blackwell.

Levy A, Lightman S. *Endocrinology: an Oxford core text.* 1997. Oxford: Oxford University Press.

Haslett C, Chilvers E, Boon N, Colledge N, Hunter J. *Davidson's principles and practice of medicine.* 2002. London: Churchill Livingstone.

Journal of Clinical Endocrinology and Metabolism

Clinical Endocrinology

Endocrinology

Endocrine Reviews

Diabetes, Diabetes Care, Diabetologia and *Diabetic Medicine*

Revision summary

You should now understand that:

1. There are three main types of hormone: amines, peptides and steroids. Remember that thyroxine is an exception to the rule and is an amine that acts as a steroid. Amines and peptides have a short half-life, and act on cell surface receptors often via a second messenger. There are three mechanisms for transmitting the signal to the cell's interior: cAMP, a rise in intracellular calcium and via receptor tyrosine kinases. Rule of thumb: peptides or amines (excluding thyroxine) act via cAMP except insulin and those containing 'growth' in their name. These act via tyrosine kinase. Steroids have a longer half-life and act on intracellular receptors and on DNA to alter gene expression.

2. In illness, thyroid hormone levels fall, along with luteinising hormone, follicle-stimulating hormone, testosterone, oestrogen and insulin. Stress hormone levels rise, such as growth hormone, ACTH, glucocorticoids, adrenaline and glucagon. Normal ranges for hormones are difficult to define because of natural fluctuations in their levels; therefore, dynamic testing is required, in the form of suppression (for suspected hormone excess) or stimulation (for suspected hormone deficiency) tests.

3. The pituitary gland is divided into the anterior (adenohypophysis) and posterior (neurohypophysis) lobes. The anterior pituitary secretes growth hormone, prolactin, follicle-stimulating hormone, luteinising hormone, thyroid-stimulating hormone, ACTH and endorphins. The posterior pituitary secretes oxytocin and antidiuretic hormone. The pituitary gland has a role in the following functions: growth, blood pressure, pregnancy and childbirth, breast milk production, sex organ function, thyroid gland function and control of metabolism and water balance. Therefore, any malfunction of the pituitary gland has implications for all these body systems.

4. Primary hypothyroidism (underactive thyroid gland) leads to raised TSH and low T_4. Secondary hypothyroidism is caused by pituitary failure: TSH is not raised, but T_4 is low. Clinical features are many, including: weight gain, dry skin, thin eyebrows, hair loss, feel cold, bradycardia, raised cholesterol, constipation, cramps. Treatment is with oral T_4. Primary hyperthyroidism (overactive gland) leads to low TSH and raised T_3. Clinical features include: weight loss, feel hot, sweaty, hair loss, tremor, agitation, tachycardia, atrial fibrillation, diarrhoea, eye signs. Treatment is with: antithyroid drugs, radioiodine or surgery.

5. It is necessary to be aware of the clinical features, investigations and treatment of abnormal adrenal gland function

   Cushing's syndrome is sustained overproduction of cortisol, with classic associated features. Causes are pituitary tumour, ectopic ACTH production, adrenal tumour, steroid treatment. Two phases to diagnosis: confirmation of cortisol overproduction and determination of cause. Treatment is surgical removal of source of cortisol.

   Primary hyperaldosteronism is an increasingly recognised cause of hypertension.

   The most common form of hypoadrenalism is Addison's disease. It is important to recognise the classical clinical features to avoid death of the patient. Diagnosis confirmed by synacthen test and treatment is with hydrocortisone and fludrocortisone.

6. Diabetes mellitus is most commonly (85%) caused by insulin resistance (type 2, maturity-onset, non-insulin-dependent); 10% caused by pancreatic failure (type 1, juvenile-onset, insulin-dependent). Presenting features include: polydipsia, polyuria, blurred vision and thrush. Type 1 diabetes requires insulin. Type 2 diabetes is treated by lifestyle modification and medication.

Gastroenterology

CONTENTS

Gastroenterology

You should be able to:

1. Gain an understanding of the anatomy, physiology and function of the gastrointestinal tract.
2. Understand the mechanisms and causes of dysphagia.
3. Understand the causes and treatment of peptic ulcer disease.
4. Understand the causes and treatment of acute upper gastrointestinal haemorrhage.
5. Understand the risk factors, symptoms and treatment of gastrointestinal malignancies.
6. Understand the diagnosis and treatment of acute pancreatitis.
7. Understand the mechanisms of digestion and nutrient absorption and recognise the causes of malabsorption.
8. Know the causes of diarrhoea and constipation and how to treat them.
9. Recognise the differences between ulcerative colitis and Crohn's disease and learn how to diagnose and treat inflammatory bowel disease.
10. Learn about the mechanisms, causes and treatment of jaundice.

1. ANATOMY AND PHYSIOLOGY OF THE GI TRACT

1.1 Oesophagus

The oesophagus is 25 cm in length and consists of outer longitudinal and inner circular muscle layers. In the upper section both layers are striated muscle, whereas in the lower section both layers are smooth muscle; the myenteric plexus lies between the two layers. The mucosa is lined with squamous epithelium.

Defences against acid damage include:

- Lower oesophageal sphincter pressure of 10–30 mmHg
- Salivary bicarbonate
- Oesophageal *bicarbonate* secretion
- Gravity
- The 'pinchcock' effect of the diaphragmatic crura.

1.2 Stomach

cleaves amino acids

There is a transition from squamous to columnar epithelium at the gastro-oesophageal junction. Total stomach secretions amount to approximately 3 litres daily. The gastric pits contain chief cells producing pepsin, and parietal cells (fuelled by H+ K+ATPase) producing hydrochloric acid and intrinsic factor. The surface cells secrete mucus and bicarbonate.

Innervation is both parasympathetic via the vagus (motor and secretory supply) *and* sympathetic via Meissner's and Auerbach's plexi (peristalsis). The blood supply is derived from the coeliac trunk.

The control of gastric acid secretion is illustrated in the figure.

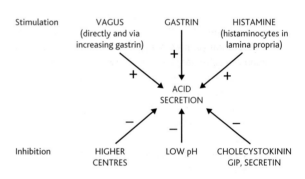

Figure 1 Control of gastric secretion

1.3 Pancreas

Pancreatic secretions amount to 1200–1500 ml per day of an alkaline fluid, containing proteins and electrolytes. 98% of the pancreatic mass is exocrine acini of epithelial cells; islets of Langerhans (source of endocrine secretion) make up the remaining 2%. Innervation is via the coeliac plexus.

- Exocrine (from acini of epithelial cells)

  - Trypsinogen
  - Chymotrypsinogen
  - Pancreatic amylase
  - Lipase

Endocrine (from islets of Langerhans)

- Glucagon from α cells
- Insulin from β cells
- Somatostatin from δ cells
- Pancreatic polypeptide

1.4 Liver

Blood supply to the liver is via the hepatic artery and portal vein (bringing blood from the gut and spleen); drainage is via the hepatic vein into the inferior vena cava.

Bile release from the gallbladder is stimulated by cholecystokinin; 250–1000 ml of bile is produced daily.

1.5 Small intestine

The small intestine is 2–3 metres in length, with an enlarged surface area created by villi and enterocytes. Its main function is absorption (6 litres daily), mostly in the duodenum and jejunum. A subsidiary function is immunity, via lymphoid aggregates, especially Peyer's patches in the ileum. Two litres of alkaline fluid is secreted daily, containing mucus and digestive enzymes. Secretion is from enterocytes of the villi, Paneth cells at the bases of the crypts of Lieberkühn and Brunner's glands.

Blood supply is via the superior mesenteric artery from mid-duodenum onwards.

1.6 Colon

The colon is 90–125 cm in length, its function being absorption of water, sodium and chloride (1–1.5 litres daily but can rise to 5 litres per day). Secretions contain mucus, potassium and bicarbonate.

Blood supply is via the superior mesenteric artery up to the distal transverse colon; the inferior mesenteric artery supplies the remainder.

Essential note

The GI tract comprises the oesophagus, stomach, pancreas, liver, small intestine and colon

1.7 Gut hormones

The response to a meal is regulated by complex hormonal and neural mechanisms. Secretion of most hormones is determined by the composition of intestinal contents.

1.8 Metabolism of haematinics

Iron

- Total body iron: 4–5 g; iron content maintained by control of absorption in the upper small intestine
- Iron intake mostly in Fe^{3+} form and approximately 5–10% of that consumed is absorbed
- Iron better absorbed from foods of animal than of plant origin.

Major gut hormones

Hormone	Source	Stimulus	Action
Gastrin	G cells in antrum	Gastric distension Amino acids in antrum	Secretion of pepsin, gastric acid and intrinsic factor
Cholecystokinin-pancreozymin (CCK-PZ)	Duodenum and jejunum	Fat, amino acids and peptides in small bowel	Pancreatic secretion Gallbladder contraction Delays gastric emptying
Vasoactive intestinal peptide (VIP)	Small intestine	Neural stimulation	Inhibits gastric acid and pepsin secretion Stimulates secretion by intestine and pancreas
Gastric inhibitory peptide	Duodenum and jejunum	Glucose, fats and amino acids	Inhibits gastric acid secretion Stimulates insulin secretion Reduces motility
Somatostatin	D cells in pancreas	Vagal and β-adrenergic stimulation	Inhibits gastric and pancreatic secretion

Factors that affect iron absorption

- Increased absorption

  - Increased erythropoiesis (eg pregnancy)
  - Decreased body iron (eg GI blood loss)
  - Vitamin C
  - Gastric acid*

- Decreased absorption

  - Partial/total gastrectomy
  - Achlorhydria
  - Disease of small intestine (eg Crohn's disease, coeliac disease)
  - Drugs (eg desferrioxamine)

*Gastric acid and vitamin C promote reduction of Fe^{3+} to Fe^{2+} which is more easily absorbed

Folate

- Recommended daily intake (RDI): 50–200 µg
- Source: green vegetables
- Absorption: duodenum and jejunum
- Deficiency: in small bowel pathology (eg coeliac disease, Crohn's disease); increased demand (eg haemolysis, pregnancy) and in patients being treated with antimetabolites such as methotrexate
- Clinical deficiency results in macrocytic anaemia; in pregnancy this can be associated with neural tube defects in the fetus.

Vitamin B_{12}

- RDI: 1–2 µg for adults daily
- Source: predominantly foods of animal origin
- Transport and metabolism: tightly protein bound; released by peptic digestion; oral B_{12} binds to intrinsic factor in the stomach and is then absorbed in the terminal ileum
- Deficiency can occur for several reasons:

  - Dietary deficiency in vegetarians or vegans
  - Post-gastrectomy (lack of intrinsic factor)
  - Atrophic gastritis (pernicious anaemia)
  - Terminal ileal disease
  - Blind loops (bacterial overgrowth utilising vitamin B_{12}).

The Schilling test

The **Schilling test** determines whether deficiency is due to malabsorption in the terminal ileum or to lack of intrinsic factor (eg post-gastrectomy, pernicious anaemia):

1. Administer orally labelled B_{12}
2. Administer intramuscular unlabelled B_{12} to saturate body binding sites
3. Assay amount of labelled B_{12} excreted in urine (>10% in normal subjects)
4. Repeat above with concurrent administration of intrinsic factor: the amount excreted will rise if B_{12} deficiency was due to lack of intrinsic factor which is now corrected.

In pernicious anaemia, autoantibodies to gastric parietal cells result in B_{12} deficiency, atrophic gastritis and achlorhydria. Approximately 1% of the population aged over 50 years is affected, with a female preponderance and a familial tendency.

Autoantibodies to gastric parietal cell are present in 90%, and autoantibodies to intrinsic factor are present in 50%. Pancytopenia may occur and other autoimmune disease may be present. The risk of gastric cancer is increased threefold.

Essential note

The GI tract also has hormonal, haematinic and calcium regulatory functions

2. DISORDERS OF THE OESOPHAGUS

Introduction

Symptoms of oesophageal disease
Oesophageal disease usually presents with dysphagia (difficulty swallowing), odynophagia (painful swallowing), retrosternal chest pain or heartburn.

Causes of dysphagia

Type of dysphagia	Symptoms	Causes
Oropharyngeal	Difficulty initiating swallow	Bulbar palsy Pseudo-bulbar palsy
Motility disorders	Dysphagia for solids and liquids – often intermittent	Scleroderma Diabetic neuropathy Oesophageal spasm Achalasia (motility and obstructive)

Causes of dysphagia

Type of dysphagia	Symptoms	Causes
Obstruction	Progressive, solids>liquids	Oesophageal stricture Oesophageal cancer Extrinsic oesophageal compression Oesophageal web (iron deficiency 'Plummer–Vinson syndrome') Pharyngeal pouch

Management of oesophageal disorders
A full history should include:

- Duration of symptoms
- Progressive or intermittent symptoms
- Dysphagia for liquids, solids or both
- Heartburn
- Weight loss
- Odynophagia
- Smoking (risk factor for cancer and reflux)
- Drugs (predisposing to reflux)
- NSAIDs
- Alcohol ingestion.

Investigation of oesophageal disease

- **Gastroscopy** – this is the most useful investigation and allows direct imaging of the oesophageal mucosa and biopsies of abnormalities
- **Barium meal** – shows outline of oesophagus and stomach and some indication of contractility
- **Videofluoroscopy** – barium study of swallowing mechanism highlighting problems with oropharyngeal component of swallowing
- **24-hour ambulatory pH monitoring** – monitoring of lower oesophageal acidity using pH probe inserted via nose with tip just above gastro-oesophageal junction
- **Oesophageal manometry** – pressure monitoring using oesophageal balloon.

2.1 Achalasia

The aetiology of achalasia is unknown. It presents with dysphagia, which may affect solids and liquids from the onset. There is abnormal peristalsis, in which the lower oesophageal sphincter fails to relax. Regurgitation, pain and weight loss may occur, and there is a risk of recurrent aspiration. Squamous carcinoma is a late and rare complication.

The incidence is approximately 1/100 000 per year, occurring at any age (usually 3rd to 5th decade) but it is rare in children.

- **Investigations**: demonstrable on manometry, endoscopy or barium studies where it is characterised by oesophageal dilation with a smooth distal 'bird's beak' stricture; chest radiograph may show an air/fluid level behind the heart
- **Treatment**: endoscopic dilatation or surgical myotomy.

2.2 Reflux oesophagitis

Acid reflux is extremely common – *approximately 40% of people experience 'heartburn' at least once per month*. The development of reflux oesophagitis depends on a number of factors.

Factors predisposing to reflux oesophagitis

GI factors	Other factors
Acid content of refluxate	Obesity
	Smoking
Mucosal defences in oesophagus	Alcohol and coffee intake
Gastric/oesophageal motility	Large meals (especially late at night)
Hiatus hernia	Drugs (most commonly theophyllines, nitrates, calcium antagonists and anticholinergics)

The correlation between symptoms and endoscopic appearances is poor; severe symptoms are compatible with a normal gastroscopy. The gold standard for diagnosis is oesophageal pH monitoring.

- The main symptom is heartburn but other symptoms include chest pain, odynophagia and dysphagia due to oesophageal dysmotility.
- Complications include strictures, haemorrhage, oesophageal ulcer, Barrett's oesophagus and carcinoma of the oesophagus (independent of Barrett's).

Treatment of reflux oesophagitis

- Lifestyle modifications (not evidence-based)
- Antacids, H_2 antagonists or proton pump inhibitors (PPI) plus pro-motility agent (metoclopramide, domperidone or erythromycin) for large volume reflux

- Surgery indicated for patients failing medical therapy, those with large volume reflux, bile reflux and those preferring to avoid long-term medical therapy
- Most fundoplication procedures are now performed laparoscopically and endoscopic anti-reflux procedures are under evaluation.

2.3 Other causes of oesophagitis

Candidal oesophagitis may occur in patients who are immunosuppressed, on antibiotics or steroids (especially inhaled corticosteroids), or suffering from diabetes mellitus. Barium swallow shows irregular filling defects in the oesophagus and white patches can be seen on endoscopy – biopsy will confirm the diagnosis.

Chemical oesophagitis may be caused by drugs such as NSAIDs, tetracycline and potassium chloride tablets.

Hiatus hernia occurs when part of the upper stomach herniates through the diaphragm into the chest; this is extremely common, especially with increasing age and obesity. The majority are asymptomatic and found incidentally during investigations. There are two types:

- Sliding 80% – may cause aspiration and acid reflux
- Rolling 20% – may obstruct or strangulate.

Hiatus hernia can be diagnosed at endoscopy, by CT scan or with barium studies and may be seen on a plain chest radiograph. Treatment is with acid suppression where necessary.

Surgical correction may sometimes be warranted.

2.4 Barrett's oesophagus

This is found in 10–20% of patients with long-standing acid reflux. There is extension of the columnar gastric epithelium into the oesophagus to replace the normal squamous epithelium. It is usually caused by chronic acid exposure and is pre-malignant. Estimates of the rate of transformation to adenocarcinoma vary from 30–100 times greater than in the normal population.

- Treatment is of the underlying reflux disease.
- Benefits of regular endoscopic screening and biopsy to detect dysplastic change are controversial but most centres undertake periodic endoscopy with multiple biopsies to detect evidence of dysplastic change.
- Photodynamic therapy and argon beam ablation are being assessed as potential cures.

2.5 Oesophageal carcinoma

Most oesophageal carcinomas are squamous carcinoma. Adenocarcinoma is rare unless arising from ectopic gastric mucosa or Barrett's oesophagus. The incidence is rising, and also increases with advancing age. Most tumours arise in the mid-thoracic portion of the oesophagus.

Risk factors and clinical features of oesophageal carcinoma

- **Risk factors**

  - Smoking
  - High alcohol intake
  - Oesophageal web (iron deficiency anaemia)
  - Achalasia
  - Barrett's oesophagus
  - Chronic reflux (independent of Barrett's oesophagus)
  - Chinese or Russian ethnicity
  - Tylosis

- **Clinical features**

  - Pain and dyspepsia
  - Progressive dysphagia for solids then liquids
  - Weight loss

Oesophageal carcinoma is often asymptomatic until a late stage, resulting in poor survival figures. Diagnosis is by endoscopy or barium swallow (this shows a stricture with irregular shouldering, unlike the smooth outline of a benign peptic stricture). CT scanning is used for staging, although the accuracy is poor especially for lymph node spread; laparoscopy may be useful. Endoscopic ultrasound is especially useful for assessing transmural extension but is not yet generally available.

Treatment of oesophageal carcinoma

- Surgery

  - Radical, high operative mortality (up to 10%)
  - Only one-third of lesions suitable for resection at presentation
  - Improves 5-year survival to approximately 10%

- Endoscopic dilatation and stenting
- Radiotherapy*
- Chemotherapy* (eg cisplatin, 5-fluorouracil)

*Used alone or in combination with surgery

Over 50% of patients have local or distant spread such that palliation is the only option. The overall 5-year survival is less than 5%.

Essential note

Disorders of the oesophagus include difficulty swallowing, acid reflux, Barrett's oesophagus and carcinoma

3. DISORDERS OF THE STOMACH

3.1 Peptic ulcer disease

- Most epidemiological data are from studies pre-dating the re-discovery and treatment of *Helicobacter pylori*.
- Incidence rates: 0.1–0.3%.
- The ratio of duodenal to gastric ulceration is 4:1.
- Males are more susceptible than females.
- Incidence peaks at approximately 60 years of age.
- Most patients treated medically with acid suppression and *H. pylori* eradication.
- Surgery limited to those with complications unresponsive to medical or endoscopic therapy (less than 5%).

Recent NICE guidelines recommend a 'test and treat' strategy for the management of dyspepsia. This will heal underlying lesions and avoid the necessity for endoscopy in many cases. Patients with 'sinister' symptoms (weight loss, iron deficiency, dysphagia, persistent vomiting or an abdominal mass) require urgent endoscopy to exclude gastric or oesophageal malignancy.

Peptic ulcer disease

- Risk factors
  - High alcohol intake
  - NSAID use
  - High-dose steroids
  - Male sex
  - Smoking (increases acid, decreases protective prostaglandins)
  - *H. pylori* colonisation
  - Zollinger–Ellison syndrome

- Clinical symptoms
  - Epigastric pain (sometimes radiating to back if posterior duodenal ulcer)
  - Vomiting
  - Symptoms often relapsing/remitting
  - Weight loss
  - Iron deficiency anaemia
  - Acute haemorrhage*

Peptic ulcer disease

*Duodenal ulcers are the most common cause of major upper GI haemorrhage

- Treatment
  - Remove precipitating factors
  - Acid-suppressing drugs
  - Eradication of *H. pylori*
  - Surgery if perforation, pyloric stenosis, or resistant haemorrhage

Upper gastrointestinal haemorrhage

This presents usually with haematemesis and/or melaena or postural hypotension.

Investigations include a full blood count (FBC) and U&Es. The (FBC) may reveal iron deficiency anaemia if there has been chronic blood loss, but haemoglobin may be normal even after a large haemorrhage prior to haemodilution.

The urea level is usually elevated in acute upper GI haemorrhage. Clotting and liver function tests (LFTs) should always be checked.

Treatment:

- Stabilisation (with fluid and blood transfusion where necessary) prior to urgent gastroscopy.
- Bleeding ulcers can be treated endoscopically with adrenaline injection or application of 'endoclips'.
- Varices can be injected or banded to control haemorrhage.

Causes of upper gastrointestinal haemorrhage

- Oesophageal
  - Varices
  - Oesophagitis
  - Oesophageal ulcer
  - Oesophageal cancer
  - Mallory–Weiss tear (mucosal tear at gastro-oesophageal junction following retching)

- Stomach
  - Gastric ulcer
  - Gastritis/erosions
  - Gastric cancer

Continued over

Causes of upper gastrointestinal haemorrhage

Continued

- **Duodenum**

  - Duodenitis
  - Duodenal ulcer
  - Ampullary tumour
  - Aorto-duodenal fistula

- **Other**

  - Large nose bleed (swallowed blood)
  - Dental extraction (swallowed blood)
  - Angiodysplasia (can occur anywhere in GI tract)
  - Hereditary haemorrhagic telangiectasia

Helicobacter pylori

This Gram-negative spiral bacillus is the primary cause of most peptic ulcer disease. Infection rates increase with age such that >50% of those over 50 years old are colonised by *H. pylori* in the gastric antral mucosa. It is detected in 70% of patients with gastric ulcer and over 90% of patients with duodenal ulcer, compared with 50% of control subjects.

Detection of *Helicobacter pylori*

- Antral biopsy at endoscopy with haematoxylin/eosin or Giemsa stain
- Urease testing – the bacillus secretes a urease enzyme which splits urea to release ammonia. A biopsy sample is put into a jelly containing urea and a pH indicator; this will thus change colour if *H. pylori* is present
- $^{13\text{ or }14}$C breath testing – the patient ingests urea labelled with $^{13\text{ or }14}$C; CO_2, produced by urease, is detected in the exhaled breath
- Serology (stays positive after treatment and NOT useful for confirming eradication)

H. pylori causes chronic gastritis and is associated with gastric carcinoma. All patients with peptic ulceration or gastritis found to be positive should undergo eradication therapy.

Effective eradication should be assessed by either repeat biopsies or breath testing in patients with complications (perforation or haemorrhage) and those with persistent symptoms.

Eradication regimes vary but usually involve triple therapy of a PPI and two antibiotics (eg amoxicillin and clarithromycin); metronidazole resistance is a problem in some areas.

3.2 Zollinger–Ellison syndrome

This is a rare condition with an incidence in the general population of 1/1 000 000.

Gastrin-secreting adenomas cause severe gastric and/or duodenal ulceration – the tumour is usually pancreatic in origin, although it may arise in the stomach, duodenum or adjacent tissues. 50–60% of cases are malignant, and 10% are multiple neoplasms. Zollinger–Ellison syndrome may occur as part of the syndrome of multiple endocrine neoplasia (MEN) type I, in which case malignancy is more likely.

Clinical signs of Zollinger–Ellison syndrome

- **Pain and dyspepsia**

  - From multiple ulcers

- **Steatorrhoea**

  - From acid-related inactivation of digestive enzymes and mucosal damage in the upper small bowel

- **Diarrhoea**

  - Due to copious acid secretion

3.3 Gastric carcinoma

- Incidence: decreasing in Western world
- Remains 6th commonest cause of cancer deaths
- Usually takes the form of an adenocarcinoma, most commonly in the pyloric region
- Incidence of carcinoma occurring in the cardia is rising
- Little early detection in the UK, unlike Japan where the extremely high incidence of the disease merits an intensive screening programme
- Most patients have local spread at the time of diagnosis, making curative resection unusual.

Gastric carcinoma

- **Risk factors**

  - Japanese
  - Hypo/achlorhydria (pernicious anaemia, chronic atrophic gastritis, partial gastrectomy)
  - Male sex
  - Dietary factors (high salt, nitrites)
  - Gastric polyps (rare)

- Clinical presentation

  - Dyspepsia (often only symptom)
  - Epigastric pain
  - Anorexia and weight loss
  - Early satiety
  - Iron deficiency anaemia
  - Haematemesis/melaena

Very few tumours are confined to the mucosa at diagnosis, but if so, cure rates are above 90%. Overall 5-year survival is below 10%. Diagnosis is by endoscopy and biopsy; endoscopic ultrasound and CT scan of the abdomen and thorax are used to determine resectability. Adjuvant chemotherapy before and after surgery may improve prognosis, although patients are often too unwell post-operatively to receive the second course.

Other gastric tumours include lymphoma (about 5%), which has a good prognosis, and leiomyosarcoma (<1%), which has a 50% 5-year survival.

3.4 Other gastric pathology

Gastroparesis

Reduced gastric motility results in vomiting, bloating and weight loss. Some cases are idiopathic, others are due to diabetes, autonomic neuropathy or following vagotomy.

- **Investigations**: Gastric distension and delayed emptying can be demonstrated using a barium meal (which is useful to exclude obstructing lesions) or isotope emptying studies (which are more useful for quantifying the amount of delay)
- **Treatment**: Pro-motility agents such as metoclopramide, domperidone or erythromycin, but if symptoms are severe or if aspiration pneumonia occurs a feeding jejunostomy may be required.

Gastric polyps

Unlike colonic polyps, most gastric polyps are rare and usually benign, occurring in about 2% of the population.

- Multiple hamartomatous polyps are occasionally found in Peutz–Jeghers syndrome and adenomata in polyposis coli, but over 90% are hyperplastic (usually arising from Brunner's glands)
- Adenomatous polyps should be removed in view of their pre-malignant potential.

3.5 Complications of gastric surgery – dumping syndrome

Gastric surgery is much less common since the advent of H_2 antagonists and PPIs, but long-term complications of previous gastric surgery are frequently encountered. **Dumping syndrome** results from an inappropriate metabolic response to eating and can occur within half an hour of eating (early dumping) or between 1 and 3 hours (late dumping).

- Symptoms include palpitations, sweating, hypotension and light-headedness.
- Early dumping is a vagally mediated response to rapid gastric emptying.
- Late dumping is due to hypoglycaemia – a rebound insulin-mediated phenomenon following transient hyperglycaemia due to a heavy carbohydrate load to the duodenum.
- Diagnosis is usually clinical, but may be confirmed by glucose, electrolyte or blood pressure monitoring during an attack.

Essential note

Stomach disease includes gastric ulcers, carcinoma, gastroparesis, polyps and Zollinger–Ellison syndrome

4. DISORDERS OF THE PANCREAS

4.1 Acute pancreatitis

This is a common and potentially fatal disease: the mortality in hospital remains at 7–10%, usually due to multi-organ failure or peripancreatic sepsis. Scoring systems, such as the APACHE II or the Glasgow score, identify high-risk patients by assessing factors such as age, urea, hypoxia and white cell count but are unreliable within the first 48 hours.

Obstruction of the pancreatic duct by gallstones accounts for over 50% of cases, most of the rest being alcohol-related; 4% are thought to have a viral aetiology, and all other causes are rare. Oxygen free radicals are thought to mediate tissue injury.

Acute pancreatitis

- **Causes**

  - Gallstones
  - Alcohol
  - Viral (eg mumps, Coxsackie B)
  - Trauma
  - Drugs (eg azathioprine, oral contraceptive pill, frusemide, steroids)
  - Hypercalcaemia
  - Hyperlipidaemia
  - Following surgery to bile duct, or after endoscopic retrograde cholangiopancreatography (ERCP)

- **Early complications**

  - Adult respiratory distress syndrome
  - Acute renal failure
  - Disseminated intravascular coagulation (DIC)

- **Poor prognostic indicators**

  - Age >55 years
  - WCC >15 × 10^9/l
  - Urea >16 mmol/l
  - pO_2 <8 kPa
  - Calcium <2 mmol/l
  - Albumin <32 g/l
  - Glucose >10 mmol/l
  - LDH >600 IU/l
  - (Severe attack if more than three factors are present)

- **Late complications**

  - Abscess
  - Pseudocyst
  - Splenic or portal vein thrombosis

- **Clinical presentation**: usually abdominal pain and vomiting with tachycardia and hypotension in more severe cases

- **Investigations**

  - Amylase (in blood, urine or peritoneal fluid) raised, usually to at least 4 times normal values
  - A plain abdominal X-ray may show a sentinel loop of adynamic small bowel adjacent to the pancreas
  - CT scan to show extent of inflammation or pseudogut ultrasound scan to look for gallstones or pseudogut

- **Treatment**: supportive with fluids and analgesia; the presence of three or more poor prognostic indicators suggests that referral to **ITU** should be considered. **Prophylactic antibiotics** reduce morbidity. In severe pancreatitis due to gallstones (where jaundice and cholangitis are present), early **ERCP** to achieve duct decompression is of proven value. Any patient with a biliary aetiology should have **cholecystectomy** during the same admission once the acute symptoms have settled.

4.2 Chronic pancreatitis

This is an inflammatory condition characterised by irreversible damage to the exocrine and later to the endocrine tissue of the pancreas. Most cases are secondary to alcohol but it is occasionally due to cystic fibrosis or haemochromatosis.

There is a male predominance, often with a long history of alcohol abuse.

Chronic pancreatitis

- **Clinical features**

  - Malabsorption and steatorrhoea
  - Abdominal pain radiating to the back, often severe and relapsing
  - Diabetes mellitus

- **Diagnosis**

  - X-ray may show speckled pancreatic calcification, present in 50–60% of advanced cases
  - CT is the most sensitive for detection of pancreatic calcification
  - ERCP shows irregular dilation and stricturing of the pancreatic ducts although magnetic resonance cholangio-pancreatogram (MRCP) is the modality of choice for diagnostic pancreatography
  - Pancrealauryl and PABA (p-aminobenzoic acid) testing are of use to assess exocrine function – both these involve ingestion of an oral substrate that is cleaved by pancreatic enzymes and can then be assayed in the urine

- **Treatment**: pancreatic enzyme supplementation, analgesia and abstention from alcohol. Antioxidants (vitamins A, C and E) are of unproven value and coeliac axis block for pain relief is now rarely performed because of poor results and surgical complications.
- **Prognosis**: 60% survive for 20 years – death is usually from complications of diabetes or alcohol.

4.3 Pancreatic carcinoma

There are >6000 deaths annually in the UK from carcinoma of the exocrine pancreas. The incidence is 110–120 per million, rising to 800–1000 per million over the age of 75 years.

70–80% arise in the head of the pancreas where there is maximal pancreatic tissue; those in the tail are often silent in the early stages and present at an advanced stage.

- Risk factors

  - Smoking increases risk 2- to 3-fold
  - ? Diabetes – suggested this is an early symptom of carcinoma rather than a risk factor
  - Alcohol does not increase the risk

- Clinical signs

  - Abdominal pain radiating through to back, weight loss and obstructive jaundice in 80–90%
  - Exocrine and endocrine functions are usually maintained
  - Pancreatic carcinoma may invade into the duodenum and this can lead to small bowel obstruction

- Investigations

  - Ultrasound and CT are both useful diagnostic tools, although ERCP is probably of most use, enabling stenting to relieve jaundice and pruritus

- Treatment

  - 10–20% of patients are suitable for surgery but peri-operative mortality is high
  - Radiotherapy and chemotherapy are under evaluation but so far have been shown to confer little survival benefit

- Prognosis

  - Median survival remains 2–3 months from diagnosis, with 1- and 5-year survival rates of 10% and 3%, respectively.

4.4 Endocrine tumours

These are very rare with an annual incidence of 4 per million. They can occur independently, or as part of MEN I syndrome.

The more important lesions include:

- Insulinoma
- Gastrinoma (**Zollinger–Ellison syndrome**, *see* Section 3.2)
- Glucagonoma
- VIPoma
- Somatostatinoma.

> **Essential note**
>
> Pancreatic disease includes acute and chronic pancreatitis, carcinoma and endocrine tumours

---

5. SMALL BOWEL DISORDERS

The small bowel is the main site of absorption of nutrients for the body, so small bowel diseases such as coeliac or Crohn's disease often result in malabsorption and malnutrition. Small bowel pathology can be difficult to diagnose because of the inaccessibility of this part of the GI tract. Special investigations, such as enteroscopy or white cell scanning, may be of use in addition to more routine tests such as gastroduodenoscopy or barium studies. Crohn's disease will be discussed further later in this chapter.

5.1 Coeliac disease

Also known as gluten-sensitive enteropathy, this common and under-diagnosed condition is caused by an immunological reaction to the gliadin fraction of wheat, barley and rye. Some 0.1–0.2% of the population are affected and the onset may be at any age, although peaks occur in babies and in the third decade.

Pathologically, gliadin provokes an inflammatory response that results in partial or total villous atrophy in the proximal small bowel; this reverses on a gluten-free diet but recurs on re-challenge.

> **Coeliac disease**
>
> - Clinical picture
>
>   - Diarrhoea
>   - Oral aphthous ulcers
>   - Weight loss
>   - Growth retardation
>   - General malaise
>   - Neurological symptoms – ataxia, weakness and paraesthesiae
>   - Amenorrhoea
>
> *Continued over*

Coeliac disease

Continued

- Complications

  - Anaemia – folate, or iron deficiency
  - Increased malignancy*
  - Hyposplenism
  - Dermatitis herpetiformis – itchy rash, improves with dapsone
  - Osteomalacia

- Diagnosis

  - Upper GI endoscopy with duodenal biopsy
  - Antiendomyseal antibody
  - Antigliadin antibody – may become negative after treatment

*There is an increased risk of all GI malignancies but especially small bowel lymphoma, occurring in approximately 6% of cases. This risk returns to almost normal with treatment of the disease

Treatment is by strict avoidance of wheat, rye and barley. The role of oats is debatable and many patients can eat oats without significant pathological or clinical effects. Patients require folate, iron and calcium supplements in the early stages of treatment. Failure to respond to treatment is usually due to non-compliance (often unwittingly) with diet. However, supervening pathology, such as lymphoma, should always be excluded and a small number of patients may require steroids to control their symptoms.

Although 10% of first-degree relatives will develop coeliac disease, routine screening is not advocated unless they have symptoms to suggest the diagnosis.

Other causes of villous atrophy:

- Whipple's disease
- Hypogammaglobulinaemia
- Lymphoma
- Tropical sprue: aetiology unknown, but likely to be infective as it responds to long-term tetracycline therapy.

5.2 Carcinoid tumours

These are relatively common; it is estimated that carcinoid tumours are an incidental finding in up to 1% of post-mortems. **Carcinoid syndrome**, however, is extremely rare.

- The tumours secrete serotonin and therefore can be detected by assay of its metabolite, 5-hydroxyindoleacetic acid (5-HIAA) in the urine.

- Carcinoid syndrome occurs only when secondaries in the liver release serotonin into the systemic circulation; any hormone from non-metastatic gut carcinoids will be metabolised in the liver.

Clinical features of carcinoid syndrome

- Diarrhoea
- Bronchospasm
- Local effect of the primary (eg obstruction, intussusception)
- Flushing
- Right heart valvular stenosis

5.3 Whipple's disease

This is an uncommon condition usually affecting middle-aged men (occasionally women and children) caused by infection with *Tropheryma whippeli*. Jejunal biopsy shows deposition of macrophages containing PAS-positive granules within villi. There is a clinical syndrome of diarrhoea, mal-absorption, arthropathy and lymphadenopathy. Whipple's disease remains poorly understood but symptoms respond to extended courses of tetracycline or penicillin.

5.4 Angiodysplasia

Although most commonly occurring in the caecum and ascending colon, angiodysplasia is included here because of the diagnostic challenge it may present when affecting the small intestine. Angiodysplasia may be found throughout the GI tract and its frequency in the population is unknown. It is a rare but significant cause of acute GI haemorrhage, but presents more frequently as occult iron-deficiency anaemia.

Diagnosis of angiodysplasia

This can be difficult, but useful investigations include:

- **Gastroscopy/colonoscopy**: may detect gastric and large bowel lesions.
- **Mesenteric angiography**: only of use if currently bleeding; if so, will localise source in approximately 40%.
- **Small bowel enteroscopy**: intubation of the upper small bowel is possible using an elongated endoscope with an overtube to provide rigidity.
- **Capsule enteroscopy**: this is the most effective method of detecting small bowel angiodysplasia and other sources of small bowel bleeding. A small (11 × 27 mm) capsule is swallowed which transmits thousands of images from the gut as it transits. Images are analysed manually and with computer assistance. The technique is not yet widely available.

Treatment of angiodysplasia

Treatment is by heat or laser coagulation at endoscopy or by embolisation of the bleeding point during angiography. Surgery may be indicated if the lesions are very numerous or if there is severe bleeding. Drug therapy with danazol is thought to reduce the risk of bleeding but is poorly tolerated by many patients.

> **Essential note**
>
> Small bowel disorders include coeliac disease, carcinoid tumours, Whipple's disease, Peutz–Jeghers syndrome and angiodysplasia

6. NUTRITION

There are three components.

1. **Intact GI tract**

   This may be compromised by resections (resulting in a short bowel syndrome) or by fistulae (such that segments of bowel are bypassed). Specific nutrients are absorbed from different parts of the gut and clinical sequelae reflect the segment of bowel affected (eg B_{12} deficiency after terminal ileal resection, iron deficiency after partial gastrectomy).

2. **Ability to absorb nutrients**

   Impairment of absorptive function may be caused by mucosal damage such as occurs in Crohn's or coeliac disease, or after radiation damage. Motility problems resulting in accelerated transit times may also reduce absorption.

3. **Adequate intake**

   This is dependent on the motivation and physical ability to maintain an adequate oral intake (often lacking in sick or elderly people), and on the composition of the diet.

Inability to maintain nutrition is an indication to provide supplementation by one of the three routes listed below. The underlying disease will determine which is appropriate.

- **Oral**: obviously the most simple form but relies on a conscious patient with an intact swallowing mechanism. High protein or carbohydrate drinks may be used to provide good nutritional intake in a small volume.
- **Enteral**: useful when swallowing impaired (eg in neurological disease) or when high volume intake is needed. May take the form of a simple nasogastric tube, or a percutaneous gastrostomy (PEG) or jejunostomy, which can be inserted endoscopically or surgically.
- **Parenteral**: this is intravenous feeding, either to supplement enteral nutrition or to provide total support in the case of complete intestinal failure. Requires short- or long-term central venous access (with associated risks of infection and thrombosis) and close monitoring of electrolyte balance and trace elements.

6.1 Diarrhoea

Medically, diarrhoea is defined as >200 ml of stool per day. In lay terms, diarrhoea is used to describe increased frequency and/or decreased consistency of motions. There are multiple causes (as illustrated below), and these result in diarrhoea by differing mechanisms.

Various classifications can be used:

- acute or chronic
- large bowel (often smaller amounts, may contain blood or mucus)
- small bowel (often voluminous, pale and fatty).

> **Causes of diarrhoea**
>
> - Infective
> - Bacterial
>   - *Salmonella*
>   - *Shigella*
>   - *Campylobacter*
>   - *E. coli*
>   - *Clostridium difficile* (antibiotic related)
>   - Cholera (small bowel infection)
> - Viral
>   - Rotavirus
>   - Norovirus
> - Amoebic
>   - Amoebic dysentery
> - Protozoan
>   - Giardiasis (chronic small bowel infection malabsorption)
> - 'Food poisoning' (bacterial toxin related diarrhoea/vomiting)
>   - *Staphylococcus aureus*
>   - *Bacillus cereus*
>
> *Continued over*

Gastroenterology

Causes of diarrhoea

Continued

- **Inflammatory**

  - Ulcerative colitis
  - Crohn's disease
  - Radiation colitis
  - Ischaemic colitis

- **Malabsorption**

  - Coeliac disease
  - Pancreatic insufficiency
  - Short bowel syndrome

- **Dysmotility**

  - Autonomic neuropathy (eg diabetes mellitus)
  - Irritable bowel syndrome (IBS)

- **Endocrine**

  - Thyrotoxicosis
  - Carcinoid syndrome
  - Hypergastrinaemia
  - VIPoma

- **Drugs**

  - Laxatives
  - Metoclopramide
  - Cisapride
  - Misoprostol
  - Cimetidine
  - Omeprazole
  - Many drugs as idiosyncratic response

- **Antibiotics**

  - Erythromycin (stimulates motility)
  - Penicillins (osmotic effect)
  - Broad spectrum antibiotics (*Clostridium difficile*)

- **Other**

  - Rectal polyp
  - Rectal cancer
  - Overflow diarrhoea secondary to constipation

Mechanisms of diarrhoea

- **Osmotic** (osmotic agents draw water into gut)

  - Osmotic laxatives (lactulose, polyethylene glycol)
  - Magnesium sulphate
  - Lactase deficiency* (poorly absorbed lactose acts as a laxative)
  - *Stops with fasting*

- **Altered motility** (altered peristalsis or damage to autonomic nervous system)

  - Irritable bowel syndrome
  - Thyrotoxicosis
  - Post-vagotomy
  - Diabetic autonomic neuropathy
  - *Stops with fasting*

- **Secretory** (failure of active ion absorption ± active ion secretion)

  - Infection (eg *E. coli*, cholera)
  - Malabsorption
  - Bile salts (increased deposition into bowel after cholecystectomy)
  - *Continues with fasting*

*Lactase deficiency may be congenital (possibly severe) or acquired, and often occurs in the setting of viral gastroenteritis or coeliac disease. Complete exclusion of lactose from diet usually not necessary – there is often a threshold below which symptoms are absent

Causes of bloody diarrhoea

- Crohn's disease
- Ulcerative colitis
- Colorectal cancer
- Ischaemic colitis
- Pseudomembranous colitis
- Schistosomiasis
- *Salmonella*
- *Shigella*
- Amoebiasis
- *Campylobacter*
- *Strongyloides stercoralis*
- Haemolytic uraemic syndrome (which can be caused by *E. coli* type O157, *Campylobacter*, *Shigella*, etc)

Management of diarrhoea

- **History** – confirm true diarrhoea, duration of symptoms, continuous or intermittent, recent foreign travel, rectal bleeding, systemic disease, drug history, steatorrhoea.
- **Examination** – stigmata of inflammatory bowel disease (IBD), dehydration, malnutrition, anaemia, abdominal tenderness, rectal examination (essential)
- **Investigation** (as indicated by symptoms) includes:

  - Stool culture to diagnose bacterial infections – including microscopy for ova and cysts
  - Full blood count (if anaemic check haematinics, raised white cell count, elevated platelets)
  - Biochemistry – hypokalaemia, elevated urea
  - Inflammatory markers – ESR, CRP, albumin (falls in severe diarrhoea), platelets (rise in IBD especially Crohn's disease)
  - Thyroid function tests
  - Coeliac antibodies
  - Sigmoidoscopy/colonoscopy with biopsies
  - Gastroscopy with duodenal biopsies if coeliac disease suspected
  - Small bowel enema/barium meal and follow-through if small bowel pathology suspected
  - Pancreatic function tests if pancreatic disease suspected
  - Breath tests – lactose intolerance, bacterial overgrowth

Treatment of diarrhoea

Treatment should be targeted at the underlying diagnosis.

Loperamide or codeine increase gut transit time and may control symptoms but should be avoided in acute colitis and bacterial diarrhoea. **Octreotide** may be useful for chronic secretory diarrhoea, short bowel symptoms and diarrhoea secondary to endocrine tumours.

6.2 Malabsorption

Causes of malabsorption

- **Structural abnormalities**

  - Coeliac disease*
  - Crohn's disease*
  - Post-surgical resections*
  - Bacterial overgrowth due to blind loops or anatomical abnormalities
  - Whipple's disease
  - Tropical sprue

- **Motility abnormalities**

  - Thyrotoxicosis
  - Drugs (eg neomycin)
  - Diabetes

- **Secretory abnormalities**

  - GI tract infection (eg *Giardia*, amoebiasis)
  - Chronic pancreatitis*
  - Cystic fibrosis

*Common causes in the UK

Bacterial overgrowth of the small bowel

This is common in patients who have undergone small bowel resections or in those with jejunal diverticulae or systemic sclerosis. These bacteria are able to metabolise vitamin B_{12} and carbohydrate but the serum folate remains normal or elevated. Patients usually have diarrhoea, and malabsorption may ensue. Treatment is with antibiotics such as metronidazole, tetracycline or ciprofloxacin, and recurrent or rotating courses of these antibiotics may be necessary.

Essential note

Adequate nutrition requires: an intact GI tract, good absorption and balanced diet

7. LARGE BOWEL DISORDERS

7.1 Crohn's disease and ulcerative colitis

Crohn's disease and ulcerative colitis are both chronic relapsing inflammatory diseases of the gastrointestinal tract.

Aetiology of inflammatory bowel disease

Undoubtedly there is a genetic predisposition, based on identification of at least five susceptibility loci in family studies, and the recent discovery of the NOD2/CARD15 gene on chromosome 16, which is clearly associated with the development of Crohn's disease. This gene codes for a protein that facilitates opsonisation of gut bacteria, and animal studies have confirmed that colitis does not develop in animals raised in a sterile environment.

The major similarities and differences between the two diseases are detailed below.

Clinico-pathology of Crohn's disease and ulcerative colitis

• Crohn's disease	• Ulcerative colitis
Affects any part of the GI tract from mouth to anus. Commonly terminal ileum (70%), colon (30%), anorectum (30%). May be 'skip lesions' of normal mucosa between affected areas	Always involves rectum and extends confluently into the colon. Terminal ileum may be affected by 'backwash ileitis' but remainder of gut unaffected

Pathology

Transmural inflammation	Mucosa and submucosa only involved
Non-caseating granulomata (in 30% only)	Mucosal ulcers
Fissuring ulcers	Inflammatory cell infiltrate
Lymphoid aggregates	Crypt abscesses
Neutrophil infiltrates	

Clinical

Abdominal pain	Diarrhoea, often with blood and mucus
Prominent and frequent fever	Fever
Diarrhoea ± blood p.r.	Abdominal pain less prominent
Anal/perianal/oral lesions	
Stricturing common, resulting in obstructive symptoms	

Clinico-pathology of Crohn's disease and ulcerative colitis

• Crohn's disease	• Ulcerative colitis

Associations

Increased incidence in smokers (50–60% smokers)	Decreased incidence in smokers (70–80% non-smokers)
Skin disorders: erythema nodosum (5–10%) pyoderma gangrenosum (0.5%) iritis/uveitis (3–10%)	Increased incidence of: primary biliary cirrhosis chronic active hepatitis sclerosing cholangitis
Joint pain/arthritis (6–12%)	Other systemic manifestations are slightly less common than in Crohn's disease
Cholelithiasis (common)	
Clubbing	
Depression	

Diagnosis

Barium studies: cobblestoning of mucosa rosethorn ulcers strictures skip lesions	Barium studies: pseudopolyps between ulcers loss of haustral pattern featureless shortened colon
Endoscopy with biopsy Isotope leukocyte scans useful to diagnose active small bowel disease	Sigmoidoscopy with biopsy may be sufficient

Complications

Fistulae: entero-enteral entero-vesical entero-vaginal perianal	Fistulae do not develop Toxic megacolon (acute colitis – usually an indication for urgent colectomy)
Carcinoma – slightly increased risk of colonic malignancy (see later)	Increased risk of carcinoma* (risk increases with time since diagnosis, extent of disease and early age of onset)
B_{12} deficiency common (decreased absorption in terminal ileal disease)	Iron deficiency anaemia
Iron deficiency anaemia	
Abscess formation	

*See section 'Carcinoma complicating inflammatory bowel disease'

Treatment of inflammatory bowel disease

Treatment is similar for both Crohn's disease and ulcerative colitis, although the latter may be more amenable to topical drug therapy. The major treatment strategies are:

- **5-ASA compounds** (sulfasalazine, mesalazine, olsalazine, balsalazide): these are used to treat mild–moderate relapses of colitis and are taken long-term to maintain remission. Oral 5-ASAs are targeted to the colon using pH-dependent or bacterial cleavage systems to release active 5-ASA from carrier molecules. Side-effects are common with sulfasalazine, and these include rash, infertility, agranulocytosis, headache, diarrhoea and renal failure. Interstitial nephritis is a rare side-effect of all 5-ASA drugs.
- **Steroids**: this is the main treatment for active disease, and is available for topical, oral and intravenous administration. Terminal ileal Crohn's disease may be treated with topically acting oral budesonide, which is metabolised in the liver and has far fewer systemic side-effects.
- **Immunosuppressants: azathioprine** is very effective as a steroid-sparing agent and in some patients who are steroid unresponsive. Its use is limited by gastrointestinal and systemic side-effects and close monitoring for evidence of marrow suppression and hepatotoxicity is necessary. Pancreatitis is an uncommon but potentially serious idiosyncratic side-effect.

  - **Methotrexate** is useful in patients with Crohn's disease but does not appear to be effective in patients with ulcerative colitis. **Intravenous ciclosporin** is sometimes effective in the treatment of acute, steroid-resistant colitis, but long-term benefit has not been established.

- **Metronidazole and ciprofloxacin**, used in treatment of perianal disease.
- **Anti-tumour necrosis factor alpha (infliximab)**: this chimeric (mouse/human) monoclonal antibody is very effective in the treatment of active Crohn's disease and many patients benefit from long-term maintenance therapy. The cost (up to £15 000/year) has to be balanced against the reduced costs of hospital admission, surgery, lost productivity and improved quality of life. In the UK its use is restricted to patients who are unresponsive to immunosuppressant therapy, have severe symptoms and who are unsuitable for surgery. Newer immunological therapies are currently under evaluation.
- **Nutritional support and treatment**: patients with IBD are often malnourished and require nutritional supplementation (enteral or parenteral), especially if surgery is planned. An elemental diet may be as effective as steroids in inducing remission in Crohn's disease.
- **Surgery**: surgical resection is very effective for symptom relief in obstructive Crohn's disease, and colectomy offers a cure to patients with ulcerative colitis. The recurrence rate for Crohn's disease after surgery is approximately 50%, although this can be reduced with post-operative azathioprine. Ileo-anal pouch surgery restores continence to patients undergoing colectomy for ulcerative colitis.

Carcinoma complicating inflammatory bowel disease

The risk of carcinoma associated with inflammatory bowel disease is increased if:

- onset occurs at less than 15 years of age
- disease duration has been longer than 10 years
- there is widespread disease (eg total colitis)
- the disease takes an unremitting course
- compliance with treatment and follow-up is poor.

The value of screening for colonic carcinoma in ulcerative colitis and Crohn's disease is controversial. Some units advise a screening colonoscopy every 3 years for patients who have had extensive disease for more than 10 years. This is certainly indicated if one or more adenomatous colonic polyps are present at sigmoidoscopy, if there is long-standing extensive ulcerative colitis, or if the patient has a family history of colonic carcinoma at a young age. In patients with long-standing and extensive colitis, prophylactic colectomy is recommended for persistent dysplasia.

7.2 Pseudomembranous colitis

This is acute colitis due to the enterotoxin of *Clostridium difficile*, usually precipitated by broad-spectrum antibiotics (particularly clindamycin). It is common in the elderly or chronically ill, and mortality may be as high as 20%. Patient-to-patient spread in hospital is common. Diagnosis is by demonstration of the toxin in stools or by endoscopy (which shows inflamed mucosa with yellow pseudomembranes). Treatment is with oral vancomycin or metronidazole.

7.3 Familial polyposis coli

This is an autosomal dominant condition, caused by mutation in the APC tumour suppressor gene, which is located on the long arm of chromosome 5. Estimates of the incidence vary from 1 in 7000–30 000 of the population in the UK. Multiple adenomata occur throughout the colon; if untreated, malignancy is inevitable, often when patients are aged only 30 or 40 years. Surveillance colonoscopy begins in adolescence and prophylactic colectomy usually follows at around age 20 years in view of the high risk of malignant change. Many patients opt for an ileo-anal pouch. Screening of family members is essential.

7.4 Peutz–Jeghers syndrome

This is an autosomal dominant condition in which multiple hamartomatous polyps occur throughout the GI tract (particularly in the small bowel). Patients may have mucocutaneous pigmentation and perioral freckles. Lesions may lead to GI haemorrhage and may undergo malignant change (carcinoma is increased 12-fold in patients with this condition).

7.5 Hereditary non-polyposis colorectal cancer (HNPCC)

This is a dominantly inherited disorder of DNA mismatch repair genes located on chromosomes 2 and 3. Malignancies such as those affecting the colon, breast, ovary and endometrium occur at a young age. Relatives of affected patients require genetic counselling and cancer screening.

7.6 Colorectal cancer

This is the second most common cause of cancer death in the UK, with an incidence of approximately 30/100 000 in the UK. Because of its frequency a national screening programme based on faecal occult blood testing and colonoscopy will be introduced in the UK in 2006. Colorectal cancer is common from the sixth decade onwards and the incidence increases with advancing age. Recent studies have suggested that non-steroidal anti-inflammatory agents (NSAIDs) may have a protective effect.

Pathologically, it is an adenocarcinoma usually arising from tubular and villous adenomatous polyps (although in inflammatory bowel disease, malignant change arises directly from the mucosa). The commonest sites are the rectum and sigmoid colon.

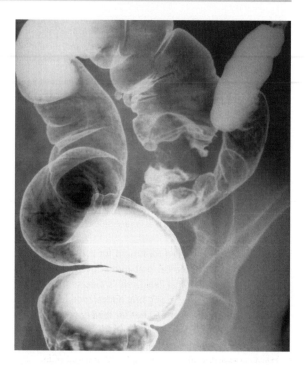

Figure 2 Radiograph of the colon of a 59 year old patient with cancer of the sigmoid colon

Credit ZEPHYR / SCIENCE PHOTO LIBRARY

Risk factors and clinical features of colorectal cancer

- Increased incidence

  - Male sex
  - Inflammatory bowel disease, especially ulcerative colitis
  - Familial polyposis coli
  - Diet low in fibre, fruit and vegetables
  - Diet high in fat and red meat
  - Cholecystectomy (bile salts 'dumped' in colon)

Risk factors and clinical features of colorectal cancer

- Genetics

  - Sporadic mutations may occur in the p53, Ras and APC genes. p53 regulates the cell cycle and causes apoptosis in the event of DNA damage – its loss therefore leads to uncontrolled proliferation of cells

- Clinical signs

  - These depend on the site of the lesion; all can cause weight loss and obstructive symptoms.

Right-sided	Left-sided	Rectum
Iron deficiency anaemia	Blood p.r.	Blood p.r.
Abdominal pain	Altered bowel habit	Tenesmus
Abdominal mass	Abdominal mass	

Treatment of colorectal cancer

This consists of surgery (for cure) or symptomatic relief depending, on **Duke's staging**.

Duke's classification and prognosis of colorectal cancer	
Stage	Five-year survival
A – confined to mucosa and submucosa	80% +
B – extends through muscularis propria	60–70%
C – regional lymph nodes involved	30–40%
D – distant spread	0%

- **Radiotherapy** may be used as an adjuvant, particularly to reduce tumour bulk before surgery.
- Adjuvant chemotherapy (eg 5-fluorouracil post-operatively) has been shown to improve prognosis for patients at Duke's stages B and C, toxicity is low so quality of life tends to be good.
- Serial monitoring of carcinoembryonic antigen (CEA), a glycoprotein from gastrointestinal epithelia, may be of use in detecting recurrence.
- Some surgeons are now resecting hepatic metastases isolated to a single lobe of liver.

7.7 Irritable bowel syndrome (IBS)

This is a chronic, relapsing functional gut disorder with no recognisable pathological abnormality. In most cases the diagnosis is based on clinical presentation although symptoms presenting in older patients require investigation to exclude other pathologies. IBS affects up to 10% of the population with a ratio of 5:1 female dominance. Strict diagnosis is based on Rome II criteria requiring abdominal pain provoked by eating or relieved by defecation and a change in bowel habit occurring for at least 3 months in a year.

Full blood count, ESR, CRP, thyroid function tests (TFTs) and stool culture are useful screening investigations to exclude common pathological diagnoses, and sigmoidoscopy provides reassurance for patients and clinicians that there is no underlying pathology.

- Bloating, borborygmi, excessive flatus, belching and mucorrhoea are common gastrointestinal symptoms.
- IBS is often associated with alternating bowel habit but may also present with 'diarrhoea-dominant' or 'constipation-dominant' symptoms.

- Patients with IBS often complain of other 'functional' symptoms and have a higher prevalence of fibromyalgia, non-cardiac chest pain, tension headache, sterile cystitis, dyspareunia, back pain, anxiety and depression.
- There is a clear association with a history of childhood abuse.
- In about a quarter of cases IBS is preceded by gastrointestinal infection, raising the possibility of damage to the neuroenteric innervation in some cases.

Treatment

Treatment is usually symptomatic and includes antispasmodics, increased dietary fibre, laxatives, constipating agents, antidepressants, hypnotherapy and psychotherapy. The latter are particularly useful for patients whose symptoms occur on a background of significant psychological morbidity.

Essential note
Large bowel disorders include: Crohn's disease, ulcerative colitis, gastroenteritis, familial polyposis coli, colorectal cancer and IBS

8. GASTROINTESTINAL INFECTIONS

8.1 Gastroenteritis

Most gastrointestinal infections in the UK are viral or self-limiting bacterial infections such as *Staphylococcus aureus* or *Campylobacter*. Most patients require no treatment but oral rehydration therapy (ORT) may be required in patients who are at risk of dehydration. ORT utilises the capacity of the small bowel to absorb chloride, sodium and water via a glucose-dependent active transport channel that is not disrupted by infections. More intensive therapy is confined to those systemically unwell or immunosuppressed.

Amoebiasis

- Infection is due to *Entamoeba histolytica* with faecal–oral spread.
- The clinical spectrum ranges from mild diarrhoea to dysentery with profuse bloody stool; a chronic illness with irritable-bowel-type symptoms may also occur. Colonic or hepatic abscesses occur, the latter commonly in the setting of a severe amoebic colitis.
- Treatment is with metronidazole.

Campylobacter

This is due to a Gram-negative bacillus; spread is faecal–oral.

- Gram-negative rods.
- Clinically, patients are often systemically unwell with headache and malaise prior to the onset of diarrhoeal illness. Abdominal pain may be severe, mimicking an acute abdomen.
- Erythromycin may be indicated if symptoms are prolonged.

Cholera

- Infection is due to *Vibrio cholerae* (Gram-negative rods) which colonise the small bowel; spread is faecal–oral. A high infecting dose is needed, as the bacteria are susceptible to gastric acid.
- A severe toxin-mediated diarrhoea occurs with 'rice-water' stool which may exceed 20 litres per day. Dehydration is the main cause of death especially in young or elderly, and mortality is high without rehydration treatment.
- Tetracycline may reduce transmission.

Giardiasis

- Infection is due to *Giardia lamblia* (a flagellate protozoan) which colonises the duodenum and jejunum; spread is faecal–oral.
- Bloating and diarrhoea (not bloody) occur and may be chronic. Malabsorption may occur with small intestinal colonisation. Asymptomatic carriage is common and duodenal biopsy may be necessary to make the diagnosis in patients with chronic diarrhoea or malabsorption symptoms.
- Treatment is with metronidazole.

Salmonella

- A Gram-negative bacillus with multiple serotypes divided into two main groups: those causing typhoid and paratyphoid (enteric fever) and those causing gastroenteritis. Spread is faecal–oral.
- Diarrhoea (may be bloody) occurs, with or without vomiting and abdominal pain.
- Treatment is supportive but occasionally ciprofloxacin or trimethoprim may be required for chronic symptoms or severe illness in the very young or elderly.

Shigella

- Gram-negative rods. Spread is faecal–oral with a very low infecting dose of organisms needed owing to its high virulence.

- The clinical spectrum ranges from diarrhoeal illness to severe dysentery depending on the infecting type: *S. sonnei, S. flexneri, S. boydi, S. dysenteriae.*
- Diarrhoea (may be bloody), vomiting, abdominal pain.
- Treat if severe with ampicillin or ciprofloxacin although antibiotic resistance is widespread.

8.2 Gastrointestinal tuberculosis

This is common in developing countries, and causes ileo–caecal TB (mimicking Crohn's disease) or occasionally spontaneous TB peritonitis. Suspect TB in any patient with unexplained bowel symptoms if they have been in an endemic area.

- Clinical features are often non-specific such as malaise, fever and weight loss, as well as diarrhoea and abdominal pain.
- Ultrasound, barium studies or CT may suggest the diagnosis but biopsy, either by laparoscopy or endoscopy, is confirmative.
- Treatment is with conventional anti-tuberculous therapy.

> **Essential note**
>
> Most gastroenteritis in UK is self-limiting, requiring no treatment

9. HEPATOLOGY

9.1 Jaundice

Jaundice is one of the most common symptoms of liver disease, caused by the accumulation of bilirubin in the tissues. Bilirubin is formed as the end product of catabolism of haem-containing compounds and is clinically detectable at a level of >40 µmol/l. The formation and excretion of bilirubin is shown in the following figure.

The most common causes of jaundice in the UK are alcoholic liver disease, gallstones and tumours of the liver and pancreas.

Hyperbilirubinaemia may occur because of excess production or decreased elimination of bilirubin. Jaundice can thus be broadly divided into three categories depending on the site of the pathology.

- **Pre-hepatic**: excess production of bilirubin or failure of uptake into the liver. Bilirubin is unconjugated and insoluble thus it does not appear in the urine – acholuric jaundice.

- **Hepatic**: defect is at the level of hepatocyte. There is diminished hepatocyte function, and thus both conjugated bilirubin and urobilinogen appear in the urine.
- **Post-hepatic**: there is impaired excretion of bile from liver into the gut. Conjugated bilirubin is therefore reabsorbed which increases serum and urine levels and produces dark urine. The stools become pale due to lack of stercobilinogen; urobilinogen (produced in the gut – see accompanying figure) becomes undetectable in urine.

Causes of jaundice

Pre-hepatic	• Haemolysis causing excess haem production
	• Congenital hyperbilirubinaemia (eg Gilbert's syndrome, Crigler–Najjar syndrome)
Hepatic	• Viral infection (eg hepatitis A, B, EBV)
	• Drugs (eg phenothiazines)
	• Wilson's disease
	• Rotor and Dubin–Johnson syndromes
	• Cirrhosis
	• Multiple hepatic metastases
	• Hepatic congestion in cardiac failure
Post-hepatic	• Gallstones
	• Carcinoma of pancreas or bile ducts
	• Lymph nodes at porta hepatis (eg metastatic, lymphoma)
	• Primary biliary cirrhosis – small bile duct obliteration
	• Sclerosing cholangitis
	• Structural abnormality of the biliary tree – post-surgery, congenital (eg biliary atresia)

Essential note

Gallstones and viral hepatitis are the commonest causes of jaundice in Britain

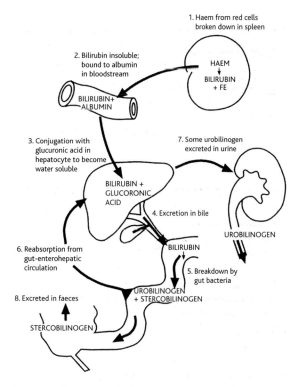

Figure 3 Enterohepatic circulation of bile

Investigation of jaundice

The following would be a typical systematic approach.

Blood tests

- **Liver function tests** may indicate if jaundice is obstructive (elevated alkaline phosphatase from cells lining canaliculi) or hepatocellular (elevated transaminases). Patients with chronic liver disease may have normal enzyme levels, but poor synthetic function (low albumin, prolonged prothrombin time) will indicate hepatic aetiology. Full blood count, reticulocyte count and blood film are useful if haemolysis is suspected.
- **Viral serology** (hepatitis A, B and C), **autoantibody titres** (antimitochondrial M2 for primary biliary cirrhosis and anti-smooth muscle for chronic autoimmune hepatitis), alpha$_1$-antitrypsin, alpha fetoprotein (AFP), ferritin and copper studies are essential when investigating unexplained jaundice or chronic liver disease.

Imaging and biopsy

- **Liver ultrasound**: is the single most useful radiological test and will identify obstruction, metastases, cirrhosis and hepatoma.
- **CT scanning**: is frequently used to complement ultrasound images, to define lesions more clearly and to diagnose lesions not seen on ultrasound.
- **ERCP**: is used to investigate obstructive jaundice and to stent obstructing tumours or remove obstructing gallstones.
- **Liver biopsy**: may be helpful in non-obstructive jaundice, but is contraindicated in the presence of uncorrected coagulation disorders and is technically difficult if ascites is present.
- **MRCP**: non-invasive magnetic resonance imaging of the biliary tree.

9.2 Gallstone disease

Gallstones are one of the commonest causes of jaundice, usually presenting with colicky upper abdominal pain and cholestatic liver function tests. Approximately 1 litre of bile is secreted by the hepatocytes each day. Half of this drains directly into the duodenum whilst the remainder is stored and concentrated in the gallbladder by removal of sodium, chloride, bicarbonate and water. Cholecystokinin (CCK) then stimulates its release.

- Stones are found in 10–20% of the population (with a female preponderance) but are asymptomatic in the majority.
- 70–90% gallstones are a mixture of cholesterol and bile pigment and 10% are pure cholesterol. Pure pigment stones are rare except with chronic haemolysis (eg sickle cell disease, spherocytosis).

Risk factors for and clinical presentation of gallstones

- Risk factors for stone formation

  - Female sex
  - Increasing age
  - Drugs (eg oral contraceptive pill, clofibrate)
  - Crohn's disease (terminal ileum)
  - Short bowel syndrome
  - Haemolysis (pigment stones)

Risk factors for and clinical presentation of gallstones

- Clinical presentation

  - Acute/chronic cholecystitis
  - Biliary colic
  - Cholestatic jaundice if duct obstruction
  - Pancreatitis
  - Cholangitis
  - Gallstone ileus → *usually in ileocaecal valve*

NB Stones may form in the common bile duct even after cholecystectomy

- **Diagnosis** in most cases may be established by ultrasound with/without ERCP. **MRCP** is replacing ERCP as a useful, non-invasive investigation but it does not allow therapeutic intervention during the procedure.
- Definitive treatment is by cholecystectomy. ERCP with sphincterotomy and balloon clearance of the common bile duct may be indicated for duct stones. Medical treatment with ursodeoxycholic acid can be used to dissolve cholesterol stones; however, this is extremely slow and should be reserved only for patients who are unfit for other treatment.

9.3 Ascites

Ascites is defined as the accumulation of free fluid within the peritoneal cavity. It can be subdivided into transudate or exudate depending on whether the protein content is less or greater than 30 g/l, respectively. The most common causes in the UK are cirrhosis and malignant disease.

Causes of ascites

- Transudate

  - Portal hypertension (in cirrhosis)
  - Nephrotic syndrome
  - Malnutrition
  - Cardiac failure
  - Budd–Chiari syndrome
  - Myxoedema (hypothyroidism)

- Exudate

  - Hepatic or peritoneal malignancy
  - Intra-abdominal TB
  - Pancreatitis

The **treatment** of ascites depends on the aetiology.

- **Transudates** respond to fluid restriction, low sodium intake and diuretic therapy, to promote sodium and water excretion via the kidneys. Paracentesis may be used for tense ascites or ascites which is not responding to diuretics. However, paracentesis may result in a further shift of fluid from the intravascular space into the peritoneal cavity with the risk of circulatory collapse. This can be reduced by supporting the circulation using intravenous albumin.
- Exudates can be safely paracentesed without protein replacement.

9.4 Viral hepatitis

The six major hepatitis viruses are described below, but further types are already postulated.

Hepatitis A

Spread: faecal–oral

Virus: RNA

Clinical: anorexia, jaundice, nausea, joint pains, fever

Treatment: supportive

Chronicity: no chronic state

Vaccine: yes.

Hepatitis B

Spread: blood-borne (eg sexual, vertical, congenital transmission)

Virus: DNA

Clinical: acute fever, arteritis, glomerulo-nephritis, arthropathy

Treatment: supportive; chronic HBV may respond to interferon (the effectiveness of antiviral agents lamivudine and famciclovir are under evaluation)

Chronicity: 5% → chronic carriage (risk of cirrhosis and hepatocellular carcinoma)

Vaccine: yes.

Hepatitis B serology

Antigens/antibodies related to viral surface (**s**), envelope (**e**) and core (**c**) are useful for determining the stages, infectivity and chronicity of hepatitis B infection:

- **HBsAg**: present in acute infection; if present longer than 6 months = chronic hepatitis
- **HBeAg**: present in acute or chronic infection; signifies high infectivity
- **HBcAg**: present in acute or chronic infection; found only in liver tissue; present for life
- **AntiHBs**: signifies immunity after vaccination or acute infection
- **AntiHBe**: signifies declining infectivity and resolving infection
- **AntiHBe IgM**: signifies recent acute infection; lasts <6 months
- **AntiHBc IgG**: is a lifelong marker of past acute or chronic infection; does not signify immunity or previous vaccination

---

Hepatitis C

Spread: blood-borne, sexual

Virus: RNA

Clinical: acute hepatitis – less severe than A or B, fulminant failure rate

Treatment: pegylated interferon alpha (interferon bound to polyethylene glycol) for chronic HCV. This may be more effective when used in combination with ribavirin

Chronicity: 60–80% develop chronic hepatitis and 20% of these progress to cirrhosis (of whom a third will develop hepatocellular carcinoma). IV-drug-related hepatitis C represents a major public health problem in the UK

Vaccine: no.

Hepatitis D (delta agent)

Spread: blood-borne (dependent on concurrent hepatitis B infection for replication)

Virus: incomplete RNA

Clinical: exacerbates established hepatitis B infection and increases risk of hepatic failure and cirrhosis

Treatment: interferon of limited benefit

Chronicity: increases incidence of cirrhosis in chronic HBV

Vaccine: no.

Hepatitis E

Spread: faecal–oral

Virus: RNA

Clinical: acute self-limiting illness, but there is a 25% mortality (fetal and maternal) in pregnancy, which increases in later stages of gestation

Treatment: supportive

Chronicity: no chronic state

Vaccine: no.

Hepatitis G

Spread: blood-borne

Virus: RNA

Clinical: doubtful relevance; 20% of patients with chronic HCV are infected with hepatitis G

Treatment: viraemia may decline with interferon

Chronicity: unknown – may cause cirrhosis and hepatocellular carcinoma

Vaccine: no.

Interferon in viral hepatitis

Interferon is predominantly of benefit in patients suffering from chronic hepatitis B and C. In hepatitis B, there is a response in 40% of chronic carriers. The response is poorer in Asian patients. The response is likely to be very poor if the patient is also infected with HIV and thus treatment is not usually indicated in this group. In hepatitis C, there is a response in 50% of chronic carriers but 50% of these will relapse despite treatment.

9.5 Drug-induced hepatitis

Many drugs can cause hepatitis. Toxicity may be due to overdose (eg paracetamol), idiosyncratic (eg flucloxacillin) or may be related to dosage or duration of therapy (eg azathioprine). Three patterns of damage can occur:

- **Cholestasis**: some drugs produce a functional obstruction to bile flow by causing bile duct inflammation and interfering with excretory transport mechanisms. The commonest examples are flucloxacillin, chlorpromazine, oral contraceptives and anabolic steroids.
- **True hepatitis**: some drugs produce direct hepatocellular damage which may be trivial or result in fulminant liver failure. Several mechanisms are responsible. Examples include statins, antituberculous drugs, immunosuppressants, ketoconazole and halothane.
- **Hepatic necrosis**: if the ability of the liver to detoxify metabolites is overwhelmed, glutathione levels fall and toxic metabolites accumulate causing liver necrosis. This

is the pattern of damage with carbon tetrachloride ingestion and paracetamol overdosage.

Other causes of acute hepatitis include:

- alcohol
- other viruses (eg Epstein–Barr, yellow fever, CMV, rubella, Herpes simplex)
- other infections (eg malaria, toxoplasmosis, leptospirosis, brucellosis).

9.6 Chronic hepatitis

Chronic hepatitis is defined as any hepatitis persisting for longer than 6 months. The main differentiation is between chronic persistent hepatitis, which is a benign condition with a good prognosis, and the more serious chronic active hepatitis.

Chronic persistent hepatitis

This is defined as a benign inflammatory reaction lasting longer than 6 months. It will remit spontaneously after several months or years. Biopsy (necessary to exclude chronic active hepatitis) shows portal fibrosis but no piece-meal necrosis. Patients are often asymptomatic; there may be hepatomegaly but signs of chronic liver disease are absent. Liver biochemistry is often normal except for elevated aspartate aminotransferase.

Causes of chronic hepatitis
<ul><li>Viral hepatitis</li><li>Drugs (eg methyldopa, isoniazid, cytotoxics)</li><li>Alcohol</li></ul>Because of its benign nature, treatment is not indicated.

Chronic active hepatitis (CAH)

This is an aggressive persistent hepatitis characterised by piecemeal necrosis on biopsy. Progression to cirrhosis with the associated risk of hepatocellular carcinoma is common.

Causes of chronic active hepatitis (CAH)
<ul><li>Hepatitis B ± hepatitis D (20% of all CAH; not responsive to steroids but may respond to interferon – see earlier)</li><li>Alpha$_1$-antitrypsin deficiency</li><li>Hepatitis C (see earlier)</li><li>Autoimmune (see below)</li><li>Wilson's disease</li></ul>

Autoimmune 'lupoid' hepatitis

This condition occurs predominantly in female patients. Other autoimmune disease is often present and patients are usually ANF and anti smooth muscle antibody positive. It responds to steroids and azathioprine but the majority progress to cirrhosis, although 90% are alive at 5 years and may be candidates for transplantation.

9.7 Cirrhosis

Cirrhosis is characterised by the irreversible destruction and fibrosis of normal liver architecture with some regeneration into nodules.

There are four stages of pathological change:

- liver cell necrosis
- inflammatory infiltrate
- fibrosis
- nodular regeneration.

Regeneration may be macronodular (eg alcohol- or drug-induced), micronodular (eg viral hepatitis) or mixed, but a more useful categorisation is according to the aetiological agent.

Causes of cirrhosis

- Alcohol (most common in the UK, approximately 30% of all cases)
- Hepatitis B or C (most common worldwide)
- Cryptogenic
- Primary biliary cirrhosis
- Haemochromatosis
- Wilson's disease
- Alpha$_1$-antitrypsin deficiency

Evidence of chronic liver disease may or may not be present

Essential note

Alcohol is the most common cause of cirrhosis in the UK

Clinical features

Clinical features related to hepatic insufficiency (liver failure):

- **Confusion/encephalopathy**: due to failure of liver to metabolise ammonium salts and portal hypertension diverting intestinal blood away from liver.
- **Haemorrhage**: bruising/bleeding/petechiae secondary to deficiency in factors II, VII, IX and X, and thrombocytopenia.
- **Oedema**: secondary to hypoalbuminaemia.
- **Ascites**: due to portal hypertension, hypoalbuminaemia and secondary hyperaldosteronism.
- **Jaundice**: failure to metabolise and/or excrete bilirubin.
- **Other features of chronic liver disease include**: palmar erythema, leuconychia, Dupuytren's contracture, spider naevi, splenomegaly (due to portal hypertension), caput medusae and ascites.

Diagnosis

Cirrhosis may be suspected on ultrasound scanning but biopsy is required to confirm this and to help identify the aetiology. Ultrasound guided biopsy is mandatory as the liver is often very small. Rarely, a transjugular biopsy is attempted, particularly if clotting is markedly deranged.

Treatment

Treatment is aimed at the removal of causal factors such as alcohol. Specific treatments include interferon for viral hepatitis and ursodeoxycholic acid for primary biliary cirrhosis.

Transplantation is the best hope but many patients are not suitable.

Contraindications for liver transplantation
Contraindications include:

- poor cardiac reserve
- co-morbidity such as HIV infection or severe respiratory disease
- failure to abstain from alcohol.

Indications for liver transplantation
There is no definitive cut-off regarding age but patients over 70 years are less likely to be suitable.

- **Fulminant hepatic failure**

  - (eg due to hepatitis C or paracetamol toxicity)

- **Primary biliary cirrhosis**
- **Hepatitis B**

  - Although frequent recurrence after transplant – reduce using pre-transplant treatment with interferon

- Cholangiocarcinoma

  - If unresectable at presentation

- Alcohol

  - Following psychological review and if abstained for more than 6 months

- Wilson's disease
- Haemochromatosis
- Hepatocellular carcinoma

  - If not multifocal, if <5 cm and no evidence of vascular invasion

9.8 Portal hypertension and varices

Portal hypertension occurs as a result of increased resistance to portal venous flow. Pressure in the portal vein rises and is said to be pathological when >12 mmHg, although pressures of up to 50 mmHg may occur. The spleen enlarges and anastomoses may open between the portal and systemic circulation. Some of the collaterals, which most commonly occur at the oesophagogastric junction, umbilicus and rectum, may become very large with a risk of bleeding. A variety of conditions may cause portal hypertension; in the UK the single most common is cirrhosis secondary to alcohol.

Causes of portal hypertension

- Cirrhosis due to any cause
- Portal vein thrombosis (congenital malformation, pancreatitis, tumour)
- Budd–Chiari syndrome (thrombosis or obstruction of hepatic vein due to tumour, haematological disease or the oral contraceptive pill)
- Intrahepatic tumours such as cholangiocarcinoma or hepatocellular carcinoma
- Constrictive pericarditis
- Right heart failure

Variceal haemorrhage

Thirty per cent of patients with varices will bleed at some point with a mortality of 50% for that episode. The majority of survivors will rebleed with a mortality of 30%. Bleeding is often catastrophic as many patients also have coagulopathy as a result of their underlying liver disease.

Primary prevention of haemorrhage

All patients with cirrhosis of the liver should have upper GI endoscopy to determine the presence or absence of varices. If there are none, or only very small varices, no treatment is required except regular endoscopic review every 2–3 years. Larger varices in patients with no history of variceal haemorrhage should be treated with prophylactic beta-blockade (or nitrates if beta-blockers are contraindicated). This reduces portal pressure and significantly reduces the risk of haemorrhage.

Treatment of variceal haemorrhage

After resuscitation and correction of any coagulopathy the treatment of choice is early gastroscopy with band ligation of the varices (now shown to be superior to injection sclerotherapy).

Temporary balloon tamponade (Sengstaken–Blakemore tube) may be useful if endoscopy is not immediately available or if bleeding cannot be stopped endoscopically.

Vasoactive drugs, such as terlipressin (Glypressin®), are widely used but should not be viewed as a substitute for endoscopy and banding.

Secondary prevention of haemorrhage

Patients should undergo repeated band ligation until varices are eradicated. Beta-blockade should be given as this reduces the risk of rebleeding by up to 40%.

9.9 Hepatic encephalopathy

Hepatic encephalopathy is a neuropsychiatric syndrome, which may complicate acute or chronic liver disease from any cause. Symptoms include confusion, falling level of consciousness, vomiting, fits and hyperventilation. Renal failure may often supervene – the chance of recovery from hepatorenal failure is poor. The underlying mechanisms are complex but the absorption of toxins such as ammonia from bacterial breakdown of proteins in the gut is thought to play a major part. Porto-systemic shunting of blood occurs – toxins thus bypass the liver and cross the blood–brain barrier.

The most common causes of **acute hepatic encephalopathy** are fulminant viral hepatitis and paracetamol toxicity, which are potentially fully reversible. Indicators of poor prognosis are:

- worsening acidosis
- rising prothrombin time
- falling Glasgow Coma Scale.

These patients should be referred to a specialist centre as they may need transplantation.

Chronic hepatic encephalopathy may supervene in chronic liver disease of any type. It is often precipitated by:

- alcohol
- drugs
- GI haemorrhage
- infections
- constipation
- diuretics.

It is characterised by a flapping tremor, decreased consciousness level and constructional apraxia.

Treatment of hepatic encephalopathy

- Screen for and treat sepsis aggressively – if ascites is present consider bacterial peritonitis and perform a diagnostic ascitic tap. There should be a low threshold for prescribing ciprofloxacin
- Strict fluid and electrolyte balance
- Low protein diet
- Laxatives to clear the gut and thus reduce toxin absorption; neomycin is now rarely used
- Remove or treat precipitants

Mortality is high, and if renal failure supervenes then the mortality exceeds 50%.

9.10 Primary biliary cirrhosis

Primary biliary cirrhosis accounts for approximately 5% of deaths due to cirrhosis. The cause is unknown although factors point to an autoimmune aetiology, especially the strong association with other autoimmune disease such as rheumatoid arthritis, Sjögren's syndrome and CREST syndrome. Histologically, progressive inflammation and destruction of small intrahepatic ducts lead to eventual cirrhosis. Ninety per cent of patients are female, often in middle age. There are four stages of primary biliary cirrhosis:

1. Destruction of interlobular ducts
2. Small duct proliferation
3. Fibrosis
4. Cirrhosis.

Primary biliary cirrhosis

- Clinical features
  - Cholestatic jaundice
  - Xanthelasma due to hypercholesterolaemia
  - Skin pigmentation
  - Clubbing
  - Hepatosplenomegaly
  - Portal hypertension ± varices
- Diagnosis
  - Antimitochondrial (M2) antibody present in 95%
  - Predominantly raised alkaline phosphatase – often raised in advance of symptoms/signs
  - Raised IgM
  - Liver biopsy showing the features listed above

Treatment is symptomatic; cholestyramine relieves pruritus. Ursodeoxycholic acid is widely used but it is doubtful whether this agent either improves the prognosis or delays time to liver transplantation. Rising bilirubin levels are an indication that the disease is approaching end stage and, as liver transplantation remains the only hope of cure, patients should be assessed for this later treatment at an appropriate stage of their disease process.

9.11 Other causes of chronic liver disease

- **Haemochromatosis**: this is an autosomal recessive disorder of iron metabolism leading to deposition in the liver, pancreas, pituitary and myocardium.
- **Wilson's disease**: this is an autosomal recessive disorder of copper metabolism causing deposition in the liver, basal ganglia and cornea (Kayser–Fleischer ring).

9.12 Parasitic infections of the liver

Hydatid disease

This is caused by *Echinococcus granulosus* (a dog tapeworm), and is most common in areas of sheep and cattle farming. Ingestion results from eating contaminated vegetables or as a result of poor hand hygiene. The parasitic embryos hatch in the small intestine and enter the bloodstream via the portal venous circulation to the liver, but there may also be spread to lung or brain. Hydatid cysts in the liver may be over 10 cm in diameter.

Schistosomiasis

This affects about 250 000 000 people worldwide. It is caused by *Schistosoma mansoni* (Africa, South America) or *Schistosoma japonicum* (Asia) – liver flukes. Infection occurs when the parasite penetrates the skin during swimming or bathing in infected water contaminated by the intermediate host – the freshwater snail. The parasite migrates to the liver via the portal venous system where it matures, migrates back along the portal (and mesenteric) veins and produces numerous eggs, which penetrate the gut wall and are excreted to continue the cycle. A chronic granulomatous reaction occurs in the liver leading to periportal fibrosis and cirrhosis.

- Early symptoms are related to the site of entry of the organism (swimmer's itch) and systemic effects including malaise, fever, myalgia, nausea and vomiting.
- Diagnosis is confirmed by detecting ova in stool or liver biopsy. Liver function tests show raised alkaline phosphatase, and there is an eosinophilia.
- Treatment is with praziquantel.

9.13 Hepatic abscesses

Pyogenic abscesses most commonly occur following intra-abdominal sepsis but they can occur spontaneously. The commonest organism isolated is *E. coli* but *Enterococcus*, *Proteus*, *Staphylococcus aureus* and anaerobes are recognised.

- Patients present with swinging pyrexia, weight loss, right upper quadrant pain and anorexia. Septic shock or jaundice may develop.
- Diagnosis is confirmed by liver ultrasound which is used to guide aspiration or insertion of a drain.
- Broad-spectrum antibiotics are given until sensitivities are available; occasionally surgical resection is required.

Amoebic abscesses are caused by *Entamoeba histolytica*, which spreads from the gut (where it can cause an acute diarrhoeal illness) via the portal system to the liver. Single or multiple cysts may be found on ultrasound and treatment is with metronidazole.

9.14 Hepato-biliary tumours

There are a number of types of primary hepatic malignancy, all of which are rare. Secondary tumours, however, are common, typically metastasising from the stomach, colon, breast and lung.

Treatment of metastatic tumours is usually not indicated as the disease process is far advanced, although chemotherapy may slow progression in selected patients.

Hepatocellular carcinoma

This is rare in the UK (1–2/100 000 population) but the incidence is increased 20–30 times in Africa, Asia and Japan.

Incidence is increased by:

- hepatitis B (commonest cause worldwide) and hepatitis C virus
- cirrhosis from any cause, particularly hepatitis B, C and haemochromatosis
- aflatoxin – a carcinogen from the mould *Aspergillus flavus* which may contaminate food
- long-term oral contraceptive use
- androgenic steroids

Raised serum AFP suggests the diagnosis and, in association with ultrasound, has been suggested as an appropriate annual screening for patients with cirrhosis.

Prognosis of hepatocellular carcinoma	
Treatment	**Prognosis**
No treatment	5-year survival <25%
Resection	Only 5–15% are suitable, with 20% operative mortality; 5-year survival <30%
Transplant	Very few patients are suitable – they should have single tumours smaller than 5 cm with no vascular or metastatic spread; 5-year survival 90%
Chemotherapy/ ethanol injection into tumour/ embolisation	Palliative with little survival benefit

Cholangiocarcinoma

This is an uncommon adenocarcinoma arising from the biliary epithelium.

Predisposing factors:

- sclerosing cholangitis
- choledochal cyst or other biliary tract abnormality
- schistosomiasis
- Carolli's disease (dilation of the intrahepatic bile ducts predisposing to infection and stone formation).

Treatment	Prognosis
No treatment	Average survival 2 months
Resection	Fewer than 20% of patients are suitable; average survival approximately 3 years
Transplant	Very few patients are suitable but this gives the best prognosis

Carcinoma of the gall bladder

This adenocarcinoma occurs in the elderly but is uncommon. It has usually invaded locally or metastasised by the time of diagnosis.

Benign hepatic adenoma

The incidence of this is increased in patients who have been taking oral contraceptives for longer than 5 years and also with the use of anabolic steroids. It is usually asymptomatic but may rarely cause intraperitoneal bleeding or right upper quadrant pain.

Hepatic haemangioma

This is common, and is often an incidental finding on ultrasound. It is benign but may occasionally rupture.

Further revision

Royal College of Physicians at http://www.rcplondon.ac.uk/index.asp

British Society of Gastroenterology at http://www.bsg.org.uk/

Gut Online at http://gut.bmjjournals.com/

CORE, Fighting gut and liver disease at http://www.digestivedisorders.org.uk/

Kumar PJ, Clark ML. *Clinical medicine*, 5th edn. Philadelphia: WB Saunders, 2002.

Revision summary

You should now:

1. Be familiar with the anatomy of the gastrointestinal tract including the blood supply and the relationship between structure and function.
2. Recognise the different types of dysphagia and be familiar with the symptoms associated with oropharyngeal, motility-related and obstructive dysphagia.
3. Recognise the association between *Helicobacter* infection and peptic ulcers, be familiar with the other common risk factors and understand the actions of drug therapy.
4. Recognise the symptoms of upper gastrointestinal haemorrhage and understand the principles of management.
5. Be familiar with the common gastrointestinal malignancies including the risk factors, treatment, prognosis and the principles of screening for colorectal cancer and oesophageal cancer in patients with Barrett's oesophagus.
6. Recognise the symptoms and signs of acute pancreatitis and know the common causes and treatment of this condition.
7. Be familiar with the roles of the small intestine and pancreas in digestion and understand the causes, investigation and treatment of malabsorption.
8. Be familiar with the common causes of change in bowel habit and know the basic investigations and treatment for constipation and diarrhoea.
9. Be able to distinguish between Crohn's disease and ulcerative colitis and understand the roles of steroids, 5-ASAs and immunosuppressants in the treatment of inflammatory bowel disease.
10. Be familiar with bilirubin metabolism and the enterohepatic circulation and be able to distinguish between pre-hepatic, hepatocellular and post-hepatic jaundice.

Genetics

CONTENTS

Revision objectives

You should:

1. Understand the organisation of the human genome into the nuclear and mitochondrial chromosomes, and the basic processes of DNA replication, transcription and translation
2. Understand the concept of normal human variation, the different forms of mutation that can result in human disease, and the concept of genetic heterogeneity

3. Understand the chromosomal basis of inheritance, the potential implications of chromosome rearrangements, and the basis of common chromosomal imbalances
4. Understand Mendelian patterns of inheritance, and pedigree construction
5. Be aware of unusual mechanisms of inheritance and non-Mendelian disorders

Continued over

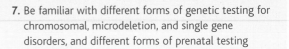

6. Be aware of the basis and phenotypes associated with common single gene disorders

7. Be familiar with different forms of genetic testing for chromosomal, microdeletion, and single gene disorders, and different forms of prenatal testing

1. THE HUMAN GENOME

The human nuclear genome is made up of around 30 million base pairs (30 megabases) of DNA organised into 23 pairs of chromosomes. It contains about 30 000 genes. One member of each nuclear chromosome pair is inherited from each parent. Humans also have a mitochondrial genome made up of 16 500 base pairs (16.5 kilobases) of DNA organised into a single circular chromosome. The mitochondrial genome is almost exclusively maternally derived.

Essential note

The human genome consists of 23 pairs of nuclear chromosomes, and multiple copies of a mitochondrial chromosome

2. MOLECULAR GENETICS BACKGROUND

2.1 DNA (deoxyribonucleic acid) structure, transcription and translation

DNA is a **double-stranded** molecule composed of nucleotides, which are purine (adenine + guanine) and pyrimidine (cytosine and thymine) bases bound to a pentose sugar called deoxyribose and linked by a backbone of covalent phosphodiester bonds between the sugar residues. The two anti-parallel strands are held together by hydrogen bonds, which can be disrupted by heating and re-form on cooling:

- **Adenine (A) pairs with thymine (T)** by two hydrogen bonds
- **Guanine (G) pairs with cytosine (C)** by three hydrogen bonds.

When DNA replicates, the double strands separate and a new complementary strand is synthesised on each.

Genes are composed of exons, introns and regulatory sequences. The DNA nucleotide sequence in the exons determines the amino acid sequence in the polypeptide chain it encodes. The exons are interspersed by introns which do not contain amino acid encoding sequence. DNA is **transcribed** in the nucleus into messenger RNA (mRNA) during which the introns are removed and the exons are joined together by a process called splicing. Introns may be involved in gene regulation, and they facilitate the production of different protein isoforms through alternative splicing. The mRNA migrates to ribosomes in the cytoplasm where it is **translated** into a polypeptide chain. Each amino acid is specified by a particular combination of three adjacent nucleotides called a codon. The positions along the mRNA where translation begins and ends are denoted by the initiator (or start) and termination codons respectively. RNA differs from DNA in that it is:

- **Single stranded**
- Thymine is replaced by **uracil**
- The sugar that the base is bound to is **ribose**.

2.2 Mutations and polymorphisms

Mutations are DNA sequence changes that have a deleterious effect on the gene product, usually a protein. Sequence changes can be categorised as insertions, deletions, substitutions or splice-site mutations. Mutations in regulatory sequences can result in altered gene expression.

Essential note

Mutations are sequence variants that are associated with alterations in the quantity or function of the product (usually a polypeptide) they encode, which in turn results in phenotypic abnormality

For most genetic conditions, the mutations within the causative gene are family specific. However, for some conditions many individuals share a common mutation, an example being the ΔF508 mutation in cystic fibrosis.

Throughout the genome there are harmless variations in the DNA sequence between individuals called **polymorphisms**. Some are within exons but are silent (do not result in an amino acid change), while others cause amino acid variants and hence protein polymorphisms that may be detectable biochemically, for example fast and slow isoniazid acetylators and α_1-antitrypsin variants (PiM and S). Many polymorphisms lie within introns or regulatory sequences or the stretches of DNA between genes. Polymorphisms have proved invaluable for mapping genes by a process called linkage (a statistical method based on the principle that the closer a polymorphism is to a mutant gene, the more likely it is to segregate with the disease in a family). Linkage can also be used to provide testing in a family with a known genetic condition where the causative family-specific mutation cannot be found.

> **Essential note**
>
> Genes contain many harmless sequence variations, called polymorphisms, which do not have any deleterious effect on the product the gene encodes

3. CHROMOSOME BACKGROUND

Within the nucleus of somatic cells there are 22 pairs of autosomes, and 1 pair of sex chromosomes called X and Y. The normal chromosome complement of 46 chromosomes is known as **diploid**. Normal male and female karyotypes are 46,XY and 46,XX respectively. Genomes with a single copy of each chromosome or three copies of each are known respectively as **haploid** and **triploid**. A karyotype with too many or too few chromosomes, where the total is not a multiple of 23, is called **aneuploid**.

Chromosomes are divided by the centromere into a short 'p' arm ('petit') and a long 'q' arm. **Acrocentric** chromosomes (13, 14, 15, 21, 22) have the centromere at one end.

Lyonisation is the process whereby in a cell containing more than one X chromosome, only one is active. Selection of the active X is usually random and each inactivated X chromosome can be seen as a Barr body on microscopy.

Mitosis occurs in somatic cells and results in two **diploid** daughter cells with nuclear chromosomes that are genetically identical both to each other and the original parent cell.

Meiosis occurs in the germ cells of the gonads and is also known as '**reduction division**' because it results in four **haploid** daughter cells, each containing just one member (homologue) of each chromosome pair and all genetically

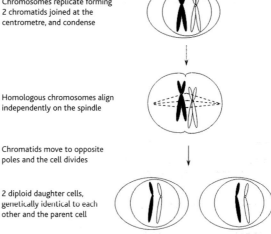

Chromosomes replicate forming 2 chromatids joined at the centrometre, and condense

Homologous chromosomes align independently on the spindle

Chromatids move to opposite poles and the cell divides

2 diploid daughter cells, genetically identical to each other and the parent cell

Figure 1 Mitosis

different. Meiosis involves two divisions (**meiosis I and II**). The reduction in chromosome number occurs during meiosis I and is preceded by exchange of chromosome segments between homologous chromosomes called **crossing over**. In males the onset of meiosis and spermatogenesis is at puberty. In females, replication of the chromosomes and crossing over begins in fetal life but the oocytes remain suspended prior to the first cell division until just before ovulation.

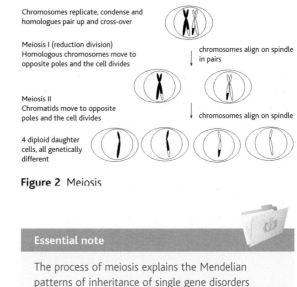

Chromosomes replicate, condense and homologues pair up and cross-over

Meiosis I (reduction division) Homologous chromosomes move to opposite poles and the cell divides

chromosomes align on spindle in pairs

Meiosis II Chromatids move to opposite poles and the cell divides

chromosomes align on spindle

4 diploid daughter cells, all genetically different

Figure 2 Meiosis

> **Essential note**
>
> The process of meiosis explains the Mendelian patterns of inheritance of single gene disorders

4. CLINICAL GENETICS

4.1 Constructing a family tree (pedigree)

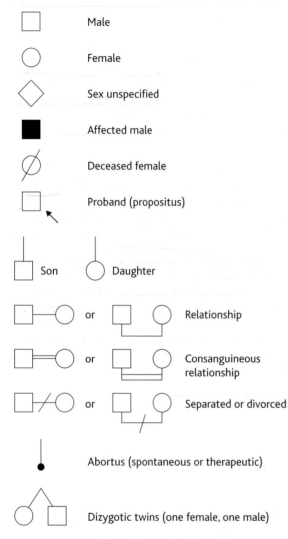

☐	Male
○	Female
◇	Sex unspecified
■	Affected male
⊘	Deceased female
☐	Proband (propositus)
☐ Son	○ Daughter
☐—○ or ☐ ○	Relationship
☐═○ or ☐ ○	Consanguineous relationship
☐╫○ or ☐ ○	Separated or divorced

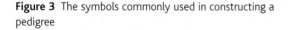

Abortus (spontaneous or therapeutic)

Dizygotic twins (one female, one male)

Monozygotic female twins

Figure 3 The symbols commonly used in constructing a pedigree

5. CHROMOSOME DISORDERS

5.1 Chromosome testing (karyotyping)

Chromosome testing is performed on lymphocytes. The cells are stimulated to divide in culture and mitosis is arrested at metaphase. For standard karyotyping the chromosomes are stained with Giemsa which causes them to take on a specific pattern of stripes called G-bands. They are then examined using light microscopy. The highest resolution generally obtainable is about five megabases.

5.2 Translocations

Individuals carrying a balanced chromosome translocation usually have a normal phenotype, but may be predisposed to having offspring with chromosome imbalance. The commonest is the Robertsonian translocation between chromosomes 14 and 21 associated with an increased risk of offspring with Down's syndrome. Rearrangements of the chromosomes are called translocations. There are two types:

- **Reciprocal**: exchange of a chromosome segment between non-homologous chromosomes.
- **Robertsonian**: fusion of two acrocentric chromosomes at their centromeres, eg (14;21).

They may be:

- **Unbalanced**: if chromosomal material has been lost or gained overall.
- **Balanced**: if no chromosomal material has been lost or gained overall.

Carriers of balanced translocations are usually pheno-typically normal but are at increased risk for having off-spring with chromosomal imbalance.

Carriers of a Robertsonian translocation involving chromosome 21 are at increased risk of having offspring with translocation Down's syndrome but they can also have offspring with normal chromosomes, or offspring who are balanced translocation carriers like themselves (see Figure 4).

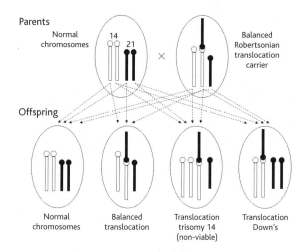

Figure 4 Robertsonian translocation

5.3 Common sex chromosome aneuploidies

Turner's syndrome (karyotype 45,X)

This affects 1 in 2500 live-born females but it is a frequent finding amongst early miscarriages. Patients are usually of normal intelligence. They have streak ovaries which result in failure of menstruation, low oestrogen with high gonadotrophins, and infertility. Normal secondary sexual characteristics may develop spontaneously or be induced with oestrogens. Short stature throughout childhood with failure of the pubertal growth spurt is typical. Final height can be increased by early treatment with growth hormone. Other features may include:

- Webbed or short neck
- Low hairline
- Shield chest with widely spaced nipples
- Cubitus valgus (wide carrying angle)
- Cardiovascular abnormalities particularly aortic coarctation in 10–15%
- Renal anomalies (eg horseshoe kidney, duplicated ureters, renal aplasia) in one-third
- Non-pitting lymphoedema in one-third.

Individuals with Turner's syndrome may be mosaic, which means they have a mixture of body cells with a 45,X karyotype and cells with another karyotype, eg 46,XX or 47,XXX. In these individuals, the clinical features may be milder and they may be fertile.

Triple X syndrome (karyotype 47,XXX)

These female patients show little phenotypic abnormality but tend to be of tall stature. Whilst intelligence is typically reduced compared to siblings it usually falls within normal or low–normal limits, however mild developmental and behavioural difficulties are more common. Fertility is normal but the incidence of early menopause is increased.

Klinefelter's syndrome (karyotype 47,XXY)

This affects 1 in 600 newborn males. Phenotypic abnormalities are rare prepubertally other than a tendency to tall stature. At puberty, spontaneous expression of secondary sexual characteristics is variable but poor growth of facial and body hair is common. The testes are small, in association with azoospermia, testosterone production around 50% of normal and raised gonadotrophins. Gynaecomastia occurs in 30% and there is an increased risk of male breast cancer. Female distribution of fat and hair and a high pitched voice may occur but are not typical. Intelligence is generally reduced compared to siblings but usually falls within normal or low–normal limits. Mild developmental and behavioural problems are more common.

47,XYY males

These males are phenotypically normal but tend to be tall. Intelligence is usually within normal limits but there is an increased incidence of behavioural abnormalities.

5.4 Common autosomal chromosome aneuploidies

Down's syndrome (trisomy 21)

Down's syndrome affects 1 in 700 live births overall and is usually secondary to meiotic non-disjunction during oogenesis, which is commoner with increasing maternal age. Around 5% of patients have an underlying Robertsonian translocation, most commonly between chromosomes 14 and 21. Around 3% have detectable **mosaicism** (a mixture of trisomy 21 and karyotypically normal cells) usually resulting in a milder phenotype. Phenotypic features include:

- Brachycephaly (shortening of the antero-posterior diameter of the head)
- Upslanting palpebral fissures, epicanthic folds, Brushfield spots on the iris

- Protruding tongue
- Single palmar crease, 5th finger clinodactyly, wide sandal gaps between 1st and 2nd toes
- Hypotonia and moderate mental retardation.

The following are more common in patients with Down's syndrome:

- Cardiovascular malformations in 40%, particularly atrioventricular septal defects (AVSD)
- Gastrointestinal abnormalities in 6%, particularly duodenal atresia and Hirschprung's disease
- Haematological abnormalities, particularly acute lymphoblastic leukaemia (ALL), acute myeloid leukaemia (AML) and transient leukaemias
- Hypothyroidism
- Cataracts in 3%
- Alzheimer's disease in the majority by 40 years of age.

Edwards' syndrome (trisomy 18)

This typically causes intrauterine growth retardation, a characteristic facies, prominent occiput, overlapping fingers (2nd and 5th overlap 3rd and 4th), rockerbottom feet (vertical talus) and short dorsiflexed great toes. Malformations, particularly congenital heart disease, diaphragmatic hernias, renal abnormalities and dislocated hips, are more common. Survival beyond early infancy is rare but associated with profound mental handicap.

Patau syndrome (trisomy 13)

Affected infants usually have multiple malformations including CNS abnormalities, scalp defects, microphthalmia, cleft lip and palate, post-axial polydactyly, rockerbottom feet, renal abnormalities and congenital heart disease. Survival beyond early infancy is rare and associated with profound mental handicap.

5.5 FISH testing

FISH (fluorescent in situ hybridisation) is a cytogenetic technique for assessing the copy number of specific DNA sequences in one genome, using fluorescently labelled complementary DNA probes.

- Rapid trisomy screening (for chromosomes 21, 13, 18)
- Rapid sexing
- Detection of specific microdeletion syndromes.

5.6 Microdeletion syndromes

These are caused by chromosomal deletions that are too small to be seen by light microscopy. They usually involve two or more adjacent genes. They can be detected using specific FISH probes.

Examples of microdeletion syndromes:

- **DiGeorge syndrome** (parathyroid gland hypoplasia with hypocalcaemia, thymus hypoplasia with T-lymphocyte deficiency, congenital cardiac malformations particularly interrupted aortic arch and truncus arteriosus, cleft palate, learning disability) due to microdeletions at 22q11. There appears to be an increased incidence of psychiatric disorders, particularly within the schizophrenic spectrum.
- **Williams syndrome** (supravalvular aortic stenosis, hypercalcaemia, stellate irides, mental retardation) due to microdeletions involving the elastin gene on chromosome 7.

6. SINGLE GENE DISORDERS

These disorders result from an altered DNA sequence within a gene.

6.1 Autosomal dominant (AD) conditions

These result from mutation of one copy of a gene carried on an autosome. All offspring of an affected person have a 50% chance of inheriting the mutation. Within a family the severity may vary (**variable expression**) and known mutation carriers may appear clinically normal (**non-penetrance**). Some conditions, such as achondroplasia and neurofibromatosis-1 (NF1), frequently begin de novo through new mutations arising in the egg or (more commonly) sperm.

Essential note

Autosomal dominant conditions can arise de novo from new mutations, and may be associated with variable expression

Example of autosomal dominant (AD) conditions

Achondroplasia
Familial adenomatous polyposis coli
Familial breast–ovarian cancer (BRCA1, BRCA2)
Huntington's chorea
Marfan's syndrome
Myotonic dystrophy
Neurofibromatosis types 1 and 2 (NF1, NF2)
Tuberous sclerosis

6.2 Autosomal recessive (AR) conditions

These result from mutations in both copies of an autosomal gene. Where both parents are carriers each of their offspring has a 1 in 4 (25%) risk of being affected, and a 50% chance of being a carrier. The new mutation rate for autosomal recessive disorders is very low. Apart from rare exceptions, the parents of a child with an autosomal recessive disorder must be carriers for it.

> **Essential note**
>
> The mutations underlying autosomal recessive conditions are generally ancient. As a result, the parents of a child with an autosomal recessive condition are almost invariably carriers for the condition, and the prevalence of some autosomal recessive disorders varies according to ethnic group

> **Examples of autosomal recessive (AR) conditions**
>
> - β-Thalassaemia
> - Congenital adrenal hyperplasia (21-hydroxylase deficiency)
> - Cystic fibrosis
> - Galactosaemia
> - Homocystinuria
> - Haemochromatosis
> - Mucopolysaccharidoses (all except Hunter's)
> - Oculocutaneous albinism
> - Phenylketonuria
> - Sickle-cell anaemia
> - Spinal muscular atrophy

Most metabolic disorders are autosomal recessive – remember the exceptions.

AR disorders are observed more commonly in children whose parents are consanguineous. That is because cousins share ancestors and hence genes (eg first cousins share one set of grandparents and on average one-eighth of their genes). As a result they are more likely to both be carriers for the same AR disorder than a couple who are unrelated to each other.

Some AR disorders are more common in particular populations because the carrier frequency is increased:

- Cystic fibrosis in North European Caucasians (carrier frequency 1 in 25)
- Tay–Sachs disease in Ashkenazi Jews
- b-Thalassaemia in Mediterranean and Asian populations
- Sickle-cell anaemia in African and African-Caribbean populations

6.3 X-linked recessive (XLR) conditions

These result from a mutation in a gene carried on the X chromosome and affect males because they have only one copy of the x-chromosome and hence just one gene copy. Females are usually unaffected but may have mild manifestations as a result of lyonisation. This form of inheritance is characterised by the following:

- NO MALE-TO-MALE TRANSMISSION (an affected father passes his Y chromosome to all his sons)
- All daughters of an affected male are carriers (an affected father passes his X chromosome to all his daughters)
- Sons of a female carrier have a 50% chance of being affected and daughters have a 50% chance of being carriers.

> **Essential note**
>
> X-linked disorders often arise as new mutations. Female carriers of an X-linked recessive disorder may manifest some features as a result of unfavourable Lyonisation. X-linked disorders are not transmitted from father to son, but all the daughters of an affected man will be carriers

> **Examples of X-linked recessive (XLR) conditions**
>
> - Becker muscular dystrophy
> - Duchenne muscular dystrophy
> - Fabry's disease
> - Favism (glucose-6-phosphate dehydrogenase deficiency)
> - Haemophilias A and B (Christmas disease)
> - Hunter's syndrome (MPS II)
> - Lesch–Nyhan disease

6.4 X-linked dominant (XLD) conditions

These are caused by a mutation in one copy of a gene on the X chromosome but both male and female mutation carriers are affected. Because of lyonisation females are usually more mildly affected and these disorders are frequently lethal in males. For the reasons outlined above:

- There is no male-to-male transmission
- All daughters of an affected male would be affected
- All offspring of an affected female have a 50% chance of being affected.

Examples of X-linked dominant (XLD) conditions

- Rett syndrome
- Vitamin D resistant rickets

7. UNUSUAL GENETIC MECHANISMS

7.1 Trinucleotide repeat disorders

These conditions are associated with genes containing stretches of repeating units of three nucleotides and include:

- Fragile X syndrome   XL
- Myotonic dystrophy   AD
- Huntington's chorea   AD
- Friedreich's ataxia   AR.

In normal individuals the number of repeats varies slightly but remains below a defined threshold. Affected patients have an increased number of repeats, called an **expansion**, above the disease-causing threshold. The expansions may be unstable and enlarge further in successive generations causing increased disease severity and earlier onset, known as 'anticipation', **eg myotonic dystrophy**, particularly congenital myotonic dystrophy following transmission by an affected mother.

Essential note

Triplet repeat expansions are the basis of the anticipation observed in families affected by myotonic dystrophy or Huntington's disease – with successive generations affected, individuals develop the disease at an earlier age and the disease is more severe.

Fragile X syndrome

This causes mental retardation, macroorchidism (large testes) in adults, and seizures, and is often associated with a cytogenetically visible constriction ('fragile site') on the X chromosome. The inheritance is X-linked but complex. Among controls there are between 6 and 55 stably inherited trinucleotide repeats in the FMR1 gene. People with between 55 and 230 repeats are said to be premutation carriers but are unaffected. During oogenesis in female premutation carriers, the triplet repeat is unstable and may expand into the disease-causing range (230 to >1000 repeats) known as a full mutation which is methylated, effectively inactivating the gene. All males and around 50% of females with the full mutation are affected. The premutation does not expand to a full mutation when passed on by a male.

7.2 Mitochondrial disorders

Mitochondria are **maternally inherited**, since they derive from those present in the cytoplasm of the ovum. They contain copies of their own **circular 16.5-kilobase chromosome** carrying genes for several respiratory chain enzyme subunits and some of the components required for translation, eg transfer RNA (tRNA) and ribosomal RNA (rRNA) molecules. The mitochondrial genome differs from the nuclear genome in that it:

- is circular
- the genes do not contain introns
- the amino acid specified by some of the codons is different
- there are multiple copies of the mitochondrial genome within each cell
- it is only maternally derived.

Essential note

Disorders caused by mutations in the mitochondrial genome are associated with maternal transmission

Within a tissue there may be a mixed population of normal and abnormal mitochondria known as **heteroplasmy**. Different proportions of abnormal mitochondria may be required to cause disease in different tissues, known as a **threshold effect**. Disorders caused by mitochondrial gene mutations include:

- **MELAS** (**m**itochondrial **e**ncephalopathy, **l**actic **a**cidosis, **s**troke-like episodes)
- **MERRF** (**m**yoclonic **e**pilepsy, **r**agged **r**ed **f**ibres)
- mitochondrially inherited diabetes mellitus and deafness

7.3 Genomic imprinting

For most genes both copies are expressed, but for some genes either the maternally or paternally derived copy is preferentially used, a phenomenon known as genomic imprinting. The best examples are the Prader–Willi and Angelman syndromes, both caused by either cytogenetic deletions of the same region of chromosome 15q or by **uniparental disomy** of chromosome 15 (where both copies of chromosome 15 are derived from one parent with no copy of chromosome 15 from the other parent).

		Prader–Willi	*Angelman*
Clinical		Neonatal hypotonia and poor feeding	'Happy puppet', unprovoked laughter/clapping
		Moderate mental handicap	Microcephaly, severe mental handicap
		Hyperphagia + obesity in later childhood	Ataxia, broad-based gait
		Small genitalia	Seizures, characteristic EEG
Genetics		Majority have a deletion on the paternal chromosome 15	Majority have a deletion on the maternal chromosome 15
		The remainder mostly have maternal uniparental disomy (ie no paternal contribution)	A small proportion have paternal uniparental disomy (ie no maternal contribution)
			Remainder due to more subtle mutations or unknown

8. POLYGENIC DISORDERS

Many conditions have a genetically determined susceptibility, but do not follow simple Mendelian patterns of inheritance. They are believed to result from an interaction between different genes and, in some cases, environmental factors. Examples include:

- Type 1 diabetes
- Type 2 diabetes
- Ischaemic heart disease
- Hirschsprung's disease
- Isolated talipes equinovarus
- Neural tube defects
- Cleft lip and palate.

For many of these conditions, studies have been undertaken to document the average chance of recurrence in couples who have had an affected child, and these empiric risks are used for genetic counselling.

Essential note

Many common diseases and single malformations are believed to result from the cumulative effect of mutations in several genes (polygenic) together with environmental factors, known as multifactorial inheritance

8.1 Genetic heterogeneity

This term is used for conditions that can be caused by more than one gene.

For example, tuberous sclerosis can result from a mutation in TSC1 gene on chromosome 9, which encodes hamartin, or from a mutation in TSC2 gene on chromosome 16, which encodes tuberin.

Conversely, different mutations within a single gene can result in different clinical phenotypes. For example, different mutations in the dystrophin gene can result in Duchenne or Becker muscular dystrophy.

9. IMPORTANT GENETIC TOPICS

9.1 Cystic fibrosis

This results from mutations in the **CFTR** (cystic fibrosis transmembrane conductance regulator) gene and the **ΔF508** mutation accounts for 75% of mutations in Caucasians. Testing in most laboratories now identifies 90% of Caucasian cystic fibrosis mutations, but a much smaller proportion in many other ethnic groups. Therefore, negative molecular testing cannot exclude a diagnosis of cystic fibrosis.

9.2 Duchenne and Becker muscular dystrophy

These result from different mutations within the dystrophin gene on chromosome Xp21. Important distinguishing features are as follows:

	Duchenne	Becker
Immunofluorescent dystrophin on muscle biopsy	Undetectable	Reduced/abnormal
Wheelchair dependence	95% at <12 years	5% at <12 years
Mental handicap	20%	Rare

9.3 Neurofibromatosis (NF)

There are two forms of NF which are clinically and genetically distinct:

	NF1	NF2
Major features	≥6 café-au-lait patches (CALs)	Bilateral acoustic neuromas (vestibular schwannomas)
	Axillary/inguinal freckling	Other cranial and spinal tumours
	Lisch nodules on the iris	
	Peripheral neurofibromas	
Minor features	Macrocephaly	CALs (usually <6)
	Short stature	Peripheral schwannomas
		Peripheral neurofibromas
Gene	Chromosome 17	Chromosome 22
Protein affected	Neurofibromin	Schwannomin

9.4 Tuberous sclerosis (TS)

There are at least two separate genes which cause TS, on chromosomes 9 and 16.

	Clinical features
Skin/nails	Ash-leaf macules
	Shagreen patches (especially over the lumbosacral area)
	Adenoma sebaceum (facial area)
	Subungual/periungual fibromas
Eyes	Retinal hamartomas
Heart	Cardiac rhabdomyomas, detectable antenatally, usually regressing during childhood
Kidneys	Renal cysts
Neurological	Seizures
	Mental handicap
Neuro-imaging	Intracranial calcification (periventricular)

9.5 Marfan's syndrome

This results from mutations in the fibrillin gene on chromosome 15. Intelligence is usually normal.

	Clinical features
Musculoskeletal	Tall stature with disproportionately long limbs
	Arachnodactyly
	Pectus carinatum or excavatum
	Scoliosis
	High, narrow arched palate
	Joint laxity, pes planus (flat feet)
Heart	Aortic root dilatation and dissection
	Mitral valve prolapse
Eyes	Lens dislocation (typically up)
	Myopia
Skin	Striae
Lung	Pneumothorax

9.6 Homocystinuria

This is most commonly due to cystathione-β-synthase deficiency and causes a Marfan-like body habitus, lens dislocation (usually down), mental handicap, thrombotic tendency and osteoporosis. Treatment includes a low methionine diet ± pyridoxine.

9.7 Achondroplasia

A short-limb skeletal dysplasia resulting from autosomal dominant mutations in the FGFR3 (fibroblast growth factor receptor 3) gene on chromosome 4. There is a high new mutation rate. Important complications are hydrocephalus, brainstem or cervical cord compression resulting from a small foramen magnum, spinal canal stenosis, kyphosis and sleep apnoea.

9.8 Potter sequence

Oligohydramnios as a result of renal abnormalities, urinary tract obstruction or amniotic fluid leakage may lead to secondary fetal compression with joint contractures (arthrogryposis), pulmonary hypoplasia and squashed facies known as the Potter sequence.

9.9 Teratogenic disorders

Teratogens are agents that harm the developing fetus causing miscarriage or abnormalities of organogenesis. Examples of teratogens are infectious agents (particularly cytomegalovirus, *Toxoplasma*, rubella), drugs (such as warfarin, valproate), and other substances (such as alcohol, cocaine). Some maternal illnesses are associated with a higher rate of fetal abnormality, such as maternal diabetes.

9.10 Genetic testing

Diagnostic

Testing for mutations in a gene known to underlie the condition which the patient is suspected to have on clinical grounds.

Example: Testing for Fragile X in a boy with learning disability.

Predictive

Testing an asymptomatic individual for a genetic change, which will reveal whether they are likely to develop the clinical features of a genetic condition or not.

Example: Testing for myotonic dystrophy in an asymptomatic person whose father has the condition.

Carrier

Testing an asymptomatic individual to see if they are heterozygous for an autosomal recessive or X-linked recessive disorder.

Predictive testing should not be undertaken without written informed consent after formal counselling, usually over more than one session. National UK guidelines recommend that predictive testing and carrier testing for disorders that will not have implications until adulthood should not be undertaken in children.

Example: Testing for cystic fibrosis in a healthy adult whose sibling was affected.

9.11 Prenatal testing

Prenatal testing is appropriate where the unborn baby is known to be at increased risk for being affected by a genetic disorder. For example:

- Prenatal testing for cystic fibrosis in a fetus whose parents are both known to be carriers.
- Prenatal testing for chromosomes in a fetus whose mother is known to carry a balanced Robertsonian translocation.
- **CVS or CVB** (chorionic villus sampling or biopsy): a small piece of placenta is taken either transabdominally or transvaginally. CVS testing can be safely performed from 10–11 weeks of gestation.
- **Amniocentesis**: amniotic fluid is taken, containing cells derived from the surfaces of the fetus and amniotic membranes. Amniocentesis is usually performed from 15–16 weeks of gestation.
- **Cordocentesis**: a method of obtaining fetal blood which can be performed from 18 weeks of gestation.

Chromosome and DNA testing can be performed on any of the above types of sample. Each carries a small risk of miscarriage.

9.12 Pre-implantation genetic diagnosis (PIGD)

This technique is being pioneered for couples whose offspring are at risk of a specific genetic disorder, where the family mutation(s) or chromosome rearrangement is known, and where prenatal testing with termination of affected fetuses is not acceptable to them. Embryos are generated by in vitro fertilisation (IVF). At the 8- to 16-cell stage a single cell is removed for testing. Only embryos predicted to be unaffected are re-implanted into the mother. PIGD is technically difficult, is not routine, the rate of achieving viable pregnancies is lower than for routine IVF, and availability in the UK is restricted to a small number of conditions.

PIGD is available for a limited number of conditions, for example, sex selection in X-linked disorders, chromosome imbalance in offspring of people with balanced translocations, and cystic fibrosis for parents carrying the ΔF508 mutation.

Further revision

Kingston HM. *ABC of clinical genetics.* 2002. London: BMJ Books. ISBN 0-7279-1627-0. This is an excellent, well-illustrated paperback introduction covering everything from the structure of DNA, through common chromosome and single gene disorders, through laboratory testing from a clinical perspective.

Baraitser M, Winter RM. *A colour atlas of clinical genetics.* 1988. New York: Wolfe Medical Publications Ltd. ISBN 0 7234 1547 1. This is an excellent, paper-back atlas of dysmorphology illustrating many chromosomal and single gene syndromes.

Websites I would recommend are:

DNA from the beginning (introductory genetics tutorials) at http://vector.cshl.org/dnaftb

The West Midlands Regional Genetics Service Website, which has links to a wide variety of useful websites, at http://www.bwhct.nhs.uk

Revision summary

You should now:

1. Understand the structure of DNA, how it replicates, how it is organised into genes, and how they encode polypeptide chains.
2. Understand the concept of polymorphisms and linkage and their value in tracking and mapping genes. Understand the concept of dominant and recessive mutations, newly arising (de novo) mutations, and the different types of mutation that can result in genetic disorders in humans (including single base changes, insertions, deletions, splicing mutations, expansions of triplet repeats). Understand that one gene can underlie different clinical disorders, and that some clinical disorders can be caused by more than one gene (genetic heterogeneity). Understand the concepts of variable expression and non-penetrance.
3. Understand meiosis and how it relates to Mendelian inheritance. Know the clinical relevance of chromosome translocations, particularly pertaining to Down's syndrome. Should be familiar with the common chromosome aneuploidies and microdeletion syndromes and with the concept of mosaicism.
4. Be familiar with common pedigree symbols and be able to perform simple risk calculations for autosomal dominant, autosomal recessive and X-linked disorders.
5. Be aware of the genetic basis of anticipation, as well as the concepts of mitochondrially inherited disorders and disorders of genetic imprinting. Should understand the concept of polygenic and multifactorial disorders and empiric recurrence risks.
6. Be familiar with the clinical features associated with the commoner single gene disorders and how they are inherited.
7. Understand the difference between diagnostic, predictive and carrier testing for genetic disorders, and be familiar with methods of prenatal genetic testing. Should understand broadly how testing for chromosome, microdeletion and single gene disorders is performed.

Genito-urinary medicine and AIDS

CONTENTS

Revision objectives

You should have:

1. An awareness of the major bacterial sexually transmitted infections.
2. A basic understanding of the biology and modes of transmission of the HIV virus.
3. An overview of the clinical stages of HIV disease and serological diagnosis.
4. An understanding of the clinical presentation and diagnosis of major opportunistic infection in advanced HIV.
5. An awareness of the principles of monitoring and treatment with HAART in HIV disease.

1. SEXUALLY TRANSMITTED INFECTIONS (STIs)

1.1 Bacterial STIs

Gonorrhoea

Male symptoms are purulent urethral discharge and dysuria. Transmission is primarily sexual. In the UK penicillin is the most appropriate treatment for susceptible organisms. However, resistance is present in 10% of cases and quinolones or ceftriaxone can be used depending on anti-microbial sensitivities.

Disseminated (bacteraemic) infection is unusual but is more common in women. Responsible strains are nearly always highly susceptible to penicillin. Pharyngeal and rectal infection is often asymptomatic. Ophthalmia neonatorum is treated with systemic anti-microbials, and appropriate eye drops.

Syphilis

Transmission is primarily sexual, congenital or, rarely, by blood transfusion. Penicillin is the drug of choice, or alternatively tetracycline. **Concurrent HIV infection may increase the risk of neurosyphilis**, and extended courses of treatment are required. Diagnosis is by:

- **Clinical assessment**: ano-genital ulceration in primary syphilis, mucocutaneous lesions including skin rash and oral ulceration in secondary syphilis. In late symptomatic syphilis involvement is primarily neurological and cardiovascular.
- **Dark ground microscopy**: of **fresh** material from chancres or lesions of secondary syphilitic rash to identify the treponeme.
- **Serology**

Early syphilis

- Positive treponemal enzyme immunoassay (EIA)
- Positive treponemal haemagglutination assay (TPHA)
- Elevated rapid plasma reagin (RPR) or venereal disease research laboratory (VDRL) titres

Late syphilis

- Positive treponemal assay (EIA)
- Positive treponemal haemagglutination assay (TPHA)
- Negative or weakly reactive raised rapid plasma reagin (RPR) or venereal disease research laboratory (VDRL) titres

EIA and TPHA are specific treponemal antibody tests, and that VDRL and RPR are non-specific treponemal antibody tests.

Chlamydia infections

Non-gonococcal urethritis (NGU) due to *Chlamydia trachomatis* is the most common bacterial STI in the Western world. In symptomatic males it presents with mucoid urethral discharge, dysuria and urethral discomfort. It is also a major cause of pelvic inflammatory disease in women (frequently silent) and prostatitis/epididymitis in men. Neonatal conjunctivitis and, more rarely, diffuse interstitial pneumonia are both complications of serovars D to K; infection is acquired by passage through an infected birth canal. Serovars are antigenic determinants that confer distinct clinico-pathological features. IE D-K serovars cause urethritis and pelvic inflammatory disease, whereas LI-L3 serovars cause lymphogranuloma venereum.

- **Trachoma** (corneal scarring) is caused by serovars A, B and C.
- **Lymphogranuloma venereum (LGV)** is due to serovars L1, L2 and L3.

Both pneumonia and conjunctivitis need systemic treatment with erythromycin. Tetracycline or azithromycin is the drug of choice for adults.

> **Essential note**
>
> The main bacterial STIs are: gonorrhoea, syphilis and *Chlamydia*.

2. BASIC EPIDEMIOLOGY AND VIROLOGY OF HIV/AIDS

2.1 Epidemiology

HIV/AIDS is a global disease. Of the estimated 44 million people infected with HIV, 30 million are from sub-Saharan Africa. In the UK the cumulative incidence of HIV in 2002 was approximately 54 000; of AIDS, 19 000.

The following are the estimated routes of transmission in the current UK HIV population:

- Sexual intercourse between men (30%)
- Sexual intercourse between men and women (50%) – mainly acquired abroad
- Injecting drug abuse (7%)
- Blood and blood products (5%).

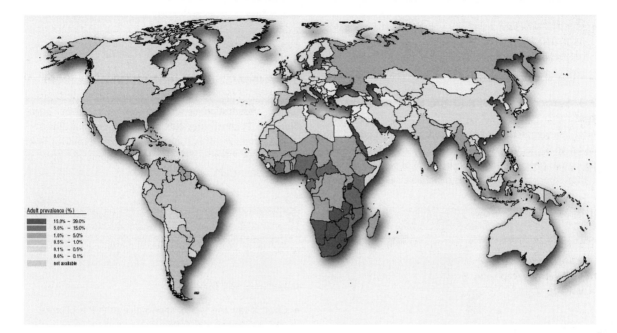

Figure 1 The worldwide epidemiology of HIV/AIDS
Source *World Health Organization (WHO)*

Risk factors facilitating sexual transmission include:

- Seroconversion and advancing stage of disease
- Concurrent STIs, particularly ulcerative disease of the genitalia.

Materno–fetal transmission occurs in 15–20% of non-breast-fed and 33% of breast-fed infants of patients with HIV/AIDS.

> **Essential note**
>
> Heterosexual intercourse is now the most common route of HIV transmission in the UK.

The risk of transmission from mother to baby can be reduced to only 1–2% with medical intervention:

- Anti-retroviral therapy
- Avoidance of breast-feeding
- Delivery by Caesarean section.

> **Essential note**
>
> HIV transmission from mother to baby can effectively be reduced from 20% to 1% with full medical intervention.

2.2 The virus

- **HIV-1**: (previously known as HTLV III) prevalent world-wide
- **HIV-2**: common in West Africa.

Pathogenesis

The HIV virus has tropism for the following CD4 cells:

- T-helper lymphocytes
- B-lymphocytes
- Macrophages
- CNS cells.

It causes progressive immune dysfunction, characterised by CD4 cell depletion. Impairment of immunity is primarily cell-mediated, but as the disease progresses there is general immune dysregulation.

The following laboratory markers are associated with disease progression:

- Decreased CD4 lymphocyte count (normal >500/mm³ or 0.5×10^9/l)

121

- High HIV viral load, using HIV polymerase chain reaction (PCR) assay (note that CD4 and HIV viral load are the only markers monitored in clinical practice that help to predict progression as well as the response to treatment).

2.3 Seroconversion and the HIV antibody test

After inoculation the window or seroconversion period can be up to 3 months; HIV antibody may not be detectable during this time. Approximately 60–90% of patients develop clinical seroconversion illnesses of variable severity.

Seroconversion illnesses

- Fever
- Diarrhoea
- Meningo-encephalitis
- Rash

2.4 Center for Disease Control (CDC) classification of HIV/AIDS

The CDC classification is adopted in the USA and most developed countries. HIV infection is not synonymous with AIDS; the latter is a stage of severe immunodeficiency characterised by opportunistic infections and/or tumour.

CDC classification of HIV/AIDS

- Stage 1

  - Primary seroconversion illness

- Stage 2

  - Asymptomatic

- Stage 3

  - Persistent generalised lymphadenopathy

- Stage 4a

  - AIDS-related complex (ie advanced HIV disease, but having none of the features of stages 4b–d)

- Stages 4b–d

  - AIDS: patient may have opportunistic infection or tumours, which are termed 'AIDS indicator' illnesses

3. RESPIRATORY DISEASES ASSOCIATED WITH HIV/AIDS

3.1 *Pneumocystis carinii* pneumonia (PCP)

Pneumonia is the most common opportunistic infection and clinical presentation of AIDS. *Pneumocystis carinii* pneumonia (PCP) constitutes 40% of all AIDS-defining illness.

The symptoms of PCP include dry cough, dyspnoea, fever and malaise. There are remarkably few abnormal signs on chest examination.

Essential note

PCP is the most common clinical presentation of AIDS

Investigations for PCP

- **Chest X-ray**: the typical appearance of PCP is bilateral mid- and lower-zone interstitial shadowing.
- **Pulse oximetry**: hypoxia with low/normal $p\mathrm{CO}_2$ is typically seen in moderate to severe infection.
- **Identification of pneumocystis cysts**: samples obtained by inducing sputum or from broncho-alveolar lavage (BAL) can be stained with silver or immunofluorescent antibody.

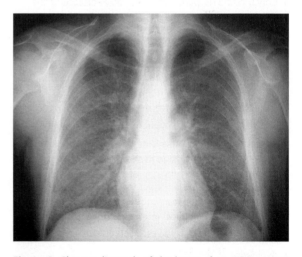

Figure 2 Chest radiograph of the lungs of an AIDS patient with pneumocystis pneumonia
Credit ISM / SCIENCE PHOTO LIBRARY

- The combination of an HIV-positive person (usually with CD4 <200/mm^3) who is not taking PCP prophylaxis and who has a typical radiological appearance and hypoxia is sufficient for a confident diagnosis to be made. Empirical treatment with cotrimoxazole should be started. It is now unusual to have to resort to lung biopsy for PCP diagnosis.

Poor prognostic features in PCP include poor response to treatment, co-infection, requirement for assisted ventilation and pneumothorax.

Treatment for PCP

- Treatment is with high-dose cotrimoxazole, or intravenous pentamidine for severe cases.
- Intolerance to cotrimoxazole is common, with nausea, vomiting, rash, leucopenia and thrombocytopenia.
- Steroids have been shown to improve prognosis in those with pO_2 <8 kPa (60 mmHg).

There is a 50% risk of recurrence within 12 months. **PCP prophylaxis** is always given to patients with a CD4 count <200/mm^3 and to those who have already had an episode of PCP.

3.2 Pulmonary tuberculosis

The incidence of infection depends upon the prevalence of TB in the rest of the general population and it is therefore much more common in African patients. In some areas of the UK up to a quarter of patients with TB are HIV positive.
Atypical features include:

- Extra-pulmonary involvement
- Normal or atypical appearances on chest X-ray

The infection occurs at any stage of HIV disease, and at any level of CD4 count.

- Atypical mycobacterial infections (when CD4 count <50/mm^3) – usually *Mycobacterium avium intracellulare*. The usual presenting features are fever, anaemia, anorexia; the disease is commonly extra-pulmonary.

Other causes of respiratory disease in HIV/AIDS

- **Viral**

  - Cytomegalovirus (CMV) pneumonitis

- **Fungal**

  - *Candida*
  - Histoplasmosis
  - *Cryptococcus*
  - *Nocardia*

Other causes of respiratory disease in HIV/AIDS

- **Bacterial**

  - *Streptococcus pneumoniae*
  - *Staphylococcus aureus*
  - *Mycobacterium tuberculosis*
  - *Mycobacterium avium intracellulare*

Radiological appearance of other infections

- **Cavitation**: *M. tuberculosis, Nocardia, S. aureus*
- **Consolidation**: *Streptococcus pneumoniae*, Toxoplasma
- **Effusion**: TB (Kaposi's sarcoma may also cause effusion).

4. GASTROINTESTINAL DISEASES IN PATIENTS WITH HIV/AIDS

There are four main presentations:

- Oral/oesophageal disease, ie oropharyngeal candidiasis
- Abdominal pain/diarrhoea, eg infective enteropathogens
- Biliary/pancreatic disease, eg drug toxicity, DDI (didanosine) and pancreatitis
- Ano-rectal symptoms, eg herpetic proctitis.

Essential note

There are four main GI presentations in HIV/AIDS: oral/oesophageal, abdominal pain/diarrhoea, biliary/pancreatic disease and ano-rectal symptoms.

4.1 Diarrhoea/abdominal pain

Weight loss, diarrhoea and malnutrition are very common in patients with any stage of HIV infection, and can be due to specific infection or advanced disease. Approximately 50% of diarrhoeal illnesses are infective in origin (due to specific enteropathogens or opportunistic infections).

Enteropathogens found in HIV

- **Bacterial**

  - *Salmonella*
  - *Shigella*

- **Protozoal**

  - *Giardia lamblia*

Continued over

Continued

- Viral

  - Cytomegalovirus

- Opportunistic organisms

  - Bacterial: atypical mycobacteria (*M. avium intracelluare* with CD4 <100/mm^3)
  - Protozoal: *Isospora belli*
  - Cryptosporidia (intracellular protozoan)
  - Microsporidia

Clinical presentation can be with watery diffuse diarrhoea as exemplified by *Cryptosporidium*, or abdominal pain and bloody diarrhoea (eg cytomegalovirus procto-colitis).

The investigation of infective diarrhoea includes the following:

- Identification of organisms in stool samples: microscopy and culture for pathogens, ovae and parasites
- If stool specimen negative, stain with modified Ziehl–Neelsen for *Cryptosporidium*
- Sigmoidoscopy/colonoscopy with biopsy: with culture of the specimen for viruses, mycobacteria, bacteriology and mycology.

Gastrointestinal tumours

These may also cause abdominal pain and diarrhoea.

- Kaposi's sarcoma
- Intra-abdominal lymphoma (often high-grade non-Hodgkin's B cell lymphoma).

5. HIV/AIDS-RELATED NEUROLOGICAL DISORDERS

Neurological disease is the first presentation of AIDS in 10% of HIV patients. An acute self-limiting lymphocytic meningitis may occur at the time of seroconversion.

The most common causes are:

- Direct neurotropic effect of the virus
- Opportunistic CNS infection
- Drug toxicity due to highly active anti-retroviral therapy (HAART).

Clinical presentation may be:

- **Focal**: hemiparesis, fits
- **Generalised**: drowsiness, confusion, behavioural change
- **Asymptomatic**: in early HIV disease.

Patients may also develop proximal myopathy, or drug-induced neuropathy (eg didanosine) and myopathy (eg zidovudine).

5.1 Direct neurotropic effects of HIV

These include:

- AIDS dementia complex
- Vacuolar myelopathy
- Neuropathy – sensorimotor or mononeuritis multiplex.

Neurotropic disorders are diagnosed with the help of:

- **CSF analysis**: raised protein, and pleocytosis
- **MRI brain scan**: cerebral atrophy
- **Nerve conduction studies**: distal symmetric sensory neuropathy.

5.2 Neurological infections

Opportunistic infections of the CNS are common.

Causes of focal neurological disease

- *Toxoplasma gondii*

  - Cerebral abscess

- *Mycobacterium tuberculosis*

  - Meningitis
  - Tuberculosis abscess

Causes of generalised neurological disease

- *Cryptococcus neoformans*

  - Meningitis
  - J.C. virus
  - Progressive multifocal leukoencephalopathy

- Cytomegalovirus

  - Encephalitis/retinitis
  - Peripheral neuropathy

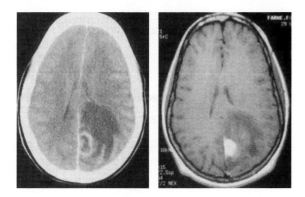

Figure 3 CT and MRI of brain lesions in patients with toxoplasmic encephalitis
Source *Toxoplasmosis: A comprehensive clinical guide*, by DHM Joynson and TG Wreghitt (2001), published by Cambridge University Press. ISBN 0 521 44328 8

Specific CNS infections

Cerebral toxoplasmosis is the most common CNS infection (90% of focal lesions) and occurs in 10% of AIDS patients. The organism is the crescentic trophozoite form of *Toxoplasma gondii*.

- **Investigations**: CT brain scan shows solitary or multiple ring-enhancing lesions. *Toxoplasma* IgG serology is positive in >90% of cases.
- It is important to differentiate from primary CNS lymphoma causing a space-occupying lesion.

Essential note

Cerebral toxoplasmosis is the most common CNS infection in HIV/AIDS.

Cryptococcal meningitis is due to a 'budding' yeast. It occurs in 5–10% of AIDS patients, and presents with a sub-acute meningitic illness.

- Cryptococcal antigen is present in blood and CSF in most cases
- **India ink stain**: positive in 70% of CSF samples.

Neurosyphilis: the co-existence of HIV and syphilis can result in aggressive and atypical neurosyphilis. Previous syphilis infection may re-activate. The following features are recognised:

- Myelopathy
- Retinitis
- Meningitis
- Meningovascular.

Diagnosis is from syphilis serology (rising VDRL and TPHA) and CSF, although serology may be modified by immune dysfunction.

Treatment includes first-line therapy with intramuscular procaine penicillin and probenecid for 14–21 days.

5.3 Ophthalmic disorders

AIDS may affect the lids or any layer of the eye.

Ophthalmic features of AIDS

- **Molluscum contagiosum of lids**
- **Cytomegalovirus (CMV) retinitis**
- **Neuro-ophthalmic manifestations** (eg cranial nerve palsies, optic neuritis, sequelae to CNS infection or space-occupying lesion)
- **Kaposi's sarcoma of the eyelids or conjunctiva**
- **Retinal changes**: haemorrhages, cotton wool spots, oedema and vascular sheathing
- **Toxoplasmosis**: may develop acquired disease or reactivation of pre-existing disease
- **Candida endophthalmitis**

Retinitis is common and may be caused by HIV itself (non-specific micro-angiopathy which is present in 75% of HIV patients) or by CMV.

CMV retinitis usually occurs when the CD4 count is <50/mm^3. This is the most common AIDS-related opportunistic infection in the eye (occurring in 25% of patients).

- **Symptoms**: blurred or loss of vision; floaters
- **Signs**: soft exudates, and retinal haemorrhages
- **Prognosis**: initially unilateral eye involvement; ultimately both eyes are affected.

---

6. MALIGNANT DISEASE IN PATIENTS WITH HIV/AIDS

The most frequently occurring malignancies are:

- Kaposi's sarcoma (83%)
- Non-Hodgkin's lymphoma (13%)
- Primary CNS lymphoma (4%).

Essential note

Kaposi's sarcoma is the most common malignancy in HIV/AIDS.

6.1 Kaposi's sarcoma (KS)

This occurs in 10–15% of HIV patients as the first AIDS-defining presentation. The tumour is derived from vascular or lymphatic endothelial cells and is due to infection with human herpes virus type 8 (HHV8). This virus is closely related to EB virus and is transmitted sexually, vertically and via organ transplantation.

- **Clinical presentation**: Kaposi's sarcoma can be cutaneous but also can involve the viscera. Lesions appear as purple plaques or nodules. The most common systems involved are the gastrointestinal tract (30% of patients with Kaposi's sarcoma of the skin also have gastrointestinal involvement), lymph nodes and the respiratory system.
- **Diagnosis**: clinical appearance (or biopsy in difficult cases).

7. HIV/AIDS-RELATED SKIN DISEASE

Dermatological diseases are extremely common in HIV patients (affecting 75%), especially in those who have AIDS. During the acute HIV illness, patients may develop an asymptomatic maculo-papular eruption affecting the face and trunk. During seroconversion, they may also develop marked seborrhoeic dermatitis. As the disease progresses to AIDS, the development of tumours and atypical infections is seen.

Dermatological associations of HIV disease

- General inflammatory dermatoses

  - Psoriasis
  - Eczema
  - Seborrhoeic dermatitis
  - Folliculitis

- Fungal/yeast infections

  - *Pityrosporum ovale**
  - Candidiasis*
  - *Cryptococcus neoformans*
  - *Histoplasma capsulatum*

- Viral infections

  - Herpes zoster/Herpes simplex
  - Human papilloma virus*
  - Cytomegalovirus
  - Molluscum contagiosum*

Dermatological associations of HIV disease

- Bacterial infections

  - Tuberculosis
  - Syphilis
  - Bacillary angiomatosis
  - *Staphylococcus aureus*

Features marked * are common in HIV patients

Other skin diseases that are recognised include:

- **Generalised maculo-papular rash** (due to drugs): cotrimoxazole (25%), nevirapine (14%), efavirenz (4%), abacavir (5%), dapsone (5%)
- **Nail pigmentation**: zidovudine, indinavir.

8. ANTI-RETROVIRAL THERAPY

Anti-retroviral therapy is usually given as combination therapy with the following aims:

- Suppression of viral replication
- Reducing the risk of viral resistance emerging with three or more drugs
- Improving patient immunity with reduction of morbidity and mortality.

8.1 Highly active anti-retroviral treatment (HAART)

This involves combinations of at least three drugs; for example, two different nucleoside/nucleotide reverse transcriptase inhibitors (NRTI) in addition to a protease inhibitor (PI), or a non-nucleoside reverse transcriptase inhibitor (NNRTI).

There are three main classes of anti-retroviral drugs currently licensed in the UK. Their modes of action are by inhibition of the viral reverse transcriptase enzyme or by inhibition of protease enzymes.

Essential note

HAART now means that HIV infection is a chronic disease rather than fatal

Side-effects of anti-retroviral drugs

- NRTI

  - **Metabolic**: lipoatrophy, lactic acidosis and mitochondrial toxicity
  - **Neurological**: peripheral neuropathy
  - **Haematological**: bone marrow suppression, anaemia

- NNRTI

  - Hepatotoxicity
  - Skin rash/Steven–Johnson syndrome

- PI

  - Lipodystrophy syndrome
  - Drug–drug interaction via CYP 450 cytochrome enzymes
  - Hyperbilirubinaemia

8.2 Monitoring of HIV patients on treatment

- **Clinical assessment**: examination of mouth (for ulcers and candidiasis), skin, lymph nodes, chest, fundoscopy and weight
- Renal and hepatic function
- CD4 lymphocyte count
- HIV viral RNA load
- Cholesterol, blood sugar, triglycerides
- Lactate if symptoms of lactic acidosis (muscle pains, malaise, gastrointestinal symptoms, breathlessness) are present
- **Adherence to treatment**: >90–95% of therapy must be

taken to maintain adequate viral suppression and this will also reduce the chance of resistance to therapy developing. If there is evidence of virological failure (increased viral load on more than two tests) then HIV **resistance testing** is indicated.

9. PROGNOSIS OF PATIENTS WITH HIV/AIDS

The prognosis of HIV/AIDS patients has now been revolutionised by HAART (introduced in 1997) and the death rate has reduced.

- All opportunistic illnesses have been reduced dramatically; however, the incidence of **lymphoma** has increased steadily.
- The new anti-retroviral agents also significantly reduce mother-to-baby transmission of the virus from 20% to <2% (if breast-feeding is avoided).
- Individual prognosis depends on viral resistance (10% of new infections in Europe involve a resistant virus), side-effects and adherence to treatment; prognosis is worse if treatment is started when the CD4 count is below 200 cells/mm^3.
- Prognosis is worse in patients who present late with AIDS (mainly heterosexuals who may have no obvious risks); death is due to delay in diagnosis.
- Coronary heart disease, end-stage liver failure (due to co-infection with hepatitis B and C) and malignancy (lymphoma) are now common causes of death in patients with HIV/AIDS.

HIV has now become a treatable chronic illness rather than a fatal disease.

Further revision

British Association for Sexual Health and HIV at http://www.bashh.org/

ÆGiS: AIDS Education Information System at http://www.aegis.com/

AIDSMAP Information on HIV and AIDS at http://www.aidsmap.com/

AIDS.org at http://www.aidsmap.com/

NHS Guide to sexually transmitted infections at http://www.playingsafely.co.uk/

NICE policy: Better prevention, better services, better sexual health: the national strategy for sexual health and HIV at http://www.publichealth.nice.org.uk/phel_policydetails.aspx?recordid=72&o=phel.policies.search&search=true

Sexually Transmitted Diseases Journal of the American Sexually Transmitted Disease Association

Sexually Transmitted Infections at http://sti.bmjjournals.com/

International Journal of STD and AIDS at http://www.rsmpress.co.uk/std.htm

Genito-urinary medicine and AIDS

You should now

1. Understand the common clinical presentation and diagnostic tests for gonorrhoea, chlamydia and syphilis, as well as the importance of interpretation of syphilis serology.

2. Know that HIV is a retrovirus that infects the CD4 lymphocyte cell directly resulting in immunosuppression. Understand that HIV is a global disease, with heterosexual transmission being the commonest mode. Be aware that effective medical intervention can prevent mother-to-child transmission.

3. Know that the various clinical stages of HIV infection are illustrated by CDC classification, and that most patients are asymptomatic following seroconversion. Understand the significance of HIV seroconversion illness and differential such as 'flu-like illness'.

Understand that there is a 3-month window for serological HIV antibodies to develop following exposure to the virus.

4. Be aware of common HIV-associated opportunistic infections presenting as systemic disease, in particular PCP and TB in respiratory disease, cryptosporidiosis and atypical mycobacteria in GI disease, and cerebral toxoplasmosis and cryptococcus in CNS disease. Know that malignancies present in the CNS as lymphoma and cutaneously as Kaposi's sarcoma.

5. Understand the value of CD4 cell counts and HIV viral load for monitoring patients. Be aware of the main classes of HAART drugs used, their common side-effects and long-term toxicities. Understand the idea that HAART treatment and regular monitoring can effectively control HIV disease long-term.

Haematology

CONTENTS

Revision objectives

You should know that:

1. If shown a blood film then remember it has three cellular components – red cells, white cells and platelets – consider these in turn.
2. If shown a blood count concentrate first on white count, haemoglobin and platelets. If anaemia is present say whether it is macrocytic, normocytic or microcytic. If there is a leucocytosis say whether neutrophilia or lymphocytosis. Try to use descriptive terms such as pancytopenia or microcytic anaemia rather than just stating a parameter is high or low.
3. Normal ranges for pathology investigations will usually be provided but you will be expected to know the ranges for the commonest investigations such as haemoglobin, white cell count, platelets and ESR.

Haematology

1. ANAEMIA

Definition

- Reduced concentration of circulating haemoglobin.

Symptoms

- Tiredness
- Shortness of breath on exertion
- Palpitations
- Ankle swelling
- Symptoms better tolerated in the young, and in gradual onset of anaemia; worse in the elderly and in sudden onset of anaemia.

Signs

- Pallor (best seen in conjunctiva, mucous membranes)
- Tachycardia
- Other signs specific to type of anaemia.

Classification

- By **cause** (but often not known); or by **size of red cell** – macrocytic, normocytic, or microcytic depending on whether mean cell volume (MCV) is high, normal or low.

Table 1 Classification of anaemia by red cell size

Microcytic anaemia	Normocytic anaemia	Macrocytic anaemia
Iron deficiency	Haemorrhage (after haemodilution)	B_{12} deficiency
Thalassaemias	Renal failure	Folic acid deficiency
Anaemia of chronic disease	Anaemia of chronic disease	Haemolytic anaemias

1.1 Haemorrhagic anaemia

Rapid bleeding causes physiological changes of:

- tachycardia
- hypotension
- vasoconstriction of non-essential vascular beds including the peripheral circulation
- preservation of blood flow to essential organs such as the brain
- reduced urine flow.

In addition to evidence of haemorrhage, such as melaena, there is thirst and pallor. Fluid moves from the tissues into the circulation to maintain the circulating fluid volume.

Essential note

Death as a result of haemorrhage is commonly due to lack of circulating blood volume rather than lack of haemoglobin – restoration of blood volume by transfusion of crystalloid or colloid may be life saving

Immediately after haemorrhage the haemoglobin concentration will be normal. Once haemodilution has occurred, in about 24 hours, there will be a normocytic anaemia.

1.2 Haematinic deficiencies

- **Haematinics**: essential components of red cell production are **iron, B_{12}, folic acid, protein**.

Iron deficiency

Leads to a microcytic anaemia.

Signs

- As for anaemia (above) plus sore tongue, angular cheilosis (splitting at angles of the mouth), rarely koilonychia (brittle spoon-shaped nails).

Causes

- Blood loss: menorrhagia, gastrointestinal (GI) blood loss (peptic ulceration, carcinoma stomach/colon, hookworm in tropics, piles, Meckel's diverticulum)
- Dietary deficiency: red meat best source.

Essential note

Iron deficiency can be the first presenting sign of otherwise asymptomatic carcinoma of stomach or colon – in the presence of GI symptoms gastroscopy/colonoscopy should be performed

Treatment

- Oral ferrous sulphate 200 mg once daily to four times daily depending on severity of anaemia and toleration of oral iron
- In the event of side-effects (constipation, diarrhoea, indigestion, metallic taste), reduce dose and accept slower rise in haemoglobin
- Rarely required: intravenous iron sucrose.

B_{12} deficiency

Leads to a macrocytic anaemia.

Symptoms

- As for anaemia (above)
- Plus neurological problems: sub-acute combined degeneration of the cord (motor and sensory problems – classic), peripheral neuropathy, optic atrophy and dementia.

Causes

- Pernicious anaemia (*see* Box)
- Dietary deficiency: red meat, liver and fish are the main sources of B_{12} in the diet, so vegans may suffer from dietary deficiency
- Other causes: partial gastrectomy, terminal ileal resection, Crohn's disease of the terminal ileum, competitive consumption by bacteria in the small bowel (diverticulae, blind loop) or fresh water fish tape worm. Metformin may also cause malabsorption.

Treatment

- Intramuscular B_{12} hydroxocobalamin is effective and cheap
- After daily injections to replete stores, maintenance 1 mg every 3 months will gradually replete liver stores
- Oral B_{12} cyanocobalamin 50 µg daily (daily requirement 5 µg) will effectively treat dietary deficiency
- The neurological manifestations of B_{12} deficiency may take months or years to improve. If normal B_{12} absorption has not been demonstrated (*see* Schilling test, Chapter 5), it is important to confirm that normal serum levels are obtained by oral therapy to avoid irreversible neurological damage. Similarly, treating B_{12} deficiency with folic acid alone may worsen neurological problems – give both until the results of blood assays are available.

Pernicious anaemia (PA)

This is due to an autoimmune attack against the gastric parietal cells of the stomach. These normally secrete gastric acid and intrinsic factor. Intrinsic factor is responsible for binding B_{12} and transporting it to specific receptors in the terminal ileum where B_{12} is unloaded into the intestinal mucosa. Other autoimmune diseases may be present, or develop, such as myxoedema or vitiligo. Gastric acid splits iron from protein so that it can be absorbed, so iron absorption is reduced in PA and patients may become iron deficient without developing carcinoma of stomach, which is an associated disease

Antibody tests in PA

- Anti-parietal cell antibodies: usually present in PA but also present in one-third of healthy women over 60 years
- Anti-intrinsic factor antibodies: when present, have high specificity for PA, but not always found in clear cases

Schilling B_{12} absorption test in PA

See Chapter 5, Gastroenterology

Folic acid deficiency

This leads to macrocytic megaloblastic anaemia.

Causes

- **Dietary**: folic acid found in fresh fruit and vegetables (destroyed by cooking), so found in the poor and alcoholics.
- **Increased requirements**: pregnancy (folic acid supplementation in pregnancy may reduce the incidence of fetal neural tube defects), haemolysis (most folic acid in the body is in red cells), premature neonates.

- **Malabsorption**: coeliac disease, Crohn's disease, tropical sprue.

Treatment

- Oral folic acid tablets are universally effective in correcting deficiency.

1.3 Haemolytic anaemia

This refers to anaemia due to premature red cell destruction. There may be **intravascular** destruction resulting in haemoglobinaemia and haemoglobinuria, or **extravascular**, in the reticulo-endothelial system, particularly the spleen.

General features of haemolytic anaemia

- Anaemia – often macrocytic
- Jaundice – unconjugated hyperbilirubinaemia
- Reticulocytosis – >2%
- Erythroid hyperplasia
- Morphological abnormalities in red cells:
    - General: spherocytes, polychromasia
    - Indicative of cause, eg fragmented cells, elliptocytes, blister cells

Causes

Congenital

- Membrane defects, eg hereditary spherocytosis, elliptocytosis
- Haemoglobinopathies, eg sickle cell disease
- Enzyme deficiencies, eg glucose-6-phosphate dehydrogenase (G6PD) deficiency.

Acquired

- Immune
    - Warm or cold autoimmune
    - Haemolytic disease of the newborn
    - Drug associated, eg DOPA, penicillin
- Traumatic
    - Artificial heart valves
    - Microangiopathic
- Infections
    - Malaria
    - *Bartonella*.

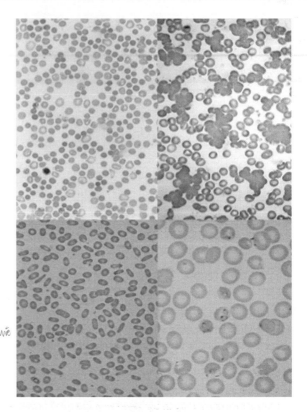

Figure 1 Blood films in four cases of haemolytic anaemia. Bottom left: hereditary elliptocytosis – many red cells are ellipsoidal in shape. Top left: hereditary spherocytosis – most red cells lack the normal central pale staining area and appear slightly smaller than normal red cells. These spherocytes have lost part of their membrane. Bottom right: malaria – many red cells contain the 'signet ring' parasites of *Plasmodium falciparum* that will eventually multiply and rupture the red cell. Top right: cold agglutinates – the red cells are clumped in an irregular haphazard way ('horse droppings') due to a cold acting complete agglutinating auto-antibody

2. LEUCOCYTOSIS

Definition

An increased total white cell count, most commonly a **neutrophilia**, less commonly a **lymphocytosis**.

Causes of neutrophilia

- Infection (usually bacterial)
- Inflammation
- Infarction
- Steroid therapy

- Necrosis of tumours
- Trauma
- Burns.

Causes of lymphocytosis

- Viral infections (particularly glandular fever)
- Whooping cough
- Chronic lymphocytic leukaemia.

Increased numbers of other types of white cells do not usually increase the total white cell count but are apparent on examining the differential white cell count:

- **Monocytosis**: recovery from chemotherapy or radiotherapy, tissue necrosis, bacterial endocarditis
- **Eosinophilia**: allergic disorders (asthma, hay fever, eczema, drug reactions), parasitic infections, Hodgkin's disease
- **Basophilia**: one of the myeloproliferative disorders.

3. LEUCOERYTHROBLASTIC BLOOD PICTURE

Definition

The presence of nucleated red blood cells AND primitive white cells of any variety in the peripheral blood.

Causes

- Very ill patient: septicaemia, trauma, acute haemolysis, shock
- Bone marrow infiltration: secondary cancer, lymphomas, myeloma, myelofibrosis, storage diseases.

NB Cancers that metastasise to bone include: breast, prostate, thyroid, kidney, lung.

4. MARROW FAILURE

Blood cells are produced by red (active) bone marrow, which lies in the axial skeleton in normal adults - skull, vertebrae, pelvis and sternum. Peripheral long bones are filled with white (fatty, inactive) marrow. At birth all bones contain active marrow.

Marrow failure is inability of the marrow to produce adequate numbers of white cells, red cells and platelets. It is usually associated with a hypocellular marrow (aplastic anaemia) or more rarely with a cellular (infiltrated) marrow. In marrow failure due to infiltration the underlying disease is treated.

4.1 Aplastic anaemia

Causes

- **Congenital**: rare – Fanconi's anaemia – often associated with other congenital abnormalities and failure of chromosome repair mechanisms
- **Acquired**
  - **Radiation** – most of the victims of Hiroshima, Nagasaki and Chernobyl died of aplastic anaemia. Total body radiation (10 Gy) is commonly used as a conditioning regimen to empty the marrow prior to bone marrow transplant
  - **Idiosyncratic drug reaction** – chloramphenicol, phenylbutazone, gold and many other drugs – stop or change if there is reported incidence of aplasia
  - **Virus infection** – all the hepatitis viruses can cause aplasia, often after the hepatitis has recovered
  - **Idiopathic** – an autoimmune attack against the patient's own stem cells.

Management

- Remove cause if known
- Blood product support for marrow failure – red cells, platelets
- Growth factors (eg granulocyte-colony stimulating factor (G-CSF)) do not affect the primitive stem cells, but by stimulating the committed myeloid precursors they can prevent death from infection while other treatments are being used
- If mild: stimulate residual marrow with anabolic steroids
- If autoimmune idiopathic: immune suppression (anti-lymphocyte globulin, steroids, ciclosporin) or bone marrow transplantation from HLA-matched donor.

5. HAEMOGLOBINOPATHIES

Haemoglobin consists of an iron-containing component (**haem**) and a protein-containing component (**globin**). Disorders of haem synthesis are the **porphyrias**: disorders of globin synthesis are the **haemoglobinopathies**. The commonest haemoglobinopathy of clinical significance is sickle cell disease.

Haematology

There are three normal haemoglobins in humans

- Fetal haemoglobin: HbF contains 2 α and 2 γ chains
- Adult haemoglobin: HbA contains 2 α and 2 β chains
- The second adult haemoglobin: HbA2 contains 2 α and 2 δ chains

During the first year of life HbF production gradually switches over to HbA. Up to 3.5% of haemoglobin in adults is HbA2.

5.1 Thalassaemias

In haemoglobin A the globin consists of two pairs of polypeptide chains – a pair of α chains and a pair of β chains. In thalassaemia, there is an inability to make these chains. Inability to synthesise α chains is α thalassaemia; inability to make β chains, β thalassaemia. The disorders may be severe (homozygous, major) or mild (heterozygous, trait).

α Thalassaemia major

- Severe suppression of α chain production
- α chains are needed for the manufacture of all three major human haemoglobins
- Incompatible with life outside the uterus.

β Thalassaemia major

- Severe suppression of β chain production
- Not apparent at birth as HbF does not contain β chains
- During the first year of life inability to make the β chains of HbA results in anaemia, stunting of growth and hepatosplenomegaly
- Marrow hypertrophy causes skeletal abnormalities such as bossing of skull, prognathism (protrusion of the bones of the mandible and maxilla – chipmonk facies) and a 'hair-on-end appearance' on the lateral skull radiograph.

Treatment of β thalassaemia major

- All these clinical problems can be ameliorated by regular life-long red cell transfusion, most patients having two or three units a month
- Regular red cell transfusion results in iron overload (the body has no way of excreting excess iron, iron balance is achieved only by controlling absorption)
- Iron overload results in endocrine failure, cardiomyopathy and cirrhosis

Treatment of β thalassaemia major

- Iron overload is prevented by administration of chelating agents such as desferrioxamine, which couple to iron and remove it in the urine. Desferrioxamine is administered by continuous subcutaneous infusion, usually by electric syringe driver on 3–6 nights a week

α Thalassaemia trait

This results in microcytic anaemia, of variable severity, depending on how many of the four genes controlling α chain production are defective.

- Common in patients of Chinese origin
- Spleen may be enlarged
- β chain production is unaffected.

The relative excess of β chains may associate together to form an abnormal haemoglobin, HbH, visible in the red cells if they are incubated with the reticulocyte stain brilliant cresyl blue ('golf-ball bodies'), and detectable by the usual methods of screening for abnormal haemoglobins.

β Thalassaemia trait

This results in microcytic anaemia, but the haemoglobin >9 g/dl is usually difficult to distinguish from iron deficiency. The red cells are often unusually small for the haemoglobin level (low MCV) and the disorder is common in persons of Mediterranean or Asian origin. The production of β chains is defective, so more HbA2 is produced as this does not require β chains.

- Elevated HbA2 level is a useful marker of β thalassaemia trait
- Autosomal recessive – patients with β thalassaemia trait usually have no clinical problems but have a 1 in 4 chance of having a child with β thalassaemia major if their partner also has β thalassaemia trait.

5.2 Sickle cell disease

Aetiology

Sickle cell disease results from the inheritance of two HbS genes (sickle cell anaemia, HbSS), or the inheritance of one HbS gene with an interacting haemoglobinopathy such as HbC (Hb S-C disease) or thalassaemia trait (HbS-thal disease). A single amino acid substitution in the β chain results in alteration in the physical and chemical properties of HbA, which is now called HbS.

The most important of these changes is precipitation of the HbS in long thin chains (tactoids) under conditions of low oxygen tension, which deform the red cell envelope into the classical sickle shape. This causes a loss in deformability of the red cell so that log-jams of sickled cells block capillaries, causing local hypoxia and more sickling. A vicious cycle builds up resulting in infarction of tissue – sickle crisis.

- Ante-natal screening for HbS and interacting haemoglobinopathies is performed in most affected areas of the UK
- Intra-uterine diagnosis by chorionic villus sampling is available.

Clinical manifestations

These depend on the organs affected.

- Most commonly infarction of red bone marrow results in simple sickle pain crisis – deep-seated bone pains requiring opiate analgesia
- Similar vaso-occlusive problems are associated with all subtypes of sickle cell disease
- Sickle pain crisis may be precipitated by hypoxia, dehydration, infection and chilling.

Treatment

- Adequate analgesia, hydration – intravenous if necessary – correction of hypoxia and antibiotic treatment of infection.
- Because patients with sickle cell disease are normal at birth – HbF protects against sickling – efforts have been made to encourage the marrow to make more HbF in adulthood
- Hydroxycarbamide, a mild cytotoxic drug used in the myeloproliferative disorders, has the side-effect of increasing HbF production and is used to ameliorate sickle cell disease in severely affected patients
- Severe complications of sickle vaso-occlusion may also be treated by exchange transfusion – replacing the patient's sicklable red cells with normal HbA-containing cells.

Essential note

The anaemia of sickle cell disease is usually well tolerated and patients do require regular transfusions as the HbS has a low oxygen affinity, easily giving up oxygen to cells that require it. Transfusion, by increasing blood viscosity, may exacerbate vaso-occlusive problems

Vaso-occlusion crisis can affect other organs – see Figure 2.

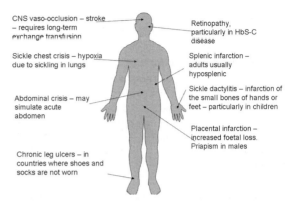

CNS vaso-occlusion – stroke – requires long-term exchange transfusion

Retinopathy, particularly in HbS-C disease

Sickle chest crisis – hypoxia due to sickling in lungs

Splenic infarction – adults usually hyposplenic

Abdominal crisis – may simulate acute abdomen

Sickle dactylitis – infarction of the small bones of hands or feet – particularly in children

Placental infarction – increased foetal loss. Priapism in males

Chronic leg ulcers – in countries where shoes and socks are not worn

ALL AREAS – INFARCTION OF RED BONE MARROW – SICKLE PAIN CRISIS

Figure 2 Consequences of sickle vaso-occlusion

Sequelae and prophylaxis

Spleen and liver

Patients with sickle cell disease infarct their spleens during childhood; therefore, most adults are hyposplenic and the usual precautions against septicaemia with capsulate organisms must be taken:

- Life-long prophylactic penicillin V
- Pneumococcal immunisation
- Meningitis C and *Haemophilus influenzae* immunisation
- Meticulous anti-malarial prophylaxis.

Hyper-haemolytic, also known as sequestration, crisis is due to sudden trapping of red cells in spleen and liver in childhood, with a higher reticulocyte count and bilirubin than normal for that patient. Mothers may be taught to feel their baby's spleens to detect this problem at an early stage. Again red cell transfusion may be life-saving.

Aplastic and hyper-haemolytic crises

Children may suffer aplastic and hyper-haemolytic crises. Aplastic crisis results from parvovirus infection of the bone marrow erythroblasts or acute folate deficiency. The patient may have a life-threatening anaemia, with a lower than normal reticulocyte count and bilirubin for that patient. Parvovirus causes a benign 'slapped cheek' infection in haematologically normal people but in patients dependent on high red cell output from their marrows to maintain a reasonable haemoglobin level, such as those with sickle cell disease, congenital haemolytic anaemias and the normal fetus, a fatal anaemia may result.

5.3 Sickle cell trait

Sickle cell trait is asymptomatic unless the patient is exposed to hypoxia or acidosis. The blood count is normal, but a little less than half the haemoglobin is HbS. This may be detected by the sickle solubility test, or usual screening methods for haemoglobinopathies. Screening for HbS is usually undertaken prior to a general anaesthetic in patients of Afro-Caribbean origin. Sickle trait protects against death from malaria, as the infected red cells become hypoxic, sickle, and are removed by the reticlo-endothelial system before protozoa multiply and burst the red cell.

---

6. POLYCYTHAEMIA

This is defined as an increase in haemoglobin, red cell count and haematocrit. The principal danger is that slow flow associated with thick viscous blood results in thrombosis, particularly stroke and myocardial infarction (MI), and the heart has to struggle to push viscous blood around the circulation resulting in hypertension. Polycythaemia is divided into **true** and **relative** types depending on the results of measurement of red cell mass and plasma volume.

Table 2 Classification of polycythaemia	
***True** – increased red cell mass*	
Primary (rubra vera): a myeloproliferative disease – see page 122	
Secondary	
Reduced O_2	Hypoxic chest disease
	Smoking
	Cyanotic congenital heart disease
	Altitude
Inappropriate increased erythropoietin secretion	Renal space-occupying lesions – cysts, tumours
	Ectopic EPO hormone production – carcinoma of kidney, hepatoma

Relative (pseudo) – reduced plasma volume	
Dehydration	
Fever, diuretics, diarrhoea, vomiting	
Stress polycythaemia	
Individuals under chronic stress run a low plasma volume	

---

7. HAEMATOLOGICAL MALIGNANCIES

These are broadly, and imperfectly, classified into four groups:

- Leukaemias
- Lymphomas
- Myelodysplasias
- Myeloproliferative disorders.

7.1 Leukaemias

These are subdivided thus:

- **Acute leukaemias**: associated with an increase in primitive undifferentiated blast cells filling the bone marrow and spilling into the blood.
- **Chronic leukaemias**: associated with an increase of relatively mature white cells in the blood.

Each of these is then subdivided into myeloid or lymphoid, depending on the type of proliferating cells. There are thus four main types of leukaemia: **acute myeloid leukaemia (AML)**, **acute lymphoblastic leukaemia (ALL)**, **chronic myeloid leukaemia (CML)** and **chronic lymphocytic leukaemia (CLL)**.

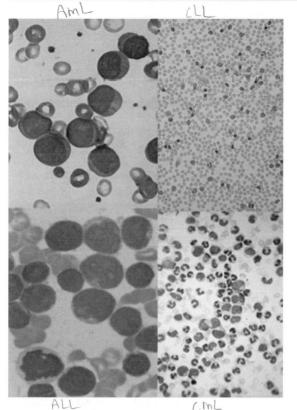
AmL   *CLL*   *ALL*   *CmL*

Figure 3 Blood films in the four main types of leukaemias. Bottom left: acute lymphoblastic leukaemia – blast cells with prominent nucleoli (including one cell in division) with other cells resembling large lymphocytes. Top left: acute myeloid leukaemia – blast cells including two whose cytoplasm contains Auer rods (pink needle-like crystals) diagnostic of AML. Bottom right: chronic myeloid leukaemia – the most common cell is the mature neutrophil granulocyte, though a few more immature cells are present. Top right: chronic lymphocytic leukaemia – the most common cell is the small mature-looking lymphocyte. These cells are fragile and some have been crushed during the spreading of the film (smear cells)

Acute myeloid leukaemia (AML)

Pathology

Primitive myeloblasts fill up the bone marrow resulting in **marrow failure** – see above – and spill into the blood. These have large nuclei, prominent nucleoli and the cytoplasm may contain **Auer rods** – a crystallisation of the normal granules found in granulocytic cells. **Auer rods are diagnostic of AML.**

Clinical features

Enlargement of lymph nodes, liver or spleen is unusual as the patients present with anaemia, neutropenia or thrombocytopenia before significant organ infiltration can occur. An exception is gum hypertrophy and skin infiltration in the monocytic varieties of AML. Although undifferentiated myeloblasts are the main feature of AML, sometimes a little differentiation occurs before the cells meet a differentiation block. When such a small degree of differentiation can be detected and ascribed to a particular cell lineage the French American British (FAB) morphological classification of AML can be applied. For example, in acute promyelocytic leukaemia (FAB type AML M3) many of the myeloblasts have differentiated to the promyelocyte stage of myeloid differentiation.

Prognostic factors

Response to the first course of chemotherapy (good to have responsive disease).

- Cytogenetics: chromosome abnormalities can be detected in the leukaemic cells in the majority of cases and sometimes these have prognostic significance.

Bone marrow transplant from an HLA-matched sibling may be employed in cases with bad cytogenetics.

Treatment

Combination chemotherapy is designed to eradicate blast cells and allow normal bone marrow to grow back. A temporary period of marrow hypoplasia is a necessary consequence of a successful remission induction. Most useful chemotherapy involves cytosine and an anthracycline such as **daunorubicin**. Remission induction (after which the bone marrow will appear normal but will still contain small numbers of residual leukaemic cells) is followed by consolidation chemotherapy designed to eradicate the disease that cannot be seen under the microscope.

Acute lymphoblastic leukaemia (ALL)

Definition/incidence

ALL is the commonest malignant disease of childhood, and, like AML, is associated with increased numbers of blast cells in the bone marrow and blood, resulting in marrow failure. Most cases in childhood can be cured by conventional chemotherapy though adults tend to have a worse prognosis.

Prognosis

This is related to age (best <10 years), degree of presenting blast cell count (ie low tumour burden), cytogenetic abnormalities in the leukaemic cells and response to chemotherapy treatment. Very sensitive techniques are now available to detect minimal residual disease in patients in morphological remission, using polymerase chain amplification (PCR) of mutations in the immunoglobulin or T-cell receptor genes characteristic of that patient's leukaemic cells. This can detect as little as 1 in 10 000 leukaemia cells, allowing adjustment of chemotherapy according to response.

Treatment

Treatment is divided into induction and consolidation phases, as in AML, but ALL benefits from a prolonged maintenance chemotherapy phase of 1–2 years, using reduced dose, mainly oral chemotherapy. Most useful chemotherapy drugs for induction are steroids, such as **dexamethasone**, and **vincristine**. Lymphoblasts have the capacity to invade the central nervous system (CNS) where they may hide behind the blood–brain barrier, so that systemically administered chemotherapy cannot kill them. Thus all cases of ALL have CNS prophylactic therapy including drugs such as methotrexate administered directly into the cerebrospinal fluid (CSF) at lumbar puncture.

Chronic myeloid leukaemia (CML)

Definition

CML may be classified as one of the leukaemias or as one of the myeloproliferative disorders, sharing features of both groups of diseases. CML is a disease of middle age, though no age is exempt.

Aetiology

The leukaemic process is driven by an abnormal tyrosine kinase enzyme, coded by an abnormal gene BCR/ABL. This gene is formed as the result of a chromosomal translocation t(9;22), when a portion of chromosome 22 becomes translocated to chromosome 9 and an even smaller bit of chromosome 9 is relocated to 22. The abnormal small chromosome 22 is the Philadelphia chromosome, characteristic of the disease, being present in more than 95% of cases.

Clinical features

Presenting symptoms are usually hypercatabolic, with weight loss and night sweats. CML may be diagnosed as an incidental finding on a blood count done for some other reason. The blood shows a massive leukocytosis, sometimes as high as (600–800) × 10⁹/l, with most white cells in the blood being mature granulocytes, including neutrophils, eosinophils and basophils. Haemoglobin and platelet count are variable. On examination there is usually significant splenomegaly, which may have been a presenting complaint. Lymph nodes are not enlarged.

Treilment

The most successful treatment is imatinib, a drug specifically designed to inhibit the abnormal tyrosine kinase enzyme present in the leukaemic cells. In the majority of cases this results in normalisation of the blood counts (haematological remission); in many, the Philadelphia chromosome can no longer be found (cytogenetic remission) and in a few the BCR/ABL genetic code can no longer be detected by PCR (molecular remission). Other, less effective, drugs may induce haematological remission, such as **interferon** and **hydroxycarbamide**, and bone marrow transplantation may be curative in resistant cases.

Chronic lymphocytic leukaemia (CLL)

Definition/incidence/pathology

Commonly CLL is diagnosed as an incidental finding on a health screening blood count. CLL is a disease of the elderly, and behaves in an indolent fashion, usually not requiring treatment in the lifetime of the patient. An early manifestation is a blood lymphocytosis. The lymphocytes are small and look relatively mature and are fragile, often being crushed during the spreading of the film ('smear cells'). The lymphocytes are of B-cell lineage in 95% of cases, though, interestingly, they usually exhibit a T-cell antigen CD5 with the B-cell markers. This is of assistance in classifying the disease by immunophenotyping.

Clinical features

A generalised lymphadenopathy is often found and in late stages enlargement of spleen and liver. Significant marrow infiltration results in marrow failure. Because B-cell maturation is deranged, patients with CLL will usually have low immunoglobulin levels and hence are predisposed to infection. Early antibiotic therapy for inter-current infection is appropriate.

Treatment

If patients have a rapid lymphocyte doubling time, significant organomegaly or marrow infiltration, treatment with single agent oral chemotherapy is usually given, the two most popular drugs being **chlorambucil** and **fludarabine**. Patients may benefit from supportive treatment such as red cell and platelet transfusions, antibiotics for infection, and immunoglobulin infusions if recurrent infections are a problem. Because antibody-mediated immunity is deranged, some patients with CLL may develop an associated auto-immune haemolytic anaemia, immune thrombocytopenia or Sjögren's syndrome. Young patients with aggressive disease may benefit from combination chemotherapy such as used in the treatment of lymphomas (see below).

7.2 Lymphomas

These are malignant proliferations of lymphoid cells commonly causing lymphadenopathy and spreading to involve other organs such as the bone marrow and blood. Major classification is into Hodgkin disease and non-Hodgkin lymphoma.

Hodgkin disease

Incidence

This commonly affects young adults, though no age is spared. Lymph node enlargement, commonly in the neck, may be the first symptom. The disease spreads to adjacent lymph node groups, and later to extra-nodal sites.

Clinical features

Clinical staging of lymphomas

Stage I: Single node group

Stage II: More than one node group, on one side of the diaphragm

Stage III: More than one node group, on both sides of the diaphragm

Stage IV: Involving extra-nodal tissues such as marrow or lung

The spleen is regarded as an honorary lymph node for this staging, ie splenic involvement is not stage IV.

Release of cytokines by the lymphomatous tissue results in symptoms of fever, night sweats and weight loss. These are termed B symptoms and if present confer a worse prognosis. Hence a patient with splenic and mediastinal nodal involvement and significant weight loss would be clinical stage IIIB. Other symptoms found in Hodgkin disease, though not classified as B symptoms, are pruritis and pain in the involved lymph nodes on consumption of alcohol.

Diagnosis

The diagnosis is established by biopsy of an affected node. The particular diagnostic feature of Hodgkin disease is the Reed–Sternberg cell. This is a giant transformed B-lymphocyte, commonly having two mirror image nuclei, containing prominent 'owl's eye' nucleoli.

Other cells in the Hodgkin disease tissue allow histological staging of disease.

- Most commonly the Hodgkin disease tissue is traversed by broad bands of fibrous tissue reacting to the Reed–Sternberg cells: nodular sclerosing Hodgkin disease.
- Sometimes small lymphocytes infiltrate the adjacent area: lymphocyte-predominant Hodgkin disease.

Prognosis

Most adults with Hodgkin disease can be cured by chemotherapy and/or radiotherapy. For those that relapse, alternative chemotherapy regimens with autografting may offer salvage.

Treatment

Earlier (eg stage I) clinical stages of Hodgkin disease are treated by radiotherapy, more advanced stages by chemotherapy. Intermediate stages may be treated by both. Where the boundaries are drawn between treatment modalities depends on national and local policies. In the UK most stages beyond stage I receive chemotherapy.

The first curative chemotherapy treatment for Hodgkin disease was **MOPP**: **m**ustine, **O**ncovin® (trade name for vincristine), **p**rocarbazine, **p**rednisolone. Mustine is very emetogenic, and so has been replaced by an alternative alkylating agent, chlorambucil, in most Western countries. Current standard chemotherapy for Hodgkin disease is **ABVD** – **A**driamycin®, **b**leomycin, **v**inblastine, **d**acarbazine.

Non-Hodgkin lymphomas (NHL)

The histological classification of NHL is complex and subject to regular change as more is learnt about these diseases. A **clinical classification** is:

- Indolent NHL – slowly progressive, has a low proliferation fraction (assessable by histopathology)
- Aggressive NHL – more rapidly progressive, less differentiated cells, higher proliferation fraction
- Very aggressive NHL – the most rapidly progressive, with proliferation fractions approaching 100%, requiring CNS prophylactic treatment as for acute lymphoblastic leukaemia – see above.

Clinical staging can be performed as for Hodgkin disease (above) but NHL is more commonly disseminated at diagnosis. For aggressive high-grade lymphomas **CHOP** is the gold-standard chemotherapy: **c**yclophosphamide, **h**ydroxydaunorubicin, **O**ncovin®, **p**rednisolone. The majority of NHL is of B-cell origin and monoclonal antibodies directed against B-cell antigens are of value in treatment, eg anti-CD20, rituximab.

7.3 Myelodysplasias

These form a group of closely related, malignant, haematological conditions characterised by dysplastic changes in the blood and marrow (eg hypogranular neutrophils, failure of neutrophil segmentation, megaloblastoid change, ring sideroblasts), cytopenias and a predisposition to transform into acute myeloid leukaemia. The disorder is usually classified by the numbers of blast cells present in the marrow:

- Refractory anaemia – no increase in blast cells but dysplastic changes.
- Refractory anaemia with ring sideroblasts – as above but with prominent ring sideroblasts in the marrow. (A ring sideroblast is a nucleated red cell precursor in the marrow in which the nucleus is surrounded by a ring of iron granules.)
- Refractory anaemia with excess blasts – indicating a high likelihood of transformation into AML.

Myelodysplasia commonly affects the elderly and is usually treated by supportive measures – red cell transfusion, platelet transfusion and antibiotics for neutropenic infection.

7.4 Myeloproliferative disorders

These disorders are associated with the overproduction of relatively mature, relatively normal-looking cells in the blood and marrow:

Table 2 Myeloproliferative disorders	
Disease	Major proliferating cell type
Primary polycythaemia (polycythaemia rubra vera, PRV)	Red cell precursors
Primary thrombocythaemia (essential thrombocythaemia, ET)	Platelet precursors
Myelofibrosis	Marrow reticulin framework
Chronic myeloid leukaemia (may also be classified as a chronic leukaemia – see above)	Myeloid precursors

The four myeloproliferative disorders share common features:

- The overproduction of (relatively) normal blood and bone marrow elements.
- Extramedullary haemopoiesis – marrow cells take up residence outside the marrow in other organs such as the spleen and liver – a form of metastasis.
- Marrow hyperplasia and hypertrophy.
- Increased marrow reticulin – the scaffolding on which the haemopoietic cells live.
- Platelet dysfunction – resulting in bleeding and/or thrombosis.
- Increased basophil count in the blood.
- Hyperuricaemia due to increased cell turnover in the marrow – sometimes present with gout.

- Clonal disorders – clonality (all cells of disease derived from one parent cell) can sometimes be shown by cytogenetic analysis (eg Philadelphia chromosome in CML – see above, Jak2 mutation in PRV – see below).
- Increased circulating stem cells able to grow in culture independently of growth factors such as erythropoietin.
- Overlapping myeloproliferative diseases – eg many cases of primary polycythaemia eventually transform into myelofibrosis.

Chronic myeloid leukaemia is dealt with above.

Primary polycythaemia (polycythaemia rubra vera)

Aetiology

There are many causes of polycythaemia, some which are shown in Table 2, page 118. In primary polycythaemia the marrow is no longer under control of erythropoietin, and levels of this hormone, if measured, are usually low. In most cases a mutation in the Jak2 gene is found, which causes over-expression of a tyrosine kinase enzyme.

Clinical features

- Plethoric complexion
- Splenomegaly – not usually found in other causes of polycythaemia
- Thrombosis – particularly arterial such as stroke and myocardial infarction
- Pruritis – not usually found in other causes of polycythaemia.

Laboratory features

- Elevated haemoglobin, red cell count and haematocrit
- Elevated neutrophil and/or platelet count
- Increased red cell mass
- Other common features of the myeloproliferative disorders – see above.

Treatment

- Venesection to reduce the haematocrit to less than 0.45.
- If the patient is taking cardiovascular drugs then this may need to be isovolaemic – with saline replacement
- Where venesection is required more than monthly then marrow red cell production is usually suppressed with hydroxycarbamide
- Treatment of thrombosis with anticoagulants and prophylaxis with aspirin or clopidogrel may be required.

Prognosis

Median survival is of the order of 10 years, but varies between 2 and 20 years. Causes of death are thrombosis, malignant transformation to acute leukaemia and bleeding.

Primary (essential) thrombocythaemia

Clinical features
The chief clinical features are bleeding/thrombosis, transient ischaemic attacks (TIAs) – microvascular occlusion, some patients bleed, some patients thrombose, some do both.

- Sometimes incidental finding of a high platelet count
- One-third of patients have splenomegaly, but some have infarcted their spleen and are hyposplenic.

Laboratory features

- Platelet count over $500\times10^9/l$ (if over $1000\times10^9/l$, usually primary)
- Giant platelets on blood film
- Abnormal platelet aggregation
- Prolonged template bleeding time
- Iron deficiency if bleeding
- White cell count high, normal or low
- Marrow shows increased numbers of megakaryocytes with clustering.

Other (secondary or reactive) causes of a high platelet count:

- Bleeding
- Acute inflammation
- Malignant disease
- Trauma
- Post splenectomy
- Iron deficiency (even when not due to bleeding).

Treatment
The platelet count should be reduced with hydroxycarbamide, anagrelide, interferon. The platelet function will then improve.

- If thrombosis is a problem, inhibit platelet activation: aspirin, clopidogrel, anticoagulants.

Prognostic indicators
Not all patients with essential thrombocythaemia require cytoreduction therapy. Factors in favour of treatment are:

- history of thrombosis
- age over 60
- other cardiovascular risk factors – diabetes, hypertension
- very high platelet count ($>1500\times10^9/l$).

Myelofibrosis

Definition
Increase in reticulin and collagen in marrow cavity.

Clinical features

- 20% have history of previous polycythaemia rubra vera/essential thrombocythaemia

- Massive splenomegaly – commonly seen in practical exams! Like CML, can have splenic infarcts
- Marrow failure – anaemia ± thrombocytopenia, neutropenia.

Laboratory features

- Leucoerythroblastic anaemia (see above) with *teardrop poikilocytes* in the blood
- Dry tap bone marrow aspirate, with increased reticulin on bone marrow trephine biopsy
- White blood cell count (WBC) and platelets may be high, normal or low
- Sometimes low folate due to increased requirement by marrow cells.

Treatment

- Regular blood transfusion
- Folic acid supplements
- Splenectomy (but caution as high operative risk)
- Splenic irradiation – technically difficult
- Hydroxycarbamide when in early cellular phase.

8. HAEMOSTASIS

Normal haemostasis involves:

- Blood vessel constriction
- Platelet adhesion, activation, aggregation
- Activation of clotting factors and formation of fibrin clot.

Platelets

- Smallest cells in peripheral blood
- Discus shaped
- Surface membrane contains openings connecting with internal canalicular system
- Contain granules and coagulation proteins essential for haemostasis
- Short lifespan = 7–10 days

Essential note

There is massive over-capacity in haemostasis – although the normal platelet count is $140\times10^9/l$ spontaneous bleeding is rare above a platelet count of $20\times10^9/l$.

8.1 Thrombocytopenia

Causes of thrombocytopenia

Congenital (rare)

Acquired

- Peripheral consumption of platelets:

    - Immune (idiopathic) thrombocytopenia
    - Disseminated intravascular coagulation (see below)
    - Hypersplenism
    - Thrombotic thrombocytopenia purpura/haemolytic uraemic syndrome (rare).

In peripheral consumption thrombocytopenia the platelets are relatively young, large and fit so bleeding is less than in marrow underproduction thrombocytopenia for an equivalent platelet count.

- Marrow underproduction of platelets:

    - Aplastic anaemia (chemotherapy, radiotherapy)
    - Marrow infiltration – leukaemia, lymphoma, myeloma.

8.2 Idiopathic thrombocytopenia (ITP)

Immune-mediated destruction of platelets, mainly in the spleen. Most cases are primary idiopathic but ITP may be associated with:

- After viral infection, particularly in children
- Systemic lupus erythematosus
- Chronic lymphocytic leukaemia
- Anti-phospholipid antibodies (Hughes' syndrome)
- Drugs – particularly quinine
- HIV infection
- Acquired common variable immune deficiency.

Most cases of ITP in childhood are of rapid onset and resolve spontaneously without treatment. In adults ITP more often becomes chronic, requiring immunosuppressive treatment. Steroids, splenectomy and other immunosuppressants such as azathioprine and high-dose intravenous immunoglobulin are most often used.

8.3 Coagulation factor deficiencies

Figure 4 is a diagram of the coagulation system. Extrinsic and intrinsic systems share a final common pathway resulting in the production of a fibrin clot. The three common screening tests of coagulation are the prothrombin time (PT), which tests the extrinsic and final common pathways, the activated partial thromboplastin time (APTT), which

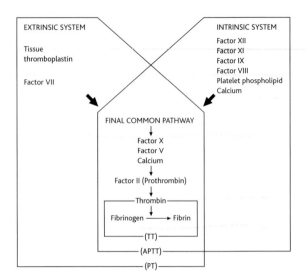

Figure 4 The coagulation system

tests the intrinsic and final common pathways, and the thrombin time (TT), which tests the final part of the final common pathway. Three boxes superimposed on the diagram represent the three coagulation screening tests. Reduction in the factors in an individual box will prolong the relevant coagulation test.

Causes of prolonged coagulation tests

Causes of a prolonged APTT

- Congenital

    - Coagulation factor deficiencies: XII, XI, IX, VIII, X, V, II, I

- Acquired

    - Liver disease, vitamin K deficiency, by reducing factors II, VII, IX and X
    - Disseminated intravascular coagulation – by consumption of all coagulation factors
    - Massive blood transfusion – dilutional effect
    - Unfractionated heparin (monitoring based on APTT, aiming for 1.5–2.5 times the control value)
    - Lupus anticoagulants – prolong the coagulation times in vitro, but paradoxically cause thrombosis in vivo

Causes of a prolonged prothrombin time

- Congenital

  - Coagulation factor deficiencies: VII, X, V, II, I

- Acquired

  - Liver disease, vitamin K deficiency (II, VII, IX, X), obstructive jaundice, haemorrhagic disease of the newborn
  - Disseminated intravascular coagulation
  - Massive blood transfusion – see page 127
  - Warfarin (monitoring test, International Normalised Ratio (INR), based on PT)
  - Gross over-heparinisation, some lupus anticoagulants

Causes of a prolonged thrombin time

- Low fibrinogen/dysfunctional fibrinogen
- Inhibitor of fibrinogen > fibrin conversion

  - Heparin
  - High fibrin degradation products (FDPs)

Disseminated intravascular coagulation (DIC)

DIC is characterised by consumption of all coagulation factors and platelets, usually due to the release into the circulation of a thromboplastin, which triggers coagulation. The clots, once formed, are rapidly dissolved (hyperfibrinolysis), so bleeding is the main clinical problem.

- All clotting tests are prolonged, platelets are low.

Causes of DIC

- Infections

  - Bacterial
  - Viral
  - Protozoal

- Malignancy

  - Metastatic carcinoma
  - Leukaemia particularly acute promyelocytic leukaemia
  - Obstetric – placental abruption, septic abortion, amniotic fluid embolus, intra-uterine death

Causes of DIC

- Tissue damage

  - Extensive trauma
  - Burns
  - Haemolytic transfusion reaction

Management of DIC

- Eliminate the precipitating cause(s)
- Avoid/correct exacerbating features

  - Hypotension, hypoxia, acidosis, hypothermia

- Control the haemorrhagic state

  - Maintain intravascular volume with fluids/red cells
  - Correct coagulation tests by administration of fresh frozen plasma
  - Treat thrombocytopenic bleeding by administration of platelet concentrate

Liver disease

The aetiology of coagulopathy and bleeding risk associated with liver disease has a multifactorial aetiology:

- Impaired synthesis of coagulation factors
- Impaired clearance of activated clotting factors
- Platelet function defect ± thrombocytopenia
- Increased fibrinolysis.

Dilutional coagulopathy

This is associated with massive blood transfusion (more than one blood volume in 24 hours) or excess blood loss/large volumes of IV fluids causing clotting factor dilution.

- All coagulation screening tests prolonged
- Platelets reduced
- FDPs normal.

Haemophilias

Classical haemophilia is factor VIII deficiency, haemophilia B is factor IX deficiency, but both are clinically the same. The disorders are congenital, with sex-linked inheritance – males affected, females carriers.

Investigation: APPT is prolonged, PT normal, TT normal, platelets normal; factor VII or IX is low.

Presentation is with deep muscular haematomas and haemarthroses or bleeding after operation (eg circumcision). If untreated, ankylosis of joints and deformity can occur.

Treatment:

- Factor VIII or IX coagulation factor concentrates – heat and detergent treated to inactivate viruses.
- Recombinant coagulation factors becoming available – no risk of infectious disease transmission.
- Severe haemophilias (< 1% of normal factor level) given prophylactic treatment.

Von Willebrand's disease

This is the commonest inherited coagulopathy (autosomal dominant); males and females affected.

- Von Willebrand factor (vWF) has two functions – allows platelets to adhere, acts as protective carrier for factor VIII.

Investigation: Normal PT, TT, platelet count, sometimes prolonged APTT because of low factor VIII.

- Clinically presentation is with 'platelet type bleeding' – superficial muco-cutaneous, purpura, nosebleeds or menorrhagia.
- Treatment – desmopressin acetate (DDAVP®), factor VIII concentrates (vWF goes with factor VIII).

9. THROMBOSIS AND ANTI-COAGULATION

9.1 Aetiology of thrombosis

Classical causes of thrombosis are embraced in Vircow's triad:

- Factors in the blood constituents; for example, increased platelets, increased coagulation factors (as found in pregnancy, oral contraception and inflammatory states) and polycythaemia.
- Factors in the blood flow; for example, stasis caused by immobility, operation, venous obstruction (by tumour, thrombosis or the pregnant uterus), slow flow in polycythaemia.
- Factors in the vessel wall; for example, atheromatous plaque which ulcerates, releasing pro-coagulants.

9.2 Prophylaxis of thrombosis

- Early mobilisation post-surgery
- Stop oral contraceptives pre-surgery
- Elastic stocking to compress superficial veins, increasing flow in deep venous system
- Devices to cause calf compression, eg pneumatic gaiters
- Prophylactic anticoagulants.

9.3 Treatment of thrombosis

Thrombosis that is not immediately life-threatening is treated with anticoagulant drugs which prevent the formation of further thrombus and allow the natural fibrinolytic system to dissolve the clot in most cases. When thrombotic events are immediately life-threatening, eg myocardial infarction due to coronary artery thrombosis or massive pulmonary embolism, then fibrinolytic dugs such as streptokinase or tissue plasminogen activator are commonly used.

Essential note

Treatment with heparin is started when a deep venous thrombosis is strongly suspected on clinical grounds even if diagnostic Doppler ultrasound scan is not immediately available

Anticoagulants

Conventional unfractionated heparin

- **Action**: immediate inhibition of thrombin and activated factor X
- **Administration**: parenterally
- **Control**: by maintaining APPT ratio between 1.5 and 2.5 the control value
- **Unwanted effects**: bleeding, thrombocytopenia
- **Duration of action**: 4–6 hours
- **Antagonist**: protamine sulphate should be given in cases of haemorrhagic emergency.

Low molecular weight heparin

- **Action**: immediate, particularly by anti-Xa effect
- **Administration**: by subcutaneous injection
- **Control**: not required unless administered for longer than a month – then measurement of Xa level used. Conventional coagulation tests will be normal unless it accumulates, eg in renal failure
- **Duration of action**: 12–24 hours – once daily administration allows out-patient treatment of thrombosis/embolus
- **Antagonist**: none available – await natural decay and do not use immediately before likely surgery.

Warfarin

- **Action**: after 2–3 days therapy (maintain anticoagulation with heparin meanwhile), reduced levels of active coagulation factors II, VII, IX and X
- **Administration**: oral
- **Control**: by INR, a derivative of the prothrombin time. For DVT/PE and AF maintain INR 2–3, for artificial heart valves and recurrent thrombosis on therapy INR 3–4.5
- **Duration of action**: days
- **Antagonist**: vitamin K or in haemorrhagic emergency fresh frozen plasma or prothrombin complex concentrate.

10. TRANSFUSION

10.1 Cardinal rules of ABO compatibility

The plasma of adults contains antibodies against A and/or B antigens NOT present on their red cells. These antibodies will destroy transfused A or B antigen, causing a haemolytic transfusion reaction.

Transfusing blood involves giving red cells ONLY – plasma is effectively removed from donor units to make plasma products.

- Group O is universal donor
- Group AB is universal recipient.

10.2 Unwanted effects of transfusion

- Transmission of infectious diseases

  - Viral – HIV, hepatitis
  - Protozoal – malaria
  - Prion – vCJD
  - Bacterial – cryophilic organisms contaminating blood

- Immunisation against antigens

  - Red cells – atypical red cell antibodies, eg anti-Kell, anti-Duffy making transfusion more difficult
  - White cells – HLA antibodies causing febrile non-haemolytic transfusion reactions. In patients with chronic renal failure, these unwanted antibodies can make future renal transplantation more difficult. Rarer now that red cells are leuco-depleted by filtration after donation
  - Platelets – HLA antibodies may cause refractoriness to random platelet transfusions, requiring HLA-matched platelet donors

- Transfusional iron overload – see thalassaemia major above
- Physical effects

- Volume overload, particularly in the elderly, or in patients with megaloblastic anaemias or cardiac failure. Avoided by giving blood as plasma reduced red cells, transfusing slowly, giving diuretics
- Thrombophlebitis, irritation at the site of cannulation, with or without infection, resulting in painful clotting of superficial vein. Prevented by regular change of cannulation site, use of central lines.

10.3 Commonly used blood products

- Red cells: correction of anaemia and haemorrhage
- Fresh frozen plasma: correction of multiple coagulation factor deficiencies
- Cryoprecipitate: source of fibrinogen and factor VIII/vWF
- Platelet concentrate: underproduction thrombocytopenia
- Albumin: nephrotic syndrome/liver failure
- Immunoglobulin: immunodeficiency, short-term immunosuppressant
- Coagulation factor concentrates, eg factor VII for haemophilia A
- Specific antibodies, eg anti-D, anti-zoster Ig.

Essential note

Transfusion of one unit of red cells in an adult raises the haemoglobin level by approximately 1 g/dl. So if you need to raise the haemoglobin from 5 g/dl to 10 g/dl then you will need to transfuse five units of red cells.

10.4 Compatibility testing

Patients who may receive transfusion have blood group typing performed (both red cell and plasma group) and **antibody screen**. The latter involves mixing recipient's plasma with mixtures of test group O red cells (incorporating all the common minor red cell antigens) and looking for evidence of a reaction, agglutination, haemolysis or a positive reaction, when anti-human globulin is added to washed red cells, indicating that antibody from the recipient's plasma has attached itself to the test red cells. Positive reactions are then investigated with a panel of group O red cells to determine the specificity of the atypical red cell antibody. Finally, when red cells are issued for a patient, a sample of the donor's red cells is incubated with the recipient's plasma and then evidence of a reaction is looked for (the 'cross-match').

10.5 Direct and indirect antiglobulin (Coombs') tests

Direct antiglobulin test looks for antibody coating on the patient's red cells.

Indirect antiglobulin test looks for antibody in the patient's plasma, which attaches itself to the red cells under test. The commonest reason for an indirect antiglobulin test is the cross-match procedure outlined above.

Further revision

Comprehensive texts of haematology

Hoffbrand V, Pettit J, Moss P. *Essential haematology.* 4th edn. London: Blackwell, 1992.

Hoffbrand AV, Pettit J. *Clinical haematology illustrated: an integrated text and colour atlas.* New York: Mosby-Year Book, 1987.

Pictures of blood films and haematology patients similar to those found in MB practical exams

Bain BJ. *Haematology.* New York: Churchill Livingstone, 1998.

Linch D, Yates A. *Colour aids to haematology.* London: Harcourt, 1986.

Commercial web-based basic explanation of cells found on the blood film http://en.wikipedia.org/wiki/Blood_film

Good article on the use of the blood film in diagnosis will become available on internet, currently in the library

Bain BJ. Diagnosis from the blood smear. N Engl J Med 2005;353:498–507 at PMID 16079373.

Undergraduate course material in Haematology including useful pictorial presentations from Queen's University Ontario http://meds.queensu.ca/medicine/deptmed/ hemonc/ugrad.htm

Comprehensive blood education site, mostly postgraduate and research advances http://www.bloodmed.com/home/

Revision summary

1. Anaemia is the commonest haematological disorder in the general population. You should be able to differentiate diagnoses associated with microcytic, normocytic and macrocytic varieties.
2. Be aware of the disparate causes of haemolysis. It is a relatively rare cause of anaemia but is a common examination question!
3. Much of the work of junior doctors in haematology units is caring for patients with marrow failure, usually as a result of chemotherapy or radiotherapy. You should be aware of the causes and management of marrow failure, one cause of which is aplastic anaemia.
4. You should know the aetiology, clinical manifestations and treatment of sickle cell disease – the most important of the haemoglobinopathies. Patients with sickle crisis are commonly managed in general medical wards.
5. Haematological malignancies are specialist haematological diseases – you should have an understanding of the basic classification and general principles of management.
6. Know the cardinal rules of ABO compatibility and be aware of the unwanted effects of transfusion and the commonly used blood products.

Immunology

CONTENTS

Revision objectives

You should know about:

1. Humoral immunity (non-cellular)
2. Cells involved in the immune system
3. Hypersensitivity.

1. COMPLEMENT

The complement system is a group of plasma protein cascades with important immunological actions in protecting against infection. There are three complement pathways: classical, alternative and the lectin binding pathway. Each is activated by a different mechanism but the final effects are similar.

Activation

- **Classical** – activated by immune complexes
- **Alternative** – activated by bacterial cell wall components
- **Lectin binding** – activated by bacterial cell wall components

Immunology

1.1 Actions

- Opsonisation – coating cells with C3b to facilitate phagocytosis
- Chemotaxis – mediated by C3a, C5a
- Inflammation – mediated by C3a, C5a
- Cell lysis – due to a complex of C5, C6, C7, C8, C9.

1.2 Regulation

The complement cascade slowly 'ticks over' and is never completely inactive. Regulatory proteins play an important role in keeping complement activity suppressed in normal circumstances. Deficiency of regulatory components can allow overactivity of the system and produce tissue damage. Examples are given below.

Hereditary angio-oedema

This is caused by a deficiency of C1 inhibitor, and is characterised by acute episodes of non-inflammatory oedema – swelling of the face, tongue and upper airway which can be life threatening. It is mediated by vasoactive fragments of C2.

Paroxysmal nocturnal haemoglobinuria

There is an inability to bind regulatory proteins on red cell surfaces, causing spontaneous complement-mediated lysis of red blood cells that results in haemolytic anaemia and free haemoglobin in the urine.

1.3 Complement deficiency

Complement factor deficiencies are common and usually asymptomatic. Most deficiency is genetic but inflammatory disorders such as lupus nephritis can lead to low levels of C3 and C4. Problems only occur if a complement factor is completely absent or levels are very low:

- **C2 or C4 deficiencies**: SLE-like disorders
- **C3 deficiency**: life-threatening infections by encapsulated organisms (eg pneumococci)
- **C5, C6, C7, C8 or C9 deficiencies**: impaired response to Neisserial infections.

2. IMMUNOGLOBULINS

Immunoglobulins are produced by B-lymphocytes and are secreted by plasma cells. They are made up of two identical light chains and two identical heavy chains.

Functions of immunoglobulins

- Complement activation
- Stimulation of phagocytic cells
- Precipitation of antigen

Essential note

B-lymphocytes and plasma cells can produce immunoglobulins but only plasma cells can secrete free immunoglobin.

2.1 Immunoglobulin isotypes

There are five isotypes:

Essential note

There are 5 immunoglobulin isotypes: IgG, IgA, IgM, IgD and IgE.

IgG

IgG is the commonest immunoglobulin in internal body fluids; it is important in the secondary immune response.

IgA

IgA is the major immunoglobulin of seromucous secretions, and is produced in mucosal-associated lymphoid tissue.

IgM

IgM is a pentameric molecule and is important in the primary immune response.

IgD

IgD is present on B-cell surfaces; it is involved in B-cell activation.

IgE

IgE is found on mast cells and is responsible for immediate (type I) hypersensitivity reactions.

2.2 Cryoglobulins and cold agglutinins

These are immunoglobulins that agglutinate cells or precipitate when cold. They can cause Raynaud's phenomenon, cyanosis of digits or vasculitis in the small cool blood vessels of the peripheries.

Cryoglobulins

- IgM, IgG or IgA
- Precipitate when cooled to 4°C, and re-dissolve when reheated
- Occur in lymphoma, myeloma, hepatitis C, SLE.

Cold agglutinins

- Only IgM
- Agglutinating red blood cells between 0°C and 4°C
- Found in lymphoma, viral infections, mycoplasma infection.

3. CELLS AND THE IMMUNE SYSTEM

3.1 Polymorphonuclear cells

Essential note

Polymorphonuclear cells include neutrophils, eosinophils and basophils.

Neutrophils

- Stored in the bone marrow and released into the bloodstream in response to infection
- Surface receptors for IgG, IgA and complement components
- Phagocytosis and destruction of bacteria.

Basophils and mast cells

- Basophils circulate and mast cells are tissue bound
- Surface receptors for C3, C5 and IgE
- Produce histamine, prostaglandins, leukotrienes and proteases
- Involved in the immune response to parasites
- Interaction of antigen with mast-cell-bound IgE produces immediate hypersensitivity.

Eosinophils

- Commonly increased in patients with allergic disease
- Surface receptors for IgG, C3 and C5
- Phagocytose antigen–antibody complexes.

3.2 Lymphocytes

Lymphocytes arise from precursors in the bone marrow and then mature in other sites. They have important roles in both cell-mediated and antibody-mediated (humoral) immunity. B-lymphocytes and T-lymphocytes have different functions and can be identified by cell surface glycoproteins. T-lymphoctyes carry the cell surface marker CD3, but can be further divided into those carrying CD4 (helper cells) and CD8 (suppressor or cytotoxic cells).

CD4 can interact with major histocompatibility complex (MHC) class II antigens (HLA-D), which are found on antigen-presenting cells. It is present on the cell surface of monocytes as well as T-helper cells.

CD8 interacts with MHC class I antigens (HLA-A, -B, -C) found on target cells. It allows cytotoxic T-cells to bind to and destroy, for example, viral-infected cells.

T-lymphocytes

- Mature in the thymus
- 70–80% of the total lymphocyte population
- Intracellular infections, tumour surveillance and graft rejection
- CD3 (part of the T-cell receptor) is present on all T-cells.

CD4+ (helper) T-cells
The normal CD4 count is 600–1500 cells per microlitre. They are responsible for cell-mediated immunity (mainly TH_1 cells), and B-cell differentiation (mainly TH_2 cells).

CD8+ (Cytotoxic) T-cells
The normal CD8 count is 300–1000 cells per microlitre. They are responsible for cell-mediated immunity, and are important in eliminating viral infected cells.

B-lymphocytes

- Mature in the spleen and lymph nodes
- Express immunoglobulin on their surface
- Differentiate into plasma cells which secrete antibody
- Activation requires both antigen and T-helper cells.

4. TRANSPLANT IMMUNOLOGY

The recognition of self is mediated by HLA antigens on cell surfaces. The closer the HLA antigens of donor and recipient are matched the more likely a transplant is to survive. In kidney transplants HLA-DR and HLA-B matching are the most important. After these, matching for HLA-A or HLA-C produces only small improvements in graft survival. Heart and liver grafts survive well with immunosuppression with only limited matching (eg at one HLA site).

Essential Note

HLA antigens on cell surfaces mediate recognition of 'self'. Transplants *must* be blood group compatible.

Immunology

Privileged sites exist where rejection is rarely a problem even when there is no MHC matching:

- **Cornea**: avascular and does not sensitise the patient
- **Bone and artery**: even if the grafts die, they provide a structure for host cells to colonise.

5. HYPERSENSITIVITY

Hypersensitivity reactions are immune responses with excessive or undesirable consequences. There are five types.

- **Type I: Anaphylactic or immediate**

  - Antigen + IgE on mast cells and basophils

This involves release of histamine and leukotrienes. Reactions occur within 30 min of exposure to antigen.

  - Clinical significance: asthma, atopy, some acute drug reactions.

- **Type II: Antibody-dependent cytotoxicity**

  - Cell-bound antigen + circulating IgG or IgM

This results in complement activation, phagocytosis, killer cell activation and cell lysis.

  - Clinical significance: transfusion reactions, rhesus incompatibility, Goodpasture's syndrome, immune thrombocytopenia.

- **Type III: Immune-complex-mediated or Arthus reaction**

  - Free antigen + free antibody

This involves complement activation, platelet aggregation and inflammation.

  - Clinical significance: in *antibody excess* antigen–antibody complexes precipitate close to the site of entry and cause localised disease, as in farmer's lung, pigeon fancier's lung and pulmonary aspergillosis
  - Clinical significance: in *antigen excess* the complexes remain soluble and produce distant or systemic disease as in glomerulonephritis and serum sickness.

- **Type IV: Cell-mediated or delayed type hypersensitivity**

  - Antigen + sensitised (memory) T-cells

This results in lymphokine release and T-cell activation Reactions take 24 hours to develop.

  - Clinical significance: tuberculin reaction, contact dermatitis, graft versus host disease, transplant rejection.

- **Type V: Stimulatory**

  - Antibody + cell surface receptor

One example of this type is anti-thyroid stimulating receptor antibody in Graves' disease.

> **Essential note**
>
> There are 5 types of hypersensitivity reaction.

6. CYTOKINES

Cytokines are soluble low-molecular-weight peptides produced by cells, which act as signals to coordinate processes such as cell differentiation and activation. They play an extremely important role in processes such as inflammation. Cytokines include interleukins (IL), interferons (IFN) and colony-stimulating factors. Actions include production of fever, C-reactive protein (CRP), thrombocythaemia and cell activation.

Patterns of cytokine production

Immune response	Important cytokines	Produced by
Acute phase response	IL-1, IL-6, tumour necrosis factor alpha (TNFα)	Macrophage
Cell-mediated	IL-2, IFNγ	TH$_1$ helper cells
Antibody-mediated	IL-4, IL-5, IL-6, IL-10	TH$_2$ helper cells

Therapeutic uses of cytokines

- Antiviral activity (eg hepatitis B or C)
- Bone marrow stimulation
- Multiple sclerosis
- Malignancy

7. AUTOANTIBODIES IN DIAGNOSIS

7.1 Rheumatoid factor
Rheumatoid factor is an antibody against human IgG. It is positive in 70% of rheumatoid arthritis (RA) patients, and is associated with extra-articular features and more severe articular disease. It is also present in other chronic inflammatory conditions.

7.2 Antinuclear antibodies
Antinuclear antibodies can be detected in conditions such as systemic lupus erythematosus (SLE), drug-induced lupus, scleroderma, Sjögren's syndrome, mixed connective tissue disease and polymyositis. There is a low titre in the normal population.

Staining patterns

- **Homogeneous staining**: suggests SLE
- **Speckled staining**: suggests mixed connective tissue disease
- **Nucleolar staining**: suggests scleroderma
- **Centromere staining**: suggests CREST (see Rheumatology chapter) syndrome

Anti double-stranded DNA is present in approximately 80% of patients with SLE. When in high titre it is specific for SLE.

Extractable nuclear antigens

- **Anti-Ro**: Sjögren's syndrome, congenital heart block
- **Anti-La**: Sjögren's syndrome
- **Anti-Sm**: SLE, renal lupus
- **Anti-RNP**: mixed connective tissue disease, SLE
- **Anti-Jo 1**: polymyositis
- **Anti-Scl-70**: scleroderma
- **Anti-centromere**: CREST syndrome.

7.3 Anti-neutrophil cytoplasmic antibodies (ANCA)

- **cANCA** (anti-PR3)

These are present in Wegener's granulomatosis and microscopic polyangiitis (MPA). The titres may reflect disease activity.

- **pANCA** (anti-MPO)

These can be detected in vasculitis (eg Wegeners and MPA), ulcerative colitis, autoimmune hepatitis and SLE.

7.4 Autoantibodies in gastrointestinal and liver disease

- **Anti-mitochondrial**: primary biliary cirrhosis
- **Anti-smooth muscle**: auto-immune hepatitis, cryptogenic cirrhosis
- **Gastric parietal cell antibodies**: pernicious anaemia
- **Intrinsic factor antibodies**: pernicious anaemia
- **Anti-tissue transglutaminase**: coeliac disease
- **Anti-gliadin**: coeliac disease.

7.5 Autoantibodies in thyroid disease
Thyroid antibodies, especially anti-TPO in high titre, increase the chance of progressing to hypothyroidism.

- **Anti-thyroglobulin (anti-Tg)**: autoimmune thyroiditis
- **Anti-thyroid peroxidase (anti-TPO)**: autoimmune thyroiditis, low titres in Grave's disease
- **Anti-thyroid stimulating hormone receptor (Anti-TSHR)**: most Graves' disease patients and some with autoimmune thyroiditis.

7.6 Antiphospholipid antibodies
These antibodies may be measured directly (as anticardiolipin antibodies) or by their effects on clotting (as lupus anticoagulant). Though they can prolong the activated partial thromboplastin time (APTT) in vitro, their clinical effect is to promote thrombosis.

Associations with anti-phospholipid antibodies:

- Arterial or venous thrombosis
- Fetal loss
- Livido reticularis
- Thrombocytopenia.

8. PRIMARY IMMUNODEFICIENCY

8.1 Neutrophil disorders

- Recurrent infections with pyogenic bacteria, and fungi such as *Candida*
- May present with failure to thrive
- Example: chronic granulomatous disease.

8.2 B-cell disorders

- Hypogammaglobulinaemia or agammaglobulinaemia
- Recurrent infections with pyogenic bacteria, or fungi such as *Candida*.
- Maternal IgG crosses the placenta so infections are rare before 6 months of age

- Example: IgA deficiency (commonest isolated Ig deficiency in the UK (1 in 700), often asymptomatic.

8.3 T-cell disorders

- Increased susceptibility to viruses, mycobacteria and fungi
- Measles, vaccinia or even BCG immunisation can be fatal
- Common bacterial infections do not cause problems
- Malignancy is more common
- Example: Di George syndrome.

8.4 Combined B- and T-cell disorders

- Rare but severe life-threatening disorders
- Example: severe combined immunodeficiency.

8.5 Acquired immunodeficiency

The immune response can be impaired by a variety of factors.

- Malnutrition impairs cell mediated immunity
- Cytotoxic drugs and corticosteroids impair cell mediated and humoral responses
- Lymphoproliferative disorders may affect antibody production (eg myeloma) or cell mediated immunity (eg Hodgkins disease)
- Common viral infections (eg chickenpox) can skew the balance between Th1 and Th2 producing a transient increased risk of pyogenic infection
- Sarcoiosis impairs cell mediated immunity
- HIV depletes T helper cells (CD4+). When the CD4 count falls below 200 per microlitre, life threatening infection may occur with otherwise harmless organisms (eg cytomegalovirus, pneumocystis carinii), counts below 100 per microlitre are associated increased infection with toxoplasma and cryptococcus, and below 75 per microlitre with mycobacterium avium complex infections. In AIDS there is often hypergammaglobulinaemia.

9. IMMUNISATION

Immunisation may reduce the risk of developing a disease, reduce the severity of disease or reduce the risk of a disease becoming epidemic.

Active immunity: this is induced by stimulating the immune system with inactivated or live attenuated organisms or their products. Most vaccines produce their effects by stimulating the production of antibodies, although BCG promotes cell-mediated immunity. Live attenuated vaccines can be effective with a single dose but inactivated organisms or sub-unit vaccines usually need repeated doses to achieve adequate immunity.

Passive immunity: this is achieved by injection of human immunoglobulin obtained from donors. The protection is immediate but may last only a few weeks. The passage of maternal IgG across the placenta to the fetus is an example of this occurring physiologically.

9.1 Vaccines

Killed organism vaccines

Examples of these inactivated vaccines are cholera, polio (Salk), pertussis, influenza, typhoid and rabies. There is no risk of infection from the immunisation, and thus they can be used in the immunocompromised. Influenza vaccine is offered to those who would fare badly with infection, ie patients with chronic illness such as chronic obstructive pulmonary disease (COPD), heart disease, chronic renal disease, rheumatoid arthritis, and the elderly.

Live attenuated vaccines

Examples of these vaccines are BCG, mumps, vaccinia, rubella, measles and polio (Sabin). They are superior to killed vaccines because better immunological memory is produced. However, attenuation may fail and actual infection may occur, especially in the immunocompromised.

Subunit vaccines

Subunit vaccines include *H. influenzae*, *S. pneumoniae*, *N. meningitidis* and Hepatitis B. They are purified components of the infective organism and thus there is no risk of infection from the immunisation. Hepatitis B immunisation is used in high-risk groups such as health workers. Pneumococcal vaccination is important in asplenic patients.

Preformed antibody vaccines

These vaccines include tetanus, rabies, hepatitis B, varicella, botulism and diphtheria. The antibodies are prepared from donors and confer passive immunity. They have anti-toxin effects in tetanus, diphtheria and botulism. They are safe in immunocompromised patients.

Essential note

There are 4 types of vaccine: killed organism, live attenuated, subunit and preformed antibody.

For the bare bones of the subject see web site *Immunology for medical students* (Dalhousie University) at http://pim.medicine.dal.ca/home.htm.

More information can be found in the Immunology chapter of the *Merck manual of diagnosis and therapy at* http://www.merck.com/mrkshared/mmanual/home.jsp.

Wikipedia has a good straightforward section at http://en.wikipedia.org/wiki/Immune_system.

For students who would like to go to the library (or buy a book for more detailed undergraduate immunology) I would recommend Roitt I, Delves P. *Roitt's essential immunology*, 10th edn. Oxford: Blackwell, at http://www.roitt.com/default.htm.

Journals: *Clinical and Experimental Immunology; Immunology*

Revision summary

You should have an understanding of:

1. Humoral immunity
   a. Complement
      i. Activated by immune complexes or bacterial cell wall components
      ii. Actions: inflammation, opsonisation, membrane attack
      iii. Deficiency: common, mostly asymptomatic
   b. Immunoglobulins
      i. Activate complement
      ii. Stimulate phagocytic cells
      iii. Precipitate antigen
2. Cells involved in the immune system
   a. Polymorphonuclear cells
      i. Neutrophils: phagocytosis of bacteria
      ii. Basophils and mast cells: type 1 hypersensitivity
      iii. Eosinophils: increased in allergic disease
   b. Lymphocytes
      i. B-lymphocytes: immunoglobulin production
      ii. T-lymphocytes:
         - CD4+ T-helper cells
         - CD8+ cytotoxic T-cells
3. Hypersensitivity
   a. Type 1: anaphylactic
   b. Type 2: antibody-dependent cytotoxicity
   c. Type 3: immune complex mediated
   d. Type 4: cell mediated
   e. Type 5: stimulatory.

Infectious diseases and tropical medicine

Chapter 10

CONTENTS

Revision objectives

You should:

1. Gain an understanding of basic epidemiological concepts such as notifiable diseases, modes of transmission of infection, predispositions to disease and microbial virulence factors
2. Learn about host defence mechanisms, such as polymorphonuclear neutrophils, the acute phase response and the complement system (collectively known as first-line defence mechanisms), humoral immunity and cellular immunity

3. Gain knowledge of specific antimicrobial agents such as antibacterial, antituberculous, antiviral and anthelmintic drugs
4. Gain an understanding of infections in specific situations such as pregnancy, alcoholism, splenectomy and sickle cell disease
5. Learn about the infections of the major physiological systems: respiratory, neurological, gastrointestinal, cardiac and soft tissue infections
6. Learn about the major tropical infections: malaria, enteric fever, amoebiasis, schistosomiasis, leprosy and cholera

Infectious diseases and tropical medicine

1. BASIC EPIDEMIOLOGICAL CONCEPTS

1.1 Notifiable diseases

The following diseases must be notified to the local Health and Protection Authority (HPA) in England and Wales. The primary aim is to prevent further spread of these diseases, which are highly infectious. The HPA will enable rapid contact tracing of people known to have been exposed to:

Anthrax, cholera, diphtheria, food poisoning, leprosy, leptospirosis, malaria, meningitis, measles, mumps, plague, rabies, rubella, smallpox, tetanus, tuberculosis, typhoid, viral haemorrhagic fever, viral hepatitis, whooping cough and yellow fever.

It is recommended that patients suffering from these diseases should be isolated from other patients. In addition isolation of patients without notification is recommended for patients with chicken pox, *Clostridium difficile*, severely infected eczema, gonococcal conjunctivitis, hepatitis A, herpes simplex, zoster, methicillin-resistant *Staphylococcus aureus* (MRSA), rotavirus and syphilis.

Essential note

Notifiable diseases must be reported to the Health and Protection Authority in England and Wales, the primary aim being to prevent further disease spread

1.2 Modes of transmission of infection

Respiratory transmission

The major pathogens are:

- *Mycobacterium tuberculosis*
- *Haemophilus influenzae*
- *Streptococcus pyogenes*
- *Neisseria meningitidis*
- *Streptococcus pneumoniae*
- Childhood respiratory viruses (eg measles, chickenpox).

Faecal–oral transmission

This occurs when gastrointestinal pathogens from the faeces of a human (or animal) case or carrier gain access to food, water or dairy products. This direct transmission from contaminated surfaces, to hands, then mouth is possible, particularly in children. **Enteroviruses** (eg poliovirus and hepatitis A) are also transmitted by this route.

Sexual transmission

Close apposition of the genitourinary (GU) mucosa is usually required for transmission of fragile GU tract pathogens. Sometimes oro-genital contact may result in sexually transmitted disease (STD), and it can occasionally occur through oral–oral contact (eg syphilis).

Congenital transmission

This may be either transplacental or perinatal. Fetal death or deformity is a variable result of transplacental infection.

Important syndromes with particular organisms are given below.

- **Rubella**: heart, eye, CNS. The fetus is nearly always affected if infection occurs in the first 7 weeks of pregnancy.
- **Toxoplasmosis**: hydrocephalus, cerebral calcification and choroidoretinitis comprise a classic triad.
- **Chickenpox**: first trimester infection can cause limb deformities; later infections cause infant/childhood zoster.
- **Cytomegalovirus (CMV)**: at least 75% of infected babies are undamaged. The main syndromes include intracranial calcification, microcephaly, cerebral palsy, septal defects, hepatosplenomegaly, cleft palate, biliary and oesophageal atresia.
- **Listeriosis**: both transplacental and perinatal infection can occur. This can result in abortion or neonatal septicaemia.

Blood-borne transmission

Viruses comprise the most common problem, but other organisms feature in certain situations.

- **Hepatitis B (and delta agent)**: there is a 30% risk of infection from needle stick injury. In contrast, needle stick transmission is much less likely with HIV (0.3%) because of low virus concentrations.
- **CMV**: transmission in blood is of clinical importance in the immunosuppressed due to the risk of CMV-related disease in such patients (eg in transplant recipients).
- **Other blood-borne viruses**: hepatitis C, Epstein–Barr virus.

Direct contact

Infections may be transmitted by direct skin contact. Cutaneous infections include impetigo and scabies. The rash of secondary syphilis is highly infectious by direct skin contact.

Insect or animal bite

Insect bites can transmit malaria (female anopheles mosquito), leishmaniasis (sand fly), trypanosomiasis (tsetse fly), and bites from rodents and mammals can transmit eg rabies and Lassa fever.

1.3 Predispositions to disease

Host vulnerability or (conversely) resistance to disease is multifactorial. The outcome of any infection depends upon the balance struck between the **inoculum size**, the **virulence** of the pathogen and **host factors**, listed in the box.

Host factors affecting vulnerability to disease

- Immunological

  - Genetic deficiency

    - Immunoglobulin/complement/T-cell deficiencies

  - Prior immunity

    - Naturally or artificially acquired

- Other factors

  - Psychological status (now recognised as an influential factor in the common cold)
  - Nutritional status

    - (eg measles in under-nutrition)

  - Prior antibiotic therapy

    - (eg Clostridium difficile, multi-resistant Staphylococcus aureus infections)

  - Acquired deficiency

    - HIV infection; malignant disease; transplant recipients; patients receiving chemotherapy

  - Miscellaneous influences on immune status

    - (eg diabetes, pregnancy, splenectomy)

  - Foreign bodies

    - (eg catheters; artificial heart valves)

  - Behavioural factors

    - (eg smokers, alcoholics)

1.4 Microbial virulence factors

These include the ability to invade and evade **host immune** defences, often by the production of **enzymes** and **toxins**.

Invasion through a mucosal surface first requires **attachment**. This can be relatively non-specific, mediated only by the production of a polysaccharide capsule or slime. Alternatively, specific structures on the organism's surface known as **adhesins** attach to specific glycoprotein or glycolipid **receptors** on the host cell.

Toxins

These are products of pathogenic bacteria which can be classified into endotoxins and exotoxins.

- **Endotoxin**: an **integral lipopolysaccharide** component of Gram-negative cell walls. Its active component, **lipid A**, induces fever, provokes the coagulation and complement cascades, activates B lymphocytes and stimulates production of tumour necrosis factor, interleukin-1 and prostaglandins. Heavy exposure as in Gram-negative sepsis causes fever, shock and occasionally death.
- **Exotoxins**: produced by a diversity of organisms, with equally diverse effects:

  - Vibrio cholerae – secretory diarrhoea (small bowel)
  - Corynebacterium diphtheriae – cardiomyopathy, neuropathy
  - Clostridium tetani – tetanus
  - Clostridium perfringens – gangrene, secretory diarrhoea
  - Clostridium botulinum – paralysis.

2.1 Non-specific mechanisms ('first line of defence')

Polymorphonuclear neutrophils (PMNs) circulate freely in the absence of an infectious process and do not attach to capillary endothelium. Cytokines and complement fragments, which are produced at the site of an infection, make local capillary endothelium and passing PMNs 'stickier'. PMNs kill by first attaching to the pathogen and then ingesting the pathogen, to form a phagosome. Lysosomes in the PMN then discharge strong hydrolytic enzymes into the phagosome.

The **acute phase response** is initiated by cytokines released by cells of the macrophage/monocyte lineage at the site of an infection. They circulate to the liver where they trigger the release of certain proteins. These include **C-reactive protein. Transferrin** is also a major component of this response. Its major role is to mop up iron and other metals (eg zinc), thus denying them to invading bacteria.

The **complement system** provides protection in many ways but its main functions are:

- Direct lysis
- Opsonisation
- Leukocyte chemotaxis
- Promotion of the inflammatory response.

Essential note

Hosts have a variety of defences against infection: first line of defence includes polymorphonuclear neutrophils, the acute phase response and the complement system. Later defences include humoral systems (antibodies) and cellular immunity (T-cells destroying infected cells)

2.2 Humoral immunity

Specific antibodies appear within 7–10 days of primary exposure to an antigen; a significant proportion of these are of the IgM class, making measurement of this antibody useful in serological diagnosis.

Secondary exposure results in an accelerated response, primarily of the IgG class.

Antibody functions can be summarised thus:

- Opsonisation/lysis (with complement)
- Neutralisation of toxins
- Eosinophil-mediated killing

- Protective coating of host cells
- Facilitation of natural killer (NK) cell activity.

2.3 Cellular immunity

Antibodies cannot penetrate infected cells to kill an organism that may be contained within. Sensitised T-cells perform the role of destroying infected cells. They are usually of the CD8 subtype and do so by cytolytic action following direct contact with the target cell. Such contact can only occur when the target cell and effector cell share the same class I histocompatibility antigens. Sensitised T-cells can also produce lymphokines, which specifically stimulate macrophages to destroy organisms against which they are indifferent in the unstimulated state. These macrophages will then be non-specifically more active against a variety of organisms.

3.1 Antibacterial agents

Penicillins

- **Mechanism of action**: damage to bacterial cell wall by attachment to penicillin-binding proteins (PBPs) in the cell wall, inhibiting cross-linking.
- **Serious side-effects**: anaphylaxis (rare); interstitial nephritis (rare); encephalopathy.
- **Excretion**: the main excretory route of most penicillins is via the kidneys.

Cephalosporins

- **Mechanism of action**: very similar to penicillins.
- **Serious side-effects**: bronchospasm; anaphylaxis; nephrotoxicity (rare).

Quinolones

- **Mechanism of action**: inhibition of bacterial DNA synthesis.
- **Spectrum of activity**: broad, but better against Gram-negatives; poor anti-anaerobe activity.
- **Serious side-effects**: hallucinations, psychotic reactions, convulsions, photosensitivity.

Sulphonamides

- **Mechanism of action**: competitive inhibition of enzyme which converts para-aminobenzoic acid (PABA) into folic acid.
- **Spectrum of activity**: wide, including chlamydiae, toxoplasma and plasmodia, but resistance common.

- **Serious side-effects**: agranulocytosis, thrombocytopenia, leukopenia, displacement of warfarin from plasma proteins.

Tetracyclines

- **Mechanism of action**: inhibition of bacterial protein synthesis by blocking binding of tRNA to the 30S subunit.
- **Spectrum of activity**: broad, inclusive of rickettsiae, chlamydiae, mycoplasmas.
- **Serious side-effects**: photosensitivity, exacerbation of renal failure, discoloration and hypoplasia of enamel in children <8 years, depression of skeletal growth.

Macrolides (eg erythromycin)

- **Mechanism of action**: inhibition of bacterial protein synthesis by binding to the 50S ribosome.
- **Spectrum of activity**: broad, inclusive of mycoplasmas, chlamydiae and rickettsiae. Useful activity against pneumococci, also legionella. Clindamycin is particularly effective against anaerobes.
- **Serious side-effects**: thrombophlebitis, transient hearing loss, cholestatic hepatitis, pseudomembranous colitis.

Aminoglycosides

- **Mechanism of action**: inhibition of bacterial protein synthesis.
- **Spectrum of activity**: predominantly active against Gram-negative aerobic bacilli. Not active against anaerobes.
- **Serious side-effects**: ototoxicity, renal tubular damage.

3.2 Antituberculous drugs

Rifampicin

- **Mechanism of action**: inhibition of DNA-dependent RNA polymerase.
- **Spectrum of activity**: broad, inclusive of antituberculous activity. Useful prophylactic against meningococcus.
- **Serious side-effects**: hepatic toxicity (especially in alcoholics).

Isoniazid

- **Mechanism of action**: inhibition of cell wall synthesis.
- **Spectrum of activity**: exclusively antituberculous.
- **Serious side-effects**: peripheral neuropathy, psychosis, convulsions, hepatitis-like syndrome, lupus-like syndrome.

Pyrazinamide

- **Mechanism of action**: poorly understood, but works best in more acid environment, ie inside phagosomes.

- **Spectrum of activity**: exclusively antituberculous.
- **Serious side-effects**: hepatotoxicity (dose-related) and gout.

Ethambutol

- **Mechanism of action**: inhibits bacterial RNA synthesis.
- **Spectrum of activity**: good range of activity against other mycobacteria.
- **Serious side-effects**: retrobulbar neuritis, impairment of colour vision or visual acuity.

3.3 Antiviral drugs

Aciclovir

- **Mechanism of action**: selective activity against **herpes viruses** that encode a **thymidine kinase**. Viral thymidine kinase converts aciclovir into a monophosphate and then host cell kinases convert the monophosphate to a triphosphate. Aciclovir triphosphate inhibits the viral DNA-polymerase to break its cycle of replication.
- **Spectrum of activity**: very useful for *herpes simplex* and *herpes varicella-zoster* infections.
- **Serious side-effects**: renal failure, neurotoxicity with hallucinations, psychosis, convulsions and/or coma.

Ganciclovir

Similar mechanism of action, metabolism and side-effects as for aciclovir. However, ganciclovir has a greater effect against CMV; it is used to treat AIDS patients with retinitis, and also for the CMV infections which are common in transplanted patients.

Ribavirin

- **Mechanism of action**: analogue of the nucleoside guanosine; inhibits nucleoside biosynthesis.
- **Spectrum of activity**: useful as an aerosol in severe respiratory syncytial virus (RSV) infection, also for Lassa fever and one of the main drugs used to treat hepatitis C.
- **Serious side-effects**: bone marrow depression.

3.4 Anthelmintic agents

Benzimidazoles

- (eg albendazole, thiabendazole, mebendazole).
- **Mechanism of action**: reduction or paralysis of parasite motility.
- **Spectrum of activity**: broad against intestinal nematodes.

Praziquantel

Spectrum of activity: has particularly useful activity against *Schistosoma* and *Taenia*.

3.5 Other agents used to counteract infection

Immunoglobulins

Normal human immunoglobulin has many applications, particularly in passively immunising patients with humoral immunodeficiency. There are a number of specific immunoglobulins for specific situations (eg tetanus, rabies, diphtheria, hepatitis B and zoster immune globulin).

Vaccines

- **Inactivated/killed vaccines**: the predominant vaccine type for bacterial disease, eg toxoids (diphtheria, tetanus); killed cell (pertussis, typhoid); capsular polysaccharide (*Haemophilus influenza* b, meningococcal, pneumococcal).
- **Attenuated/live vaccines**: the predominant vaccine type for viral disease (with exceptions), eg attenuated (measles, mumps, rubella, yellow fever, polio); subunit (hepatitis B); inactivated (rabies, Japanese encephalitis, influenza, hepatitis A).
- **Attenuated bacterial vaccines**: BCG, oral typhoid vaccine.

Tuberculin testing is the demonstration of cell-mediated immunity to purified mycobacterial proteins. Mantoux and Heaf tests are the commonest tuberculins used. Tuberculin testing is not useful in patients previously immunised with BCG. The test may be negative in patients with HIV and miliary TB. It is most useful in children who have not received BCG and in the surveillance of contact cases.

Essential note

Specific antimicrobials are grouped into antibacterial agents, antituberculous drugs, antiviral drugs and anthelmintic agents. Vaccines are either killed bacteria or attenuated viruses or bacteria

---

4. INFECTIONS IN SPECIFIC SITUATIONS

4.1 Pregnancy

Because the fetus is antigenically different from the mother, modulation of selected aspects of the maternal immune response is necessary for the fetus to be tolerated. The placenta is responsible for this modulation.

Infections in the mother exacerbated by pregnancy

- Urinary tract infection
- *Listeria*
- Varicella (pneumonitis life-threatening, especially in third trimester)
- Candidiasis
- Pulmonary tuberculosis
- *Salmonella* spp.
- Hepatitis E (25% mortality)
- HIV disease
- Falciparum malaria (especially primigravidae in second trimester)

4.2 Alcoholism

Alcoholics are more vulnerable to a number of infections because of the **immunosuppressive effects of excessive alcohol intake**. The neutropenia of alcoholism is probably due to toxic effects on the bone marrow; studies show the neutrophils themselves are less effective and less able to phagocytose foreign particles.

Important infections to which alcoholics are particularly vulnerable

- Pulmonary tuberculosis
- *Legionella*
- Aspiration pneumonias
- *Klebsiella* pneumonia
- *Listeria*

4.3 Splenectomy

The spleen accounts for approximately 25% of the body's lymphatic tissue; absence of its function causes particular vulnerability to capsulate organisms such as:

- Pneumococcus
- *Haemophilus influenzae*
- Meningococcus
- Malaria.

4.4 Sickle cell disease

Sicklers often have infarcted spleens and a reduction in complement-mediated serum opsonising activity. This gives rise to vulnerability to:

- Pneumococcal infection (in particular)
- Other forms of bacterial sepsis
- Osteomyelitis (due to *Salmonella* spp.)
- Falciparum malaria (in contrast to AS heterozygotes who are resistant to malaria).

Essential note

Excessive alcohol intake, pregnancy and hyposplenic conditions lead to relative immunosuppression, making these groups vulnerable to specific infections

5. MAJOR CLINICAL SYNDROMES

5.1 Respiratory infections

Upper respiratory tract

Clinical symptoms of upper respiratory tract infections

- The common cold (coryza)
- Mastoiditis
- Pharyngitis (± tonsillitis)
- Otitis media
- Sinusitis
- Laryngitis
- Vincent's angina (pseudomembrane formation on tonsils and gums due to *Fusobacterium*)
- Quinsy (peritonsillar abscess)
- Epiglottitis

Both viruses and bacteria may cause infection in these sites but virus infection usually 'prepares the ground' for a bacterial infection to follow.

Viruses responsible for upper respiratory tract infections

- Rhinoviruses
- Coronaviruses
- Adenoviruses
- Parainfluenza viruses
- Coxsackie groups A+B
- Respiratory syncytial virus (RSV)

Bacteria responsible for upper respiratory tract infections

- β haemolytic Group A streptococcus
- *Haemophilus influenzae*
- *Neisseria meningitidis* (usually asymptomatic)
- *Neisseria gonorrhoeae* (as above)
- *Branhamella catarrhalis*
- *Mycoplasma pneumoniae*

Lower respiratory tract

Clinical syndromes include: tracheitis, bronchiolitis, pneumonia, bronchitis and alveolitis.

Organisms responsible for lower respiratory tract infections

- Common

  - *Streptococcus pneumoniae*
  - *Haemophilus influenzae*
  - *Streptococcus pyogenes*
  - *Legionella pneumophila*
  - *Staphylococcus aureus*
  - *Mycoplasma pneumoniae*
  - *Klebsiella pneumoniae*

- Immunocompromised

  - *Pseudomonas* spp.
  - *Pneumocystis*
  - *Aspergillus*
  - CMV

Continued over

Organisms responsible for lower respiratory tract infections

Continued

- **Hospital-acquired pneumonias**

    - Methicillin-resistant *Staphylococcus aureus* (MRSA)
    - *E. coli*
    - *Enterococcus*
    - *Pseudomonas*
    - Coliforms

- **Uncommon**

    - *Chlamydia* spp.
    - *Coxiella burnetii*
    - *Leptospira icterohaemorrhagiae*
    - *Fusobacterium necrophorum*
    - *Salmonella typhi*

- **Viral**

    - RSV
    - Influenza
    - Parainfluenza

5.2 Neurological infections

The brain and spinal cord, despite being well protected from the external environment, are prone to a large range of infections from viruses to helminths. The two main clinical syndromes are meningitis and encephalitis. Routes of access are:

- Haematogenous
- Via skull fractures/direct penetration
- Via the cribriform plate
- Via infected sinuses, mastoids or middle ear
- Via peripheral nerves.

Essential note

The two main clinical syndromes of central neurological infection are meningitis and encephalitis

The **peripheral nerves** tend to be less susceptible to direct bacterial infection (with the exception of leprosy). Most bacterial infections that affect peripheral nerves do so by the action of specific toxins (eg botulinum, diphtheria). Guillain–Barré syndrome may follow several different viral and bacterial infections. A number of viruses (particularly enteroviruses, eg poliovirus) may seriously damage peripheral nerves.

Meningitis

- **Acute bacterial causes**

    - *Common in adults*

        - Meningococcus
        - Pneumococcus
        - *Haemophilus influenzae*

    - *Common in neonates*

        - Group B streptococcus
        - *Escherichia coli*
        - *Listeria monocytogenes*
        - Syphilis

- **Chronic bacterial causes**

    - *Mycobacterium tuberculosis* (mixed lymphocytic and polymorphs)

- **Chronic fungal causes**

    - Cryptococcosis (particularly in the immunosuppressed) produces a lymphocytic meningitis

- **Acute viral causes**

    - Mumps, enteroviruses (eg polio), herpes simplex (mainly type 2), varicella all produce a lymphocytic meningitis.

Encephalitis

- **Viral causes**

    - Herpes simplex (high mortality/morbidity – mainly HSV type 1)
    - Enteroviruses, flaviviruses (eg Japanese encephalitis)
    - Varicella
    - HIV
    - Rabies.

5.3 Gastrointestinal infections

Bowel

The majority of gut infections cause diarrhoea; as a general rule, small bowel infection usually manifests toxin-mediated watery diarrhoea with no blood whilst large bowel infections (with exceptions) are invasive of colonic mucosa and cause bloody diarrhoea with mucus and sometimes pus – 'dysentery'.

Small bowel, toxin-mediated, 'secretory' infective agents

- *Salmonella* spp.
  - Can occasionally be invasive
  - Acquired mainly from eggs and chickens
- Enterotoxigenic *E. coli* (ETEC)
  - Major cause of traveller's diarrhoea
- Some campylobacters
  - With salmonellas account for most acute gastroenteritis in UK.

Large bowel, invasive infective agents

- *Shigella* spp.
- Enteroinvasive *E. coli* (EIEC)
- *Entamoeba histolytica*.

Large bowel, toxin-mediated infective agents

- *Clostridium difficile*
- Enterohaemorrhagic *E. coli* (EHEC)
  - (Typical serotype is O157) – verotoxin secreting; may lead to epidemic form of haemolytic–uraemic syndrome.

HIV-related diarrhoea

Chronic diarrhoea in the immunocompromised may be caused by *Cryptosporidium, Isospora belli, Microsporidium, Cyclospora* and *Mycobacterium avium intracellulare*. See also Chapter 7, Genito-urinary medicine and AIDS.

5.4 Cardiac infections

Infective endocarditis

Streptococcus viridans (40%), *Staphylococcus aureus*, *Enterococcus faecalis* are mainly responsible for native valve endocarditis. However, atypical organisms such as *Coxiella burnetii*, *Chlamydia*, *Legionella* and *Mycoplasma* can all cause endocarditis. Non-bacterial vegetations can also be seen in malignancy, systemic lupus erythematosus (SLE) and atrial myxoma. Bacterial endocarditis is treated with 6 weeks of intravenous therapy and may sometimes require surgical valve replacement.

Myocarditis

The commonest organisms include Coxsackie virus, echovirus, *Mycoplasma pneumoniae*, *Coxiella* and *Chlamydia*. Presentation may be acute heart failure or the patient may remain asymptomatic. Most patients recover fully.

Pericarditis

Coxsackie virus, echovirus, rheumatic fever (*Streptococcus pyogenes*) and *Mycobacterium tuberculosis* can all cause pericarditis. ECGs show widespread concave ST elevation. Echocardiography may show a pericardial fluid collection. Treatment is mainly supportive unless a specific cause is identified.

Essential note

The main cardiac infections are: infective endocarditis, myocarditis and pericarditis

5.5 Specific soft tissue infections

Staphylococcus aureus and *Staphylococcus pyogenes* are mainly responsible for community-acquired soft tissue infection in otherwise healthy patients. The latter is occasionally responsible for **necrotising fasciitis**, which requires aggressive surgical debridement as well as anti-biotics (i.v. cefotaxime, metronidazole and benzyl penicillin). Necrotising fasciitis is alternatively due to mixed **facultative anaerobes and anaerobic streptococci**. Hyperbaric oxygen may be useful in this situation.

Anaerobic soft tissue infection often arises as a complication of severe trauma with destruction of tissue. Human and animal bites may do the same. Dog and cat bites may result in *Pasteurella multocida*. Anaerobes are also the predominant organism in sepsis arising from the gastrointestinal tract, from dental and gum sepsis to peri-anal abscesses.

6. SPECIFIC TROPICAL INFECTIONS

6.1 Malaria

Four species affect humans: *Plasmodium falciparum, P. vivax, P. ovale* and *P. malariae. P. falciparum* is potentially lethal, the others are usually more benign. The acute presentation includes fever, headache, myalgia and arthralgia.

Complications of falciparum malaria

- **Cerebral malaria**: depression of consciousness is the main feature; other neurological syndromes include seizures, focal neurological disorders and acute psychosis.
- **Blackwater fever**: massive intravascular haemolysis – may lead to acute renal failure.
- **Pulmonary oedema**: similar to adult respiratory distress syndrome of Gram-negative sepsis. There is a tendency for capillaries to leak fluid. Mortality is severe (80%).

- **Severe anaemia**: partly due to haemolysis, also marrow suppression.
- **Glomerulonephritis**.
- **Hyper-reactive malarious splenomegaly**: previously known as 'tropical splenomegaly' syndrome.

Treatment of falciparum malaria comprises quinine and doxycycline, or malarone or sulphadoxine pyrimethamine (Fansidar). Chloroquine is the treatment of choice for benign malaria. Due to high levels of resistance around the world it is not used to treat falciparum malaria. Newer drugs such as artemisinin are used when patients have high parasite counts.

Drugs used for prophylaxis include doxycycline, mefloquine, malarone, chloroquine and proguanil.

6.2 Enteric fevers

Both typhoid and paratyphoid are included in this category. Blood cultures are usually positive in the first two weeks of illness, and stool cultures in the second two weeks. The Widal test is unreliable and no longer used.

Quinolones are now the treatment of choice, with most *S. typhi*, particularly from the Indian subcontinent, being chloramphenicol-resistant. High-dose steroids have been shown to be beneficial in fulminant disease, unlike other forms of Gram-negative sepsis.

6.3 Amoebiasis

Amoebiasis is endemic in many tropical areas. It is caused by *Entamoeba histolytica*. Most patients present with mild diarrhoea but severe relapsing diarrhoea or symptoms mimicking an intestinal tumour (amoeboma) can occur. Carrier states exist without obvious clinical illness.

- Diagnosis is by microscopy of fresh warm stool or by serology for invasive disease (colitis or liver abscesses). **Amoebic liver abscesses hardly ever require a drainage procedure whilst pyogenic ones usually do**.
- Treatment comprises metronidazole or tinidazole with diloxanide furoate to eradicate intestinal cyst carriage.

6.4 Schistosomiasis

This causes much morbidity worldwide. The three principal species affecting humans are:

- *Schistosoma mansoni* (bowel and liver)
- *S. haematobium* (urinary tract)
- *S. japonicum* (bowel and liver).

The adult worms tend not to inflict much damage. They release huge numbers of eggs, which make their way through the wall of the blood vessel into the surrounding tissue; the principal pathological feature is a **granuloma around the egg**. Granulomas can cause **obstructive uropathy** or **liver fibrosis** with portal hypertension. **Bladder cancer** is also a well-recognised complication of urinary schistosomiasis. Sometimes the eggs gain access to the pulmonary and systemic circulations with extra consequences such as **pulmonary hypertension**. Diagnosis is by identification of ova in the urine or faeces or in tissue biopsy. Serological diagnosis is a useful alternative. The treatment of choice is praziquantel.

6.5 Leprosy

This is a very indolent inflammatory disease of skin and nerves with a natural history measurable in years. Most infection is subclinical without progression to disease; this can be demonstrated by positive serology in asymptomatic contacts. Only 5% of healthy spouses of lepromatous leprosy patients (the most infective kind) eventually get the disease. Clinical expression in a given patient depends on the degree of T-cell-mediated immune response to *Mycobacterium leprae*. There is a spectrum of clinical expression of the disease from lepromatous (LL), with no measurable T-cell responses, to tuberculoid (TT), with brisk T-cell responses. Diagnosis is by skin biopsy. Treatment comprises rifampicin, dapsone and clofazimine and protective advice (because of anaesthetic feet, hands, etc).

6.6 Cholera

This is an acute diarrhoeal illness transmitted by the faecal–oral route. It is caused by *Vibrio cholerae* which produces an exotoxin. The toxin causes a massive secretion of fluid into the intestine, resulting in profuse watery diarrhoea described as rice water stools. Muscle cramps develop as a result of electrolyte imbalance. Hypovolaemic shock is the commonest cause of death. Management is aggressive replacement of fluid and electrolytes. Administration of doxycycline shortens the duration of the diarrhoea.

Further revision

National Center for Infectious Diseases at http://www.cdc.gov/ncidod/diseases/

World Health Organization at http://www.who.int/en/

The Health Protection Agency at http://www.phls.co.uk/

You should now know that:

1. Notifiable diseases in England and Wales are reported to the Local Health and Protection Agency, with the aim of preventing further spread. Patients with notifiable diseases are isolated and people with whom they have been in contact traced.

2. Routes of transmission for infectious agents are: respiratory, faecal–oral, sexual, congenital, blood-borne, through direct skin contact, insect or animal bite. The outcome of inoculation depends on the size of the inoculum, the virulence of the pathogen and the defence of the host to the infection.

3. Hosts have a variety of defences against infection: first line of defence includes polymorphonuclear neutrophils, which attach to the pathogen and then ingest it to form a phagosome. In the acute phase response, cytokines are recruited to trigger the liver to release C-reactive protein and transferrin, the latter mops up metals, essential for the invading bacteria. The complement system causes lysis, attracts phagocytes to bacteria through opsonisation, attracts leukocytes to the site of infection and promotes the inflammatory response. Later defences include humoral systems (antibody production) and cellular immunity (T-cells destroying infected cells).

4. Antimicrobial drugs are grouped according to the pathogen they destroy. Antibacterial agents are subdivided according to their mode of action; for example, penicillins break the bacterial cell wall whereas quinolones inhibit bacterial DNA synthesis. Other agents are also prescribed to counter infection, such as immunoglobulins and vaccines.

5. In pregnancy, the placenta modulates the mother's immune response to avoid rejecting the fetus. When pregnant, women are more susceptible to various infections, including UTIs, *Listeria*, varicella, candidiasis, pulmonary TB, hepatitis E, HIV, falciparum malaria and *Salmonella*. Excessive alcohol intake makes alcoholics immunosuppressed and neutropenic. They are particularly susceptible to pulmonary TB, *Legionella*, *Klebsiella* and aspiration pneumonia and *Listeria*.

6. Upper respiratory tract infections can be viral and bacterial, with a bacterial infection commonly following on from a viral one. Clinical syndromes include the common cold, mastoiditis, pharyngitis, tonsillitis, otitis media, sinusitis, laryngitis, Vincent's angina, quinsy and epiglottitis. Lower respiratory tract infections lead to tracheitis, bronchiolitis, pneumonia, bronchitis and alveolitis.

7. Four *Plasmodium* species cause malaria, of which *P. falciparum* is potentially lethal. Acute presentation is fever, headache, myalgia and arthralgia. Prophylaxis drugs are available. Enteric fevers include typhoid and paratyphoid, with quinolones being the treatment of choice. Amoebiasis is endemic in many tropical areas. Schistosomiasis is a major cause of morbidity worldwide. Leprosy has a range of clinical expression and most infection is subclinical without progression to disease. Treatment is with dapsone and clofazimine and protective advice. Cholera is an acute diarrhoeal illness, with hypovolaemic shock being the commonest cause of death. Management is fluid and electrolyte replacement therapy.

Metabolic diseases

CONTENTS

Revision objectives

You should:

1. Understand the main disorders of amino acid metabolism
2. Understand the main disorders of purine metabolism
3. Understand the main disorders of metals and metalloproteins
4. Understand the main disorders of lipid metabolism
5. Understand the main disorders of calcium and bone metabolism
6. Have an overview of nutritional and vitamin disorders
7. Have an overview of metabolic acid–base disturbances

1. DISORDERS OF AMINO ACID METABOLISM

Most of the inherited metabolic diseases are mendelian, single-gene defects, transmitted in an autosomal recessive manner. Disease expression requires the affected individual to be homozygous – inheriting a mutant gene from each of their parents, who are both heterozygous for the defect. Although heterozygotes may synthesise equal amounts of normal and defective enzymes, they are usually asymptomatic.

Essential note

Most inherited metabolic diseases are mendelian, autosomal recessive, single-gene defects

- Even the major inborn errors of amino acid metabolism are rare – phenylketonuria, one of the most common, has an incidence of less than 1/10 000.
- Complete penetrance is common and the onset is frequently early in life.
- The consequences of these enzyme deficiencies are varied and frequently multisystem but expression tends to be uniform.

The more common of these conditions are listed in the box below and the major inborn errors of amino acid metabolism are then discussed.

Inborn errors of amino acid metabolism

- Albinism
- Cystinosis
- Homocystinuria
- Maple syrup urine disease
- Phenylketonuria
- Alkaptonuria
- Cystinuria
- Oxalosis

Essential note

The main inborn disorders of amino acid metabolism are alkaptonuria, cystinosis, cystinuria, homocystinuria, oxalosis and phenylketonuria

1.1 Alkaptonuria (ochronosis)

This is a rare autosomal recessive disease with an incidence of 1/100 000. Homogentisic acid accumulates as a result of a deficiency in the enzyme homogentisic acid oxidase. The abnormally high plasma homogentisic acid levels overwhelm the renal tubular transport system resulting in high urinary levels and darkening of the urine on standing because homogentisic acid conversion to alkapton is accelerated in alkaline conditions (alkaptonuria).

- The homogentisic acid polymerises to produce the black–brown product alkapton, which becomes deposited in cartilage and other tissues (ochronosis).
- Classical features include pigmentation of the ears, arthritis, inter-vertebral disc calcification and dark sweat-stained clothing.

1.2 Cystinosis

In cystinosis, cystine accumulates in the reticuloendothelial system, kidneys and other tissues. There is a defect of cystine transport across the lysosomal membrane resulting in widespread intra-lysosomal accumulation of cystine. Unlike cystinuria, stones do not occur in this condition.

Clinical features of cystinosis

- Fanconi syndrome (often with severe hypophosphataemia and consequent vitamin-D-resistant rickets)
- Severe growth retardation
- Lymphadenopathy
- Bone marrow failure
- Corneal opacities and photophobia
- Hypothyroidism
- Central nervous system involvement
- Insulin deficiency resulting in diabetes
- Abnormalities of cardiac conduction

Accumulation of cystine in the renal tubules leads to generalised tubular reabsorptive failure, ie the Fanconi syndrome. This is characterised by defective reabsorption of amino acids, glucose, urate, phosphate, bicarbonate, potassium and a failure to concentrate urine resulting in polyuria and nocturia.

Onset is usually in the first year of life and the renal disease is progressive, often resulting in end-stage renal disease by the age of 10 years. Corneal or conjunctival crystals usually suggest the diagnosis, which can be confirmed by measuring the cystine content of neutrophils.

1.3 Cystinuria

Cystinuria is an autosomal recessive disorder with a prevalence of about 1/7000. The transport of cystine and the other dibasic amino acids lysine, ornithine and arginine is abnormal in the proximal renal tubule and the jejunum.

- Presentation is usually in the second or third decade of life with renal stones.
- Cystine accumulates in the urine. It is highly insoluble at acid pH and this results in the formation of radio-opaque calculi.
- Management involves maintaining a large fluid intake, alkalinisation of urine and D-penicillamine (which chelates cystine and increases its solubility).

The condition cystinosis should not be confused with cystinuria.

1.4 Homocystinuria

This autosomal recessive abnormality results from reduced activity of cystathionine β-synthase. The resulting homocysteine and methionine accumulation interferes with collagen cross-linking resulting in a Marfan-like syndrome.

Clinical features of homocystinuria

- Downward lens dislocation
- Spontaneous retinal detachment
- Osteoporosis
- Venous and arterial thromboses
- Developmental and mental retardation
- Seizures and psychiatric syndromes

1.5 Oxalosis

There are two inborn errors of metabolism that cause overproduction of oxalate, type 1 and type 2. Both are autosomal recessive and can lead to hyperoxaluria with stones and tissue deposition of oxalate.

Clinical features of oxalosis

- Oxalate renal stones
- Bone disease
- Cardiac disease
- Nephrocalcinosis
- Severe arterial disease (due to deposition of oxalate crystals in the vessel wall)

Treatment of oxalosis

This initially involves high fluid intake and the use of pyridoxine. In primary hyperoxaluria type I early diagnosis and pre-emptive isolated liver transplantation can be curative. In patients who already have advanced renal failure, dialysis therapy is appropriate.

1.6 Phenylketonuria (PKU)

The biochemical abnormality is an inability to convert phenylalanine into tyrosine due to lack of phenylalanine hydroxylase. There are several variants of PKU due to different allelic mutations. This results in hyperphenylalaninaemia and increased excretion of its metabolite, phenylpyruvic acid ('phenylketone'), in the urine. Only severe deficiency of the enzyme results in classical PKU with neurological damage. PKU affects between 1:10 000 and 1:14 000 live births.

Clinical features of PKU

- Affects children usually manifesting by 6 months of life
- Eczema
- Mental retardation
- Irritability
- Decreased pigmentation* (pale skin, fair-haired and blue-eyed phenotype)

* This is due to reduced melanin formation

Diagnosis

The Guthrie screening test is a bacterial inhibition assay. Blood from a heel-prick is applied to filter paper that is subsequently incubated with *Bacillus subtilis* in the presence of β-2-thienylalanine (an analogue that inhibits utilisation of phenylalanine).

The amount of bacterial growth is proportional to the phenylalanine concentration in the neonatal blood.

Management

Diet low in phenylalanine, with tyrosine supplementation, in infancy and childhood. PKU females should be advised to reinstitute strict dietary control prior to conception and throughout pregnancy and breast-feeding. Fish oil supplementation can also improve symptoms.

1.7 Other amino acid metabolism disorders

There are many other enzyme defects producing for example alaninaemia, ammonaemia, arginaemia, citrullinaemia, isovaleric acidaemia, lysinaemia, ornithinaemia or tyrosinaemia.

2. DISORDERS OF PURINE METABOLISM

The purine nucleotides adenine and guanine can be synthesised de novo or salvaged from the breakdown of nucleic acids of endogenous or exogenous origin. Uric acid is the product of purine metabolism. Increased de novo synthesis of purines is thought to be responsible, at least partly, for primary gout (described in Chapter 16, Rheumatology). Deficiency of hypoxanthine guanine phosphoribosyl transferase (HGPRT), which is involved in the salvage pathway, results in Lesch–Nyhan syndrome.

Essential note

Uric acid is the product of purine metabolism

Disorders of purine metabolism

- Primary gout (*See also* Chapter 16, Rheumatology)
- Secondary hyperuricaemia
- Lesch–Nyhan syndrome

2.1 Lesch–Nyhan syndrome

Lesch–Nyhan syndrome is an uncommon X-linked recessive disease (therefore seen only in males) due to complete lack of HGPRT. This results in accumulation of both hypoxanthine and guanine, both of which are metabolised to xanthine and subsequently uric acid.

Essential note

Lesch–Nyhan syndrome is only seen in males

Clinical features of Lesch–Nyhan syndrome

- Mental retardation
- Athetosis
- Gout
- Spasticity
- Self-mutilation
- Renal calculi
- Renal failure due to crystal nephropathy

- Neurological manifestations are usually present in early infancy; death from renal failure in adolescence is common.
- Carrier and pre-natal diagnosis is possible by mutation detection and linkage analysis for probands (the original person presenting with a genetic condition) and their families. Biochemical measurement of HGPRT is also possible for at-risk pregnancies.

3. DISORDERS OF METALS AND METALLOPROTEINS

Iron and copper play central roles in the function of a number of metalloproteins, including cytochrome oxidase, which is essential in cellular aerobic respiration; haem, based on iron, is the key molecule in oxygen transport. Excessive accumulation of metals can, however, promote free radical injury (eg Wilson's disease and haemochromatosis), and disorders of haem synthesis leading to overproduction of the intermediate compounds called porphyrins can result in the heterogeneous group of rare inborn errors of metabolism called the porphyrias.

Disorders of metals and metalloproteins

- Wilson's disease
- Haemochromatosis
- Secondary iron overload
- The porphyrias

3.1 Wilson's disease

This autosomal recessive disorder of copper metabolism has a gene frequency of 1/400 and a disease prevalence of approximately 1/200 000. Accumulation of copper in the liver and the basal ganglia results in cirrhosis and degenerative brain disease.

In normal subjects 50% of ingested copper is absorbed and transported to the liver loosely bound to albumin. Here copper is incorporated into caeruloplasmin, which is the principal transport protein for copper, and necessary for biliary excretion. In Wilson's disease copper absorption is normal but intrahepatic formation of caeruloplasmin is defective. Total body and tissue copper levels rise due to failure of biliary excretion, and urinary excretion of copper is increased.

Clinical features of Wilson's disease

- Onset in childhood or adolescence
- Hepatic dysfunction

  - Acute hepatitis
  - Cirrhosis
  - Chronic hepatitis
  - Massive hepatic necrosis

- Hypoparathyroidism
- Haemolysis
- CNS involvement

  - Behavioural problems/psychosis
  - Mental retardation
  - Tremor/chorea
  - Seizures

- Kayser–Fleischer corneal rings

  - Due to copper deposition in Descemet's membrane

- Fanconi syndrome (including type 2 (proximal) renal tubular acidosis)
- Arthropathy

Diagnosis

This is based on a decrease in serum caeruloplasmin and increases in hepatic copper content and urinary excretion of copper. However, biochemical diagnosis is increasingly recognised to have low sensitivity. Molecular diagnosis is now available to identify pre-symptomatic individuals. Serum copper levels are of no diagnostic value.

Essential note

Serum copper levels are of no diagnostic value in Wilson's disease

Management

Early detection permits long-term use of copper chelators (eg penicillamine) to prevent the accumulation of copper. Fulminant hepatic failure and end-stage liver disease necessitate liver transplantation, which is curative (but CNS sequelae may persist). (*See also* Chapter 5, Gastroenterology.)

3.2 Haemochromatosis

Haemochromatosis is an inherited iron overload disease resulting in cirrhosis, diabetes and iron deposition in other organs.

In the normal adult the iron content of the body is closely regulated. Primary (or idiopathic) haemochromatosis is a common autosomal recessive disorder in which iron accumulates in parenchymal cells, leading to damage and fibrosis. Haemosiderin is an insoluble iron protein complex found in macrophages (it is relatively harmless to them) in the bone marrow, liver and spleen. Secondary iron overload, which has many causes, is often referred to as haemosiderosis.

- The gene frequency is 6% and disease frequency 1/220 people, but the severity of the disease seems to vary.
- Males are affected earlier and more severely than females (as menstrual loss/pregnancy protects females).
- Heterozygotes are at greater risk of secondary haemosiderosis than non-carriers if they have a predisposing condition.
- Thirty per cent of patients with cirrhosis develop hepatocellular carcinoma. (*See also* Chapter 5, Gastroenterology.)

Clinical features of haemochromatosis

- Presentation above the age of 40 years
- Hepatomegaly preceding micronodular cirrhosis
- Chondrocalcinosis and pseudogout
- Bronze skin pigmentation
- Diabetes mellitus and (rarely) exocrine pancreas failure
- Hypopituitarism, hypogonadism and testicular atrophy
- Cardiomyopathy and arrhythmias

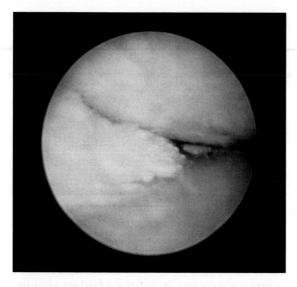

Figure 1 Arthroscope (endoscope) view of a knee affected by pseudogout or chondrocalcinosis

Credit CNRI/SCIENCE PHOTO LIBRARY

Diagnosis

Serum iron is elevated with greater than 60% transferrin saturation. Serum ferritin >500 µg/l. Liver iron concentration >180 µmol/g is also indicative of haemochromatosis. Molecular genetic diagnosis is now available.

Management

- Venesection
- Chelation therapy with desferrioxamine
- Screening of first-degree relatives (serum ferritin)
- Liver transplantation (for end-stage liver disease).

3.3 Secondary iron overload

Secondary haemochromatosis or haemosiderosis is due to iron overload which can occur in a variety of conditions. The pattern of tissue injury is similar to that in primary haemochromatosis. In the inherited haemolytic anaemias iron overload can present in adolescence; the features are often modified by the underlying disease. Treatment is with desferrioxamine.

Secondary causes of iron overload

- Anaemia due to ineffective erythropoiesis
  - Beta-thalassaemia
  - Sideroblastic anaemia
  - Aplastic anaemia
  - Pyruvate kinase deficiency
- Parenteral iron overload
  - Transfusions
  - Iron–dextran
- Liver disease
  - Alcoholic cirrhosis
  - Chronic viral hepatitis
  - Porphyria cutanea tarda
- Increased oral iron intake
  - (Bantu siderosis)

3.4 The porphyrias

The porphyrias are a group of disorders with very different manifestations resulting from the overproduction and accumulation of porphyrins – the intermediate compounds of haem biosynthesis.

Structurally porphyrins consist of four pyrrole rings and are divided into uroporphyrins, coproporphyrins or proto-porphyrins depending on the structure of their side chains. The haem metabolic pathway and the type of porphyria resulting from different enzyme deficiencies are shown in Figure 2. The accumulation of different patterns of porphyrins associated with different enzyme deficiencies results in the distinctive and varied clinical syndromes. (The two most important porphyrias are porphyria cutanea tarda and acute intermittent porphyria – these are described in more detail.)

The porphyrins can be divided by the site and excessive production – the liver (hepatic porphyrias) or bone marrow (erythropoietic porphyrias) – as well as by clinical presentation into acute and non-acute porphyrias.

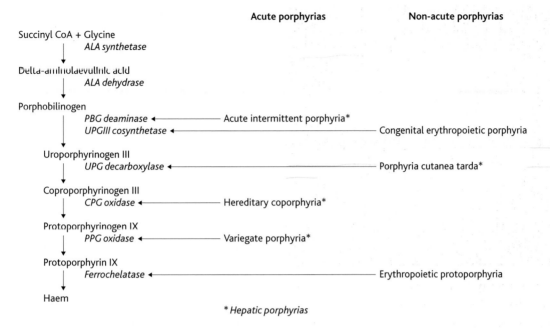

Figure 2 Haem synthesis and the porphyrias

Acute intermittent porphyria

This causes attacks of classical acute porphyria often presenting with abdominal pain and/or neuropsychiatric disorders. It is an autosomal dominant disorder.

- There is reduced hepatic porphobilinogen deaminase activity.
- The gene (and disease) frequency is between 1/10 000 and 1/50 000.
- Episodes of porphyria are more common in females (?due to the effects of oestrogens).
- There is no photosensitivity or skin rash.
- There is increased urinary porphobilinogen and aminolaevulinic acid especially during attacks.
- Urine turns dark red on standing.

Clinical features of acute intermittent porphyria

- Onset in adolescence
- Females more affected
- Polyneuropathy (motor)
- Hypertension and tachycardia
- Episodic attacks
- Abdominal pain, vomiting, constipation
- Neuropsychiatric disorders
- Chronic interstitial nephritis (CIN)

Precipitating drugs:

- Alcohol
- Benzodiazepines
- Rifampicin
- Oral contraceptives
- Phenytoin
- Sulphonamides.

Management

- Supportive: maintain high carbohydrate intake; avoid precipitating factors
- Gonadotrophin-releasing hormone analogues eg to prevent cyclical attacks
- Sertraline and other psychotropic drugs have been used without precipitating acute porphyria, but care is advisable with use of all drugs.

Porphyria cutanea tarda

This is the most common hepatic porphyria. There is a genetic predisposition but the pattern of inheritance is not established. Many sporadic cases are due to chronic liver disease, usually alcohol related.

- There is reduced uroporphyrinogen decarboxylase activity
- Uroporphyrinogen accumulates in blood and urine
- Manifests as photosensitivity rash with bullae.

Porphyria cutanea tarda is the most common hepatic porphyria

Diagnosis

Based on elevated urinary uroporphyrinogen (urine is normal in colour).

Treatment

- The underlying liver disease
- Chloroquine
- Venesection.

4. DISORDERS OF LIPID METABOLISM

Hyperlipidaemia, especially hypercholesterolaemia, is associated with cardiovascular disease.

Table 1 Cholesterol and risk of MI	
Total cholesterol (mmol/l)	Relative risk of myocardial infarct
5.2	1
6.5	2
7.8	4

Although lipid metabolism is complex, and many inherited or acquired disorders can disrupt it, the end result is usually elevated cholesterol and/or triglyceride concentrations. These can be managed by dietary and pharmacological means.

4.1 Lipid metabolism

Cholesterol and triglycerides are insoluble in plasma and circulate bound to lipoproteins. The lipoproteins consist of lipids, phospholipids and proteins. The protein components of lipoproteins are called apolipoproteins (or apoproteins) and they act as cofactors for enzymes and ligands for receptors. A schema of lipoprotein structure is shown in Figure 3.

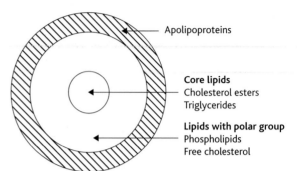

Apolipoproteins

Core lipids
Cholesterol esters
Triglycerides

Lipids with polar group
Phospholipids
Free cholesterol

Figure 3 Schema of lipoprotein structure

There are four major lipoproteins:

- **Chylomicrons**: large particles that carry dietary lipid (mainly triglycerides) from the gastrointestinal tract to the liver. In the portal circulation lipoprotein lipase acts on chylomicrons to release free fatty acids for energy metabolism.
- **Very low density lipoprotein (VLDL)**: carries endogenous triglyceride (60%), and to a lesser extent cholesterol (20%), from the liver to the tissues. The triglyceride core of the VLDL is also hydrolysed by lipoprotein lipase to release free fatty acids. The VLDL remnants are called intermediate density lipoprotein.
- **Low density lipoprotein (LDL)**: is formed from the intermediate density lipoproteins by hepatic lipase. LDL contains a cholesterol core (50%) and lesser amounts of triglyceride (10%). LDL metabolism is regulated by cellular cholesterol requirements via negative feedback control of the LDL receptor.
- **High density lipoprotein (HDL)**: carries cholesterol from the tissues back to the liver. HDL is formed in the liver and gut and acquires free cholesterol from the intracellular pools. Within the HDL, cholesterol is esterified by lecithin cholesterol acyl-transferase (LCAT). HDL is inversely associated with ischaemic heart disease (ie protective).

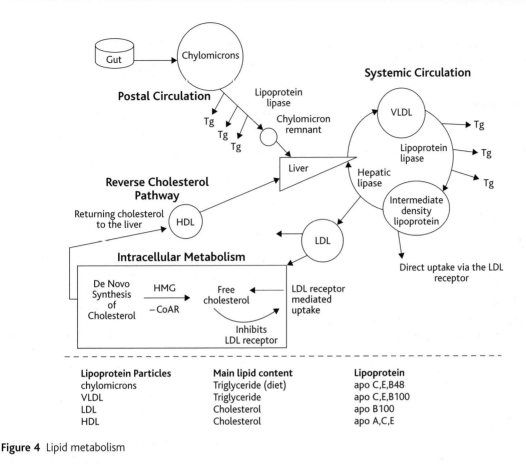

Figure 4 Lipid metabolism

The LDL receptor

Circulating LDL is taken up by the LDL receptor. Cells replete in cholesterol reduce LDL receptor expression. In contrast, inhibition of 3-hydroxy-3-methylglutaryl coenzyme A (HMG CoA) reductase (eg by statins), the enzyme that controls the rate of de novo cholesterol synthesis, leads to a fall in cellular cholesterol and an increase in LDL receptor expression.

Lipoprotein (a)

Lp(a) is a specialised form of LDL. Lp(a) inhibits fibrinolysis and promotes atherosclerotic plaque formation. It is an independent risk factor for ischaemic heart disease.

4.2 The hyperlipidaemias

Population studies have consistently demonstrated a strong relationship between both total and LDL cholesterol and coronary heart disease. HDL is protective. A total cholesterol: HDL ratio of >4.5 is associated with an increased risk. Intervention trials have now established that reduction in LDL cholesterol is associated with improvement in outcome.

Triglycerides are also associated with cardiovascular risk; very high triglycerides are also associated with pancreatitis, lipaemic serum and eruptive xanthomata. Triglycerides must be measured fasting.

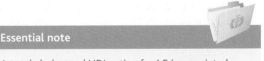

Essential note

A total cholesterol:HDL ratio of >4.5 is associated with increased risk of cardiovascular disease

The primary hyperlipidaemias can be grouped according to the simple lipid profile. Secondary causes of hyperlipidaemia need to be excluded and are discussed later.

Primary hypercholesterolaemia (without hypertriglyceridaemia)

Familial hypercholesterolaemia (FH) is a monogenic disorder resulting from LDL receptor dysfunction.

- There are many different mutations in different families all resulting in LDL receptor deficiency/dysfunction and producing isolated hypercholesterolaemia.
- Heterozygote prevalence is 1/500; these individuals have cholesterol levels of 9–15 mmol/l and sustain myocardial infarctions at about age 40 years (M = F).
- Homozygous FH is rare. Cholesterol levels are in excess of 15 mmol/l and patients suffer myocardial infarction in the second or third decades.
- Other typical clinical features are Achilles tendon xanthomata (can also occur in other extensor tendons) and xanthelasma.

In **polygenic hypercholesterolaemia** the precise nature of the metabolic defect(s) is unknown.

These individuals represent the right-hand tail of the normal cholesterol distribution. They are at risk of premature atherosclerosis. Depressed HDL levels are a risk factor for vascular disease.

Factors modifying HDL levels

- **Decreasing**

  - Familial deficiency of HDL
  - Hyperandrogenic state
  - Post-pubertal males
  - Obesity
  - Hypertriglyceridaemia
  - Diabetes mellitus
  - Sedentary states
  - Cigarette smoking

- **Increasing**

  - Familial hyper-α-lipoproteinaemia
  - Low triglyceride levels
  - Thin habitus
  - Exercise
  - Oestrogens
  - Alcohol

Primary hypertriglyceridaemia (without hypercholesterolaemia)

- **Polygenic hypertriglyceridaemia** is analogous to polygenic hypercholesterolaemia. Some cases are familial but the precise defect is not known. There is elevated VLDL.
- **Lipoprotein lipase deficiency** and **apoprotein CII deficiency** are both rare. They result in elevated triglycerides due to a failure to metabolise chylomicrons.

- These patients present in childhood with eruptive xanthomata, lipaemia retinalis, retinal vein thrombosis, pancreatitis and hepatosplenomegaly.
- Chylomicrons can be detected in fasting plasma.

Primary mixed (or combined) hyperlipidaemia

- **Familial polygenic combined hyperlipidaemia** results in elevated cholesterol and triglycerides.
- The prevalence is 1/200.
- There is premature atherosclerosis.
- **Remnant hyperlipidaemia** is a rare cause of mixed hyperlipidaemia (palmar xanthomas and tuberous xanthomas over the knees and elbows are characteristic). It is associated with apoprotein E_2. There is a high cardiovascular risk.

Secondary hyperlipidaemias are usually mixed but either elevated cholesterol or triglycerides may predominate.

Causes of secondary hyperlipidaemias

- **Predominantly increased triglycerides**

  - Alcoholism
  - Obesity
  - Chronic renal failure
  - Diabetes mellitus
  - Liver disease
  - High-dose oestrogens

- **Predominantly increased cholesterol**

  - Hypothyroidism
  - Renal transplant
  - Cigarette smoking*
  - Nephrotic syndrome
  - Cholestasis

* Cigarette smoking reduces HDL

4.3 Lipid-lowering drugs

Cholesterol and triglyceride levels should be considered in combination with other risk factors. Potential secondary causes of hyperlipidaemia should be corrected.

Dietary intervention can be expected to reduce serum cholesterol by a maximum of 30%. Dietary measures should be continued with pharmacological therapy. Table 2 shows the impact that can be expected with the various agents.

Table 2 Impact of lipid-lowering drugs			
Drug class	*↓LDL (%)*	*↑HDL (%)*	*↓TGs (%)*
HMG CoA reductase inhibitors	20–40	5–10	10–20
Fibric acid derivatives	10–15	15–25	35–50
Bile acid sequestrants	15–30	No change	No change
Nicotinic acid	10–25	15–35	25–30
Fish oil	↑5–10	No change	30–50
Fish oil	↑5–10	No change	30–50

In the majority of cases, hypercholesterolaemia will respond to dietary intervention and statin therapy, and mixed or isolated hypertriglyceridaemia to diet and a fibrate. Ezetimibe reduces cholesterol absorption through the gut, and can be used synergistically with statins in hypercholesterolaemia.

5. DISORDERS OF BONE, MINERAL METABOLISM AND INORGANIC IONS

Bone is a unique type of connective tissue that mineralises. Biochemically it is composed of matrix (35%) and inorganic calcium hydroxyapatite (65%). Bone and mineral homeostasis are tightly regulated by numerous factors, so as to maintain skeletal integrity and control plasma levels.

Essential note

Bone is 35% matrix and 65% inorganic calcium hydroxyapatite

5.1 Calcium homeostasis

Calcium homeostasis is linked to phosphate homeostasis to maintain a balanced calcium phosphate product.

- Hypocalcaemia activates parathyroid hormone (PTH) release to restore serum ionised calcium; other stimuli to PTH release include hyperphosphataemia and decreased vitamin D levels.

- Hypercalcaemia switches off PTH release.
- Vitamin D promotes calcium and phosphate absorption from the GI tract.
- Bone stores of calcium buffer the serum changes.

The metabolism and effects of vitamin D, and the actions of PTH are shown schematically in Figures 5 and 6.

5.2 Hypercalcaemia

In over 90% of cases hypercalcaemia is due to either hyperparathyroidism or malignancy. Hypercalcaemia normally suppresses PTH and so PTH is therefore the best first test to identify the cause of hypercalcaemia – if it is detectable (in or above the normal range) the patient must have hyperparathyroidism.

- Primary hyperparathyroidism is common, especially in women aged 40–60 years. It is usually due to an adenoma of one of the four parathyroid glands.
- PTH-related protein (PTH-rP) is responsible for up to 80% of hypercalcaemia in malignancy.
- PTH-rP acts on the same receptors as PTH and shares the first (N-terminal) 13 amino acids with PTH; however, they are coded from two separate genes.
- Common malignancies secreting PTH-rP are squamous cell lung tumours, and breast and kidney carcinoma.

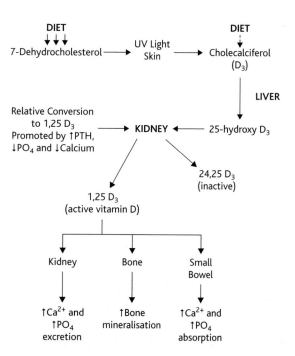

Figure 5 Metabolism and the actions of vitamin D

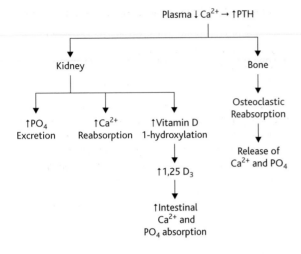

Figure 6 Control and actions of parathyroid hormone (PTH)

Causes of hypercalcaemia

- **Increased calcium absorption**

  - Increased calcium intake
  - Increased vitamin D
  - Sarcoidosis*

- **Increased bone reabsorption**

  - Primary hyperparathyroidism
  - Malignancy
  - Hyperthyroidism

- **Miscellaneous unusual causes**

  - Lithium
  - Thiazide diuretics
  - Addison's disease
  - Phaeochromocytoma
  - Familial hypocalciuric hypercalcaemia
  - Theophylline toxicity
  - Milk-alkali syndrome
  - Vitamin A toxicity

* Sarcoidosis causes hypercalcaemia due to excess production of 1,25-D_3 by macrophages in the sarcoid lesions

The symptoms of hypercalcaemia are often mild but a range of manifestations can occur as shown below.

Clinical manifestations of hypercalcaemia

- Malaise/depression
- Lethargy
- Muscle weakness
- Confusion
- Peptic ulceration*
- Pancreatitis
- Constipation
- Nephrolithiasis
- Nephrogenic diabetes insipidus
- Distal renal tubular acidosis (RTA)
- Renal failure**
- Short QT syndrome
- Band keratopathy
- Diabetes insipidus

   * Peptic ulceration is due to excess gastrin secretion
** Renal failure is due to chronic tubulo-interstitial calcification and fibrosis

The **management** of acute hypercalcaemia (serum calcium >3 mmol/l) involves:

- Adequate rehydration – 3–4 litres saline/day
- Intravenous bisphosphonates (eg pamidronate disodium)
- Identification of the cause, and its subsequent specific treatment (eg corticosteroids for sarcoid) if indicated.

5.3 Hyperparathyroid bone disease

Hyperparathyroidism has a prevalence of about 1/1000. It results in bone resorption due to excess PTH action.

Primary hyperparathyroidism is caused by a single (80% +) or multiple (5%) parathyroid adenomas or by hyperplasia (10%). Parathyroid carcinoma is rare (<2%).

Biochemically there is increased PTH, serum and urinary calcium, reduced serum phosphate and increased alkaline phosphatase. Histologically there is an increase of both osteoblasts and osteoclasts resulting in 'woven' osteoid, increased resorption cavities ('osteatitis fibrosa cystica') and marrow fibrosis. The definitive treatment of primary hyperparathyroidism is by surgical parathyroidectomy.

Secondary hyperparathyroidism is physiological compensatory hypertrophy of all four glands due to hypocalcaemia (eg renal failure, malabsorption). PTH levels are raised, calcium is low or normal. The secondary hyperparathyroidism in renal failure is controlled by phosphate restriction, phosphate binders and with use of 1-α-hydroxylated vitamin D preparations. (*See also* Chapter 12, Nephrology.)

Tertiary hyperparathyroidism is the development of autonomous parathyroid hyperplasia in the setting of long-standing secondary hyperparathyroidism – usually in renal failure. Calcium levels are raised and parathyroidectomy is the only appropriate treatment.

5.4 Hypocalcaemia

Hypocalcaemia is usually secondary to renal failure (increased serum phosphate), hypoparathyroidism or vitamin D deficiency.

Causes of hypocalcaemia

- Decreased calcium absorption

  - Hypoparathyroidism
  - Hypovitaminosis D
  - Malabsorption
  - Sepsis
  - Fluoride poisoning
  - Hypomagnesaemia*

- Acute respiratory alkalosis
- Hyperphosphataemia (by reduction in ionised calcium)

  - Renal failure
  - Phosphate administration
  - Rhabdomyolysis
  - Tumour lysis syndrome

- Deposition of calcium

  - Pancreatitis
  - Hungry bone syndrome (eg after parathyroidectomy)
  - EDTA infusion
  - Rapidly growing osteoblastic metastases

* Cause of functional hypoparathyroidism

Hypoparathyroidism can be spontaneous (autoimmune), post-surgical or due to a receptor defect (pseudo-hypoparathyroidism). Autoimmune hypoparathyroidism may be part of **autoimmune polyglandular failure type I** (mucocutaneous candidiasis, with adrenal, gonadal and thyroid failure).

Vitamin D deficiency can occur in several settings, including:

- dietary deficiency/lack of sunlight
- malabsorption
- renal failure (failure of 1-α-hydroxylation).

The symptoms of hypocalcaemia are mainly those of neuromuscular irritability and neuropsychiatric manifestations. Signs include Chvostek's (tapping the facial nerve causes twitching) and Trousseau's (precipitation of tetanic spasm in the hand by sphygmomanometer-induced ischaemia).

Clinical manifestations of hypocalcaemia

- Neuromuscular

  - Tetany
  - Seizures
  - Confusion
  - Extrapyramidal signs
  - Papilloedema
  - Psychiatric
  - Myopathy
  - Prolonged QT syndrome

- Ectodermal

  - Alopecia
  - Brittle nails
  - Dry skin

- Cataracts
- Dental hypoplasia

The **management** of hypocalcaemia involves:

- Intravenous calcium gluconate if severe (tetany/seizures)
- Oral calcium supplements
- Vitamin D (for hypoparathyroidism, vitamin D deficiency and renal failure)
- Thiazide diuretic and low-sodium diet.

5.5 Osteomalacia

Osteomalacia results from inadequate mineralisation of osteoid. The biochemical features are elevated alkaline phosphatase (95%), hypocalcaemia (50%) and hypophosphataemia (25%). The childhood equivalent is rickets. It is usually caused by a defect of vitamin D availability or metabolism.

Causes of osteomalacia

- Vitamin D deficiency*

  - Dietary
  - Sun exposure
  - Malabsorption
  - Gastrectomy
  - Small bowel disease
  - Pancreatic insufficiency

- Defective 25-hydroxylation

  - Liver disease
  - Anticonvulsant treatment**

- Loss of vitamin D binding protein

  - Nephrotic syndrome

- Defective 1-α-hydroxylation

  - Hypoparathyroidism
  - Chronic renal failure

- Defective target organ response

  - Vitamin-D-dependent rickets (type I)

- Mineralisation defects

  - Abnormal matrix
  - Osteogenesis imperfecta
  - Chronic renal failure
  - Enzyme deficiencies
  - Hypophosphatasia

- Inhibitors of mineralisation

  - Fluoride
  - Aluminium
  - Bisphosphonates

- Phosphate deficiency

  - Decreased GI intake

    - Antacids (reduce absorption)

  - Impaired renal reabsorption

    - Fanconi syndrome
    - X-linked hypophosphataemic rickets (vitamin-D-resistant rickets)

* Asian immigrants in Western countries are at increased risk because melanin in skin decreases D_3 formation; as vegans they may not benefit from dietary vitamin D and certain foods (eg chapattis) bind calcium unmasking vitamin D deficiency

** Especially phenytoin

The **management** of osteomalacia involves:

- Diagnosis and treatment of the underlying disorder
- Vitamin D therapy to correct hypocalcaemia and hypophosphataemia
- Beware iatrogenic hypercalcaemia when alkaline phosphatase begins to fall at the time of bone healing.

5.6 Paget's disease

Paget's disease is a focal (or multifocal) bone disorder characterised by accelerated and disorganised bone turnover resulting from increased numbers and activity of both osteoblasts and osteoclasts. A viral aetiology has not been confirmed.

- Rare in patients aged under 40 years
- Prevalence of 4% over the age of 40 years
- Familial clustering and HLA linkages
- Biochemically characterised by raised alkaline phosphatase, osteocalcin and urinary hydroxyproline excretion.

Paget's disease is usually diagnosed because of asymptomatic sclerotic changes (which can mimic sclerotic bone metastases) but a number of complications can arise.

Clinical manifestations of Paget's disease

- Bone pain
- Secondary arthritis
- Bone sarcoma (rare)
- High output congestive cardiac failure
- Skeletal deformity
- Fractures (and pseudofractures)
- Neurological compression syndromes*
- Hypercalcaemia (only with immobilisation)

* Including deafness, other cranial nerve palsies and spinal stenosis

Treatment is indicated for bone pain, nerve compression, disease impinging on joints and immobilisation hypercalcaemia. Options include:

- Bisphosphonates
- Calcitonin
- Mithramycin
- Surgery.

Causes of a raised bone alkaline phosphatase

- With high calcium

  - Hyperparathyroidism

- With high or normal calcium

  - Malignancy
  - Paget's disease

- With normal calcium

  - Puberty
  - Fracture
  - Osteogenic sarcoma

- With low calcium

  - Osteomalacia

Essential note

Bone loss occurs at about 1% per year after the age of 30

Aetiology of osteoporosis

- Primary

  - Type 1: post-menopausal
  - Type 2: age-related or involutional
  - Osteoporosis of pregnancy

- Secondary

  - Endocrine: premature menopause, Cushing's syndrome, hypopituitarism, hyperparathyroidism, prolactinomas, hypogonadism, hyperthyroidism
  - Drugs: steroids, heparin, ciclosporin A, anticonvulsants
  - Malignancy: multiple myeloma
  - Inflammatory: rheumatoid arthritis*, ulcerative colitis
  - GI: gastrectomy, malabsorption, primary biliary cirrhosis
  - Renal failure
  - Immobilisation: eg space flight
  - Other: osteogenesis imperfecta, homocystinuria, Turner's syndrome (oestrogen deficiency)

- Additional risk factors

  - Race: white/Asian
  - Short stature and low body mass index
  - Positive family history
  - Multiparity
  - Amenorrhoea <6 months (other than pregnancy)
  - Poor calcium and vitamin D intake
  - Excess alcohol and smoking

* In rheumatoid arthritis osteoporosis is multifactorial but corticosteroids and immobility are major contributors

5.7 Osteoporosis

A very common disorder characterised by reduced bone density and increased risk of fracture. The most common form is post-menopausal osteoporosis, which affects 50% of women aged 70. Common sites of fracture are the vertebrae, neck of femur (trabecular bone) and the distal radius and humerus (cortical bone); these fractures may occur with minimal trauma.

Diagnosis is by bone mineral densitometry not plain X-rays. The measured bone density is compared to the mean population peak bone density (ie that of young adults of the same sex) and expressed as the number of standard deviations from that mean, the T score. The bone mineralisation and serum biochemistry are normal.

- T scores down to −1 are regarded as normal
- T scores between −1 and −2.5 represent osteopenia
- T scores below −2.5 are osteoporotic.

Fracture risk

The risk of future fractures is dependent on both bone quality (strength and resilience) and the risk of falling. Fractures increase twofold with each standard deviation of the T score and independently with age by 1.5-fold per decade.

Aetiology

From the age of 30, bone loss occurs at about 1% per year. This is accelerated to about 5% per year in the five years after the menopause. Persistent elevations of parathyroid hormone will accelerate bone loss further. This occurs both in primary hyperparathyroidism but also in secondary hyperparathyroidism arising in vitamin D deficiency, or in negative calcium balance (eg hypocalcaemia, hypercalciuria).

In the absence of a recent fracture, or secondary cause of osteoporosis, bone biochemistry should be normal.

Metabolic diseases

Treatment of osteoporosis

- **General measures**
  - Correct any secondary cause
  - Weight-bearing exercise
  - Adequate dietary calcium and vitamin D intake

- **Other**
  - Fluoride (increases bone density, but can increase peripheral fractures)
  - Calcitonin

- **Specific drug treatments**
  - (These may reduce fractures by approximately 50%)
  - Oestrogens (HRT)
  - Vitamin D
  - Testosterone (in males)
  - Bisphosphonates*

* Prophylaxis with bisphosphonates is now recommended for patients receiving high-dose (eg relapsing nephrotic syndrome) or long-term (eg asthma) steroids

6. NUTRITIONAL AND VITAMIN DISORDERS

In the developed countries the most common nutritional problem is obesity (*see also* Chapter 4, Endocrinology). In contrast, in the developing countries, protein–energy malnutrition is common.

- Body mass index (BMI) = weight (kg) / (height in metres)^2.
- Obesity is defined as a BMI of >30 in males and >28.6 in females.
- Obesity is associated with increased risks of cardiovascular disease, diabetes mellitus, osteoarthritis and gall stones.
- In developed countries the long-term sequelae of fetal and childhood undernutrition are increased cardiovascular disease in adult life.

Essential note

Obesity is the most common nutritional problem in the developed world, whereas it is protein–energy malnutrition in the developing world

---

6.1 Protein–energy malnutrition (PEM)

Starvation is common in the developing world. In the developed countries PEM frequently complicates severe sepsis, cachexia, renal failure and malabsorption. In these circumstances undernutrition is a risk factor for death.

Protein–energy malnutrition in both adults and children can be divided into undernutrition, kwashiorkor and marasmus.

Wellcome Trust classification of protein–energy malnutrition

Weight (% of standard for age)	Oedema present	Oedema absent
60–80	Kwashiorkor*	Undernutrition
<60	Marasmic kwashiorkor	Marasmus

* Kwashiorkor literally means 'disease of the displaced child'

- Marasmus results from severe deficiency of both protein and calories.
- Kwashiorkor results primarily from protein deficiency (ie diet entirely of carbohydrate).
- Oedema is the cardinal sign separating marasmus from kwashiorkor; fatty liver also develops in kwashiorkor.
- Growth failure is more severe in marasmus.

6.2 Vitamin deficiencies

Multiple vitamin deficiencies frequently accompany PEM.

Isolated or grouped vitamin deficiencies (for example, of fat-soluble vitamins) can also occur in specific circumstances.

Table 3 Vitamin deficiencies

Vitamin	Causes of deficiency	Roles of vitamin	Deficiency syndromes
A	Severe PEM*	Component of visual pigment Maintenance of specialised epithelia	Night blindness Xerophthalmia** Follicular hyperkeratosis Keratomalacia***
D	Vegans[†] Elderly with poor diet Renal failure	Absorption of calcium and phosphate Bone mineralisation	Rickets Osteomalacia
E	Severe (near total) fat malabsorption[††] Abetalipoproteinaemia	Antioxidant Scavenger of free radicals	Spino-cerebellar degeneration
K	Oral antibiotics[‡] Biliary obstruction	Cofactor in carboxylation of coagulation cascade factors	Bleeding tendency

*   Although vitamin A is fat-soluble and deficiency can occur in any chronic malabsorptive state, this is rare unless there is severe protein-energy malnutrition
**   Xerophthalmia – dryness of the cornea
*** Keratomalacia – corneal ulceration and dissolution
[†]   Vitamin D_3 is produced in the skin by photoactivation of 7-dehydrocholesterol. If sun exposure is sufficient, dietary vitamin D is not essential
[††] Vitamin E deficiency is rare. It can complicate biliary atresia. In abetalipoproteinaemia (see earlier section) chylomicrons cannot be formed
[‡]   Antibacterial drugs interfere with the bacterial synthesis of vitamin K

Table 4 Deficiencies of water soluble vitamins

Vitamin	Causes of deficiency	Roles of vitamin	Deficiency syndromes
Vitamin B_1* (thiamine)	Alcoholism Dietary	Nerve conduction Coenzyme in decarboxylation	Dry beri-beri – symmetrical polyneuropathy Wernicke–Korsakoff syndrome Wet beri-beri** – peripheral vasodilatation, heart failure
Vitamin B2 (riboflavin)	Severe PEM***	Enzyme cofactor	Angular stomatitis Glossitis Corneal vascularisation
Niacin (nicotinic acid)	Carcinoid syndrome Alcoholism Low-protein diets Isoniazid[†]	Incorporated into NAD and NADP	**Pellagra** – dermatitis, diarrhoea and dementia (the three Ds)
Vitamin B_6[††] (pyridoxine)	Isoniazid Hydralazine	Enzyme cofactor	Peripheral neuropathy Dermatitis Glossitis

Continued over

Table 4 Deficiencies of water soluble vitamins (*continued*)

Vitamin	Causes of deficiency	Roles of vitamin	Deficiency syndromes
Vitamin B$_{12}$ (cyano-cobalamin)	Pernicious anaemia Post-gastrectomy Vegan diet Terminal ileal disease Blind loops	Coenzyme for DNA synthesis; coenzyme in myelin metabolism	Pernicious anaemia Subacute combined degeneration of the spinal cord
Vitamin C‡	Dietary	Redox reactions	Scurvy – bleeding, joint swelling, hyperkeratotic hair follicles, gingivitis

*   Thiamine deficiency is confirmed by reduced red cell transketolase activity
**   In alcoholics, wet beri-beri must be distinguished from alcoholic cardiomyopathy
*** Riboflavin deficiency usually occurs in association with multiple deficiencies
†   Isoniazid can lead to deficiency of pyridoxine which is needed for the synthesis of nicotinamide from tryptophan
††   Dietary deficiency of pyridoxine is extremely rare
‡   Deficiency of vitamin C is confirmed by low white cell (buffy coat) ascorbic acid levels

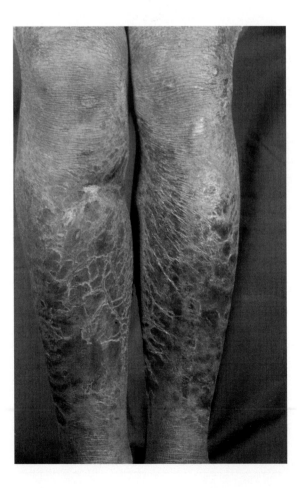

Figure 7 The cracked and inflamed skin of the legs of a patient with pellagra

Credit CNRI/SCIENCE PHOTO LIBRARY

7. METABOLIC ACID–BASE DISTURBANCES (NON-RENAL) AND HYPOTHERMIA

The kidneys and the lungs are intimately involved in the regulation of hydrogen ion concentration. Metabolic acid–base disturbances arise from abnormalities in the regulation of bicarbonate and other buffers in the blood. Acidosis results from an increase in hydrogen ion concentration and alkalosis from a fall in H$^+$. pH is the negative logarithm of H$^+$ – a small change in pH represents a large change in H$^+$ concentration – this is often poorly appreciated in clinical practice.

7.1 Metabolic acidosis
The metabolic acidoses are conveniently divided on the basis of the anion gap:

$$\text{Anion gap} = Na^+ + K^+ - (Cl^- + HCO_3^-).$$

The normal anion gap is 10–18 mmol/l and represents the excess of negative charge (unmeasured anions) present on albumin, phosphate, sulphate and other organic acids.

Relationship of metabolic acidosis to anion gaps

- Normal anion gap

  - Diarrhoea (or other GI loss)
  - Renal tubular acidosis
  - (Ureterosigmoidostemy (form of urinary diversion procedure – see below))

- Increased anion gap

  - Lactic acidosis
  - Ketoacidosis
  - Renal failure
  - Hepatic failure
  - Ingestion of methanol, aspirin, toluene, alcohol

Essential note

In clinical practice, remember that a small change in pH represents a large change in H+ concentration

Specific metabolic acidoses

Metabolic acidosis with diarrhoea

The gastrointestinal secretions (below the stomach) are relatively alkaline and have a high potassium concentration. There is usually hypokalaemia, low urinary potassium loss (<25 mmol/l) and low urine pH (<5.5). Causes include:

- Villous adenoma
- Enteric fistula
- Obstruction
- Laxative abuse.

Metabolic acidosis with ureteric diversion

This results in hyperchloraemic acidosis in 80% of ureterosigmoid diversions. The mechanism is due to urinary chloride exchange for plasma bicarbonate which is then lost in the urine.

Metabolic acidosis accompanying poisoning

Metabolic acidosis often accompanies poisoning (eg toluene, ethylene glycol, salicylates, paracetamol). These are covered in detail in Chapter 2, Clinical Pharmacology, Toxicology and Poisoning.

7.2 Metabolic alkalosis

Metabolic alkalosis is less common than metabolic acidosis because metabolic processes produce acids as by-products, and also because renal excretion of excess bicarbonate is very efficient.

Metabolic alkaloses

- Gastrointestinal hydrogen ion loss

  - Vomiting/pyloric stenosis
  - Nasogastric suction
  - Antacids (in renal failure)

- Intracellular shift of hydrogen ion

  - Hypokalaemia

- Alkali administration
- Renal hydrogen ion loss

  - Mineralocorticoid excess
  - Loop or thiazide diuretics
  - Post-hypercapnic alkalosis
  - Hypercalcaemia and the milk–alkali syndrome

- Contractional alkalosis

  - Volume depletion

Specific metabolic alkaloses

Gastric loss of hydrogen ions

In protracted vomiting (eg pyloric stenosis) or nasogastric suction there can be complete loss of up to three litres of gastric secretions per day. The gastric secretions contain:

- Hydrogen ion: 100 mmol/l
- Potassium: 15 mmol/l
- Chloride: 140 mmol/l.

Alkalosis will result but, paradoxically, acid urine is produced due to renal tubular sodium bicarbonate reabsorption to maintain plasma volume. Patients respond to volume expansion with normal saline and correction of hypokalaemia.

Milk–alkali syndrome

This is defined as the triad of hypercalcaemia, metabolic acidosis and ingestion of large amounts of calcium with absorbable alkali (traditionally for peptic ulcer pain). The hypercalcaemia increases renal bicarbonate reabsorption exacerbating the alkalosis. Clinical presentation is with symptoms of hypercalcaemia or metastatic calcification.

7.3 Hypothermia

Hypothermia is defined as a fall in core temperature to below 35°C. It is frequently fatal if the core temperature falls below 32°C.

Mild hypothermia (32–35°C) causes shivering and intense feeling of cold.

Severe hypothermia (<32°C) causes impairment in judgement and reduced awareness of the cold.

- **Clinical features of hypothermia**: include bradycardia, hypoventilation, muscle stiffness, hypotension and loss of reflexes. The pupils can be fixed and dilated in recoverable hypothermia.
- **Metabolic acidosis**: due to lactate accumulation is common, pancreatitis can complicate hypothermia.
- **Electrocardiograph changes**: include J waves, prolonged PR interval, prolonged QT and QRS complexes. Death results from ventricular arrhythmias or asystole.

Causes of hypothermia

- Elderly with inadequate heating
- Hypothyroidism
- Immersion in cold water
- Alcoholism
- Hypoglycaemia
- Exposure to low external temperatures (eg unconscious patients, mountaineers, etc)

Essential note

Hypothermia is frequently fatal if core temperature falls below 32°C

Further revision

Metabolic and Endocrine Disease Information Service at http://www.endocrine.niddk.nih.gov/

Metabolic Disease at patient UK at http://www.patient.co.uk/showdoc/431

Diabetes UK at http://www.diabetes.org.uk/

Revision summary

You should now know that:

1. The main disorders of amino acid metabolism include alkaptonuria, cystinosis, cystinuria, homocystinuria, oxalosis, phenylketonuria and others related to enzyme defects. Most of the inherited metabolic diseases are autosomal recessive, single-gene defects.
2. Disorders of purine metabolism include primary gout, secondary hyperuricaemia and Lesch–Nyhan syndrome.
3. Disorders of metals and metalloproteins include Wilson's disease, haemochromatosis, secondary iron overload and the porphyrias. Wilson's disease is an autosomal recessive disorder of copper metabolism resulting in copper accumulation in the liver and basal ganglia, hence the symptoms of cirrhosis and brain disease. Haemochromatosis is an inherited iron overload, resulting in cirrhosis, diabetes and iron deposition. The porphyrias result from overproduction and accumulation of porphyrins, which are intermediates in haem biosynthesis. Subtypes of porphyria are classed according to the site of overproduction (the liver or bone marrow) and by clinical presentation (acute and non-acute). They include: acute intermittent porphyria and porphyria cutanea tarda.
4. Hyperlipidaemia, especially hypercholesterolaemia, is associated with cardiovascular disease. Dietary and pharmacological means are used to manage the disorders. There are four lipoproteins: chylomicrons, very low density lipoproteins (VLDL), low density lipoprotein (LDL) and high density lipoprotein (HDL). There is a strong relationship between total and LDL cholesterol and coronary heart disease. HDL is protective. Triglycerides are associated with increased cardiovascular risk. Very high levels are associated with pancreatitism, lipaemic serum and eruptive xanthomata. Primary hyperlipidaemias are grouped according to lipid profile. Lipid-lowering drugs are used in management, along with dietary modification.

5. Calcium and phosphate homeostasis are linked, and controlled through vitamin D and parathyroid hormone. Most (>90%) hypercalcaemia is due to hyperparathyroidism or malignancy. Hypocalcaemia is usually secondary to renal failure, hypoparathyroidism or vitamin D deficiency. Osteomalacia (softening of the bones) is caused by inadequate mineralisation; the childhood equivalent is rickets. Paget's disease is a focal bone disorder of accelerated or disorganised bone turnover. Osteoporosis is very common and is characterised by reduced bone density and increased fracture risk.

6. In the developed world the most common nutritional problem is obesity. In the developing world, it is protein–energy malnutrition (PEM). PEM comprises undernutrition, kwashiorkor (protein deficiency) and marasmus (deficiency of protein and calories).

Oedema is the cardinal sign separating marasmus from kwashiorkor. Growth failure is more severe in marasmus.

7. The kidneys and the lungs are intimately involved in the regulation of hydrogen ion concentration. Metabolic acid–base disturbances come about through abnormal regulation of bicarbonate and other buffers. A small change in pH represents a large change in hydrogen ion concentration! The metabolic acidoses are grouped according to the anion gap ($=Na^+ + K^+ - (Cl^- + HCO_3^-)$), which is normally 10–18 mmol/l. The anion gap represents excess negative charge on albumin, phosphate, sulphate and other organic acids. Metabolic alkalosis is less common than acidosis and causes include gastric loss of hydrogen ions and milk–alkali syndrome.

Nephrology

CONTENTS

Nephrology

1. RENAL PHYSIOLOGY

The chief functions of the kidneys are:

- Excretion of water-soluble waste
- Maintenance of electrolyte balance
- Maintenance of water balance
- Acid–base homeostasis
- Endocrine: renin–angiotensin–aldosterone system, erythropoietin, vitamin D activation.

1.1 Glomerular filtration rate (GFR)

Glomerular filtration is a passive process which depends upon the net hydrostatic pressure acting across the glomerular capillaries, countered by the oncotic pressure, and also influenced by the intrinsic permeability of the glomerulus (K_f). The mean values for GFR in normal young adults are 130 ml·min^{-1}·1.73 m^{-2} (men) and 120 ml·min^{-1}·1.73 m^{-2} (women), the 1.73 m^2 being mean body surface area of young adults. However, variation between individuals is large and accepted ranges of GFR at this age are 70–140 ml·min^{-1}·1.73 m^{-2}. In health, GFR remains stable until around 40 years of age but thereafter declines at a rate of approximately 1 ml·min^{-1}·year^{-1}; by the age of 80 years the mean GFR is approximately 50% of that of a young adult.

Modification of Diet in Renal Disease

Essential note

The mean values for GFR in normal young adults are 130 ml·min^{-1}·1.73 m^{-2} (men) and 120 ml·min^{-1}·1.73 m^{-2} (women)

There are several means of calculating GFR:

- **Plasma creatinine**: creatinine is produced from muscle cells at a constant rate, and so its plasma concentration at steady state depends upon its excretion, which reflects GFR. Plasma creatinine is therefore useful to crudely assess GFR. However, when renal function is well preserved, small changes in creatinine are associated with large changes in GFR, and so plasma creatinine is an insensitive marker of early renal disease. Note that the elderly and malnourished patients may have low GFR but plasma creatinine close to the normal range.
- **Creatinine clearance**: usually calculated from a 24-hour urine collection with a consecutive blood sample. This tends to overestimate GFR, as creatinine is not just filtered but also secreted into the tubule from the post-glomerular circulation; the error increases with declining renal function.
- **Estimated GFR**: the **Cockcroft and Gault formula** and **MDRD equation** are two commonly used methods for estimating GFR, based upon sex, age and serum creatinine (and weight with the former method).

The most accurate laboratory techniques for assessing GFR are:

- **Inulin clearance**: inulin is a small molecule, freely filtered by the glomerulus, and with no tubular secretion.
- **Chromium-labelled EDTA**: the most frequently used isotopic technique.

1.2 Tubular physiology

The renal tubule has many reabsorptive and secretory functions (Figure 1); these are energy-consuming and hence tubular cells are those most vulnerable to ischaemic damage (*see* Section 4, acute tubular necrosis (ATN) of ischaemic acute renal failure).

Proximal tubule

Fifty percent of filtered sodium is reabsorbed within the proximal tubule (via Na K ATPase); 90% of bicarbonate, some chloride and all filtered glucose and amino acids are reabsorbed here. Other important characteristics are:

- Phosphate reabsorption occurs under the influence of parathormone (PTH)
- Creatinine and urate are secreted into the lumen.

Loop of Henle

The medullary concentration gradient is generated here; the medullary thick ascending limb (mTAL) is impermeable to water. Forty percent of sodium is reabsorbed here (via the Na K 2Cl co-transporter) – inhibited by loop diuretics.

Distal tubule

In this segment of the nephron 5% of sodium is reabsorbed (Na Cl co-transporter) – inhibited by thiazide diuretics.

Collecting duct

Aldosterone-sensitive sodium channels are responsible for 2% of all sodium reabsorption; spironolactone binds to the cytoplasmic aldosterone receptor. Other important collecting duct functions include:

- H^+ secreted into lumen by H-ATPase, so forming ammonia/NH_4^+ (acidifying the urine)
- Antidiuretic hormone (ADH, or vasopressin) increases water reabsorption by opening 'water channels' via insertion of **aquaporins** into the luminal membrane. The aquaporins then allow water uptake by the cell.

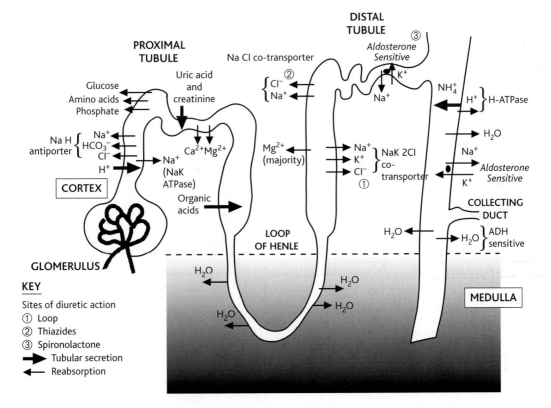

Figure 1 Schema of a nephron showing tubular physiology

Essential note

The kidney has four main non-endocrine functions: waste excretion, electrolyte balance, water balance and acid–base homeostasis

1.3 Renal endocrine function

The kidney is involved in three important endocrine functions – the metabolism of vitamin D, and the secretion of erythropoietin and renin. The first two functions are described later in this chapter.

Renin–angiotensin–aldosterone (RAA) system

This is covered in Chapter 4, Endocrinology. The RAA system has a central role in the pathogenesis of many cases of secondary renal hypertension. Intra-renal perfusion becomes critically dependent upon the RAA when hypovolaemia and hypotension supervene; this explains why patients can be vulnerable to acute renal failure induced by angiotensin converting enzyme (ACE) inhibitors (or angiotensin II receptor blocker, AIIRB) even in the absence of renovascular disease (*see* Endocrinology, Figure 3).

- Angiotensin II is also of key importance in the pathogenesis of progressive renal disease, irrespective of the primary disease aetiology (*see* section 5, Chronic renal failure (chronic kidney disease) and renal replacement therapy).
- Angiotensin is not only a vasoconstrictor – it also stimulates scarring and, indirectly (due to hyperfiltration), further nephron loss within damaged renal tissue.
- This is the reason why ACE inhibitors and/or AIIRBs are now considered to be essential therapy in patients with a variety of chronic nephropathies.

Essential note

The kidney has three important endocrine functions: the metabolism of vitamin D and the secretion of erythropoietin and renin

2. RENAL INVESTIGATION

2.1 Urinalysis

Urinary dipstick

Standard dipsticks assess the presence of protein, blood and glucose. 'Multi-stix' will also assess pH and leukocytes.

- The sticks register positive for 'blood' in the presence of erythrocytes, as well as free myoglobin (e.g. in rhabdomyolysis) and haemoglobin. Many cases of 'dipstick +ve, microscopy –ve (absence of red cells on midstream urine, MSU) haematuria' are seen, and these are presumably due to haemoglobinuria (eg exercise, low-grade haemolysis).
- Standard dipsticks do not detect Bence–Jones proteins, and so if free urinary light chains are to be identified immunoelectrophoresis of urine is necessary.
- Microalbuminuria (see below) may also not be detected.

Proteinuria

Normal urinary protein excretion is <150 mg/day, and this consists of <30 mg albumin, tubular secreted proteins (40–60 mg) such as the Tamm–Horsfall or tubular glycoprotein and immunoglobulin, and various filtered low-molecular-weight proteins.

- **Microalbuminuria**, which is the hallmark of early diabetic nephropathy but which is also prognostically important when present in hypertensive patients, is defined as albumin excretion of 30–300 mg/day.
- The urinary **albumin (mg):creatinine (mmol) excretion ratio (ACR)** is often used to quantify proteinuria in clinical practice – normal ACR <3.3, microalbuminuric range 3.3–33, nephrotic range >400.

Significant non-nephrotic proteinuria (eg dipstick + to +++, 0.2–3.5 g/24 h) is usually indicative of renal parenchymal disease (unless due to urinary tract infection). **Nephrotic** range proteinuria (>3.5 g/24 h, dipstick ++++) is always due to glomerular disease.

Non-renal causes of proteinuria:

- Fever
- Severe exercise
- Skin disease (eg severe exfoliation, psoriasis)
- Lower urinary tract infection (eg cystitis).

Orthostatic proteinuria

This describes proteinuria detectable after the patient has spent several hours in the upright posture; it disappears after recumbency, and so the first morning urine should test negative. Proteinuria is usually <1 g/24 h, there is no haematuria and renal function and blood pressure are normal. Renal biopsy samples are usually normal and nephrological consensus suggests this is a benign condition.

Urine microscopy

Microscopic examination of a fresh specimen of urine may yield many helpful pointers to intrinsic renal pathology.

- **Red cells**: >2–3/high-power field is pathological (microscopic haematuria)
- **Leukocytes**: infection, and some cases of glomerular and interstitial nephritis
- **Crystals**: eg with polarised light, uric acid
- **Casts**: there are several types of cast:
  - *Tubular cells* – acute tubular necrosis (ATN) or interstitial nephritis
  - *Hyaline* – Tamm–Horsfall glycoprotein (ie in normals)
  - *Granular* – non-specific
  - *Red cell* – glomerulonephritis or tubular bleeding
  - *Leukocytes* – pyelonephritis or ATN.

Causes of urinary discoloration

- Haematuria
- Myoglobinuria (brown)
- Beetroot consumption
- Alkaptonuria (urine brown on exposure to the air)
- Obstructive jaundice (yellow)
- Haemoglobinuria
- Drugs (eg rifampicin, para-aminosalicylic acid)
- Porphyria (urine dark brown or red on standing)

Essential note

Methods of urinalysis include measurement of protein, blood and glucose by dipstick, and visual inspection by light microscopy

2.2 Renal radiology

The essential first-line radiological investigation for acute (ARF) or chronic (CRF) renal failure, and most other nephrological conditions, is **renal ultrasound**. This will demonstrate:

- **Bipolar renal length**: in most cases of **CRF**, the kidneys are small (<8 cm) – the exceptions are polycystic kidney disease (very large with multiple cysts), and sometimes in diabetes and amyloid (normal size). In **ARF** the kidneys

are usually normal size (8.5–13.5 cm), but slight enlargement is common due to swelling. Asymmetry (>1.5 cm disparity) is seen in unilateral renal artery stenosis (RAS), but also in chronic pyelonephritis and other causes of renal atrophy

- **Obstruction**
- **Cortical scarring**: for example in reflux nephropathy or following segmental ischaemic damage
- **Calculi**: within the substance of the kidney and collecting systems
- **Mass lesions and cysts**: (eg renal tumour, polycystic disease or simple renal cysts).

Intravenous urography (IVU) is reserved for investigation of urinary tract bleeding (eg to detect urothelial tumours of the renal pelvis, ureters and bladder), urinary tract infection (UTI) and for some cases of obstructive uropathy. IVU can exacerbate ARF (*see* section 4.3 Radio-contrast nephropathy), and has very limited value in advanced CRF (eg creatinine >250 µmol/l) because of poor concentration of the dye.

Isotope renography

Two major types of renograms are commonly utilised:

- **Static scans (eg DMSA)**: demonstrates aspects of structure (eg scars in reflux nephropathy) and split function of the two kidneys.
- **Dynamic scans (eg MAG$_3$, DTPA, Hippuran)**: such scans are used to assess renal blood flow, split function and also to investigate obstruction (eg to show whether urinary tract dilatation is due to obstruction).

Renal angiography

The most frequently used techniques are **MR angiography (MRA)** (non-invasive – non-nephrotoxic gadolinium is used as the 'contrast' agent) and **CT angiography (CTA)** (risk of contrast nephropathy in renal impairment). Conventional **intra-arterial angiography** is invasive and now less frequently used.

Renal tract CT and MR

These imaging modalities are commonly used in nephro-urology in the investigation of many conditions including obstruction and masses.

Essential note

Imaging techniques used in renal investigation include ultrasound, intravenous urography (IVU), renal angiography (MRA and CTA) and CT or MR

3. ACID–BASE, WATER AND ELECTROLYTE DISORDERS

3.1 Acidosis and alkalosis

Respiratory acidosis (eg carbon dioxide retention due to chronic or acute-on-chronic lung disease) and alkalosis (eg due to hyperventilation) are common. Metabolic alkalosis and metabolic acidosis are covered in detail in Chapter 11, Metabolic diseases. The width of the anion gap can help differentiate the likely causes of a metabolic acidosis; the HCO_3 will be low, and the anion gap can be either wide (normal chloride and exogenous acid) or normal (increased chloride and, hence, hyperchloraemic acidosis). Renal failure is associated with a wide gap acidosis (due to excess ammonia and organic acids), whereas renal tubular acidosis is worth consideration as a cause of a normal gap acidosis.

> **Essential note**
>
> Renal failure is associated with wide gap acidosis; renal tubular acidosis can cause normal gap acidosis

3.2 Renal tubular acidosis (RTA)

Distal or type 1 RTA (due to impaired urinary acidification) is fairly common, and can complicate many renal parenchymal disorders, particularly those which predominantly affect the medullary regions. Proximal or type 2 RTA (due to failure of bicarbonate reabsorption in the proximal tubule) is uncommon. GFR is usually normal in both conditions. The two types of RTA can be differentiated by several parameters, but the hallmark associations are severe acidosis, hypokalaemia and renal calculi/nephrocalcinosis in distal RTA, and proximal tubular dysfunction, osteomalacia/rickets and less severe acidosis in proximal RTA.

- **Nephrocalcinosis and renal calculi formation**: urinary calcium excretion is increased in severe acidosis, and calcium salts are more insoluble in alkaline urine, and hence calculi develop frequently in distal but not in proximal RTA (which is usually associated with a lower urinary pH and less severe acidosis).

Treatment

This is usually straightforward (compared to an understanding of the condition!), and consists of oral potassium and bicarbonate replacement therapy. Close monitoring is needed to prevent major imbalances in electrolyte concentrations, especially during inter-current illness.

3.3 Polyuria

Polyuria (urine output >3 litres/day) may result from:

- Diuretic usage
- Large fluid intake (eg alcohol – inhibits ADH release)
- Cranial diabetes insipidus: osmolality high
- Nephrogenic diabetes insipidus: osmolality high; note that the polyuria (often manifest as nocturia) is often the first symptom of CRF
- Psychogenic polydipsia: osmolality usually low
- Atrial natriuretic peptide release: post-arrhythmia, cardiac failure.

The causes of cranial and nephrogenic diabetes insipidus are listed in Chapter 4, Endocrinology; hyponatraemia as well as other disorders of water balance, including syndrome of inappropriate ADH (SIADH), are also discussed in that chapter.

> **Essential note**
>
> Polyuria is often the first symptom of chronic renal failure

3.4 Hypokalaemia

Acute hypokalaemia can lead to muscle weakness and direct renal tubular cell injury (vacuolation). Chronic hypokalaemia is a cause of interstitial nephritis. The causes can be classified according to the presence or absence of hypertension with reference also to the plasma renin activity and urinary potassium excretion.

Causes of hypokalaemia	
With hypertension	**Without hypertension**
Common	*Common*
Renovascular disease	Diuretic usage
Primary hyperaldosteronism (including Conn's syndrome)	Gastro-intestinal tract losses
	Secondary hyperaldosteronism (eg cardiac or hepatic failure)
Rare	*Rare*
Cushing's syndrome	Bartter's syndrome
Renin-secreting tumour	Gitelman syndrome
Liquorice excess	
Liddle's syndrome (see text)	

Bartter's syndrome

Severe hypokalaemia is consequent upon a salt-wasting state (increased sodium delivery to the distal tubule) that is due to defective chloride reabsorption in the loop of Henle. Patients have normal or low blood pressure and severe hyper-reninaemia (with hypertrophy of the juxtaglomerular apparatus) with consequent hyperaldosteronism; GFR is usually normal.

4. ACUTE RENAL FAILURE

4.1 Pathogenesis and management of acute renal failure

Acute deterioration of renal function is seen in up to 5% of all hospital admissions. The incidence of severe ARF (eg creatinine >500 µmol/l) increases with age.

Clinical presentation

Patients usually present soon after the precipitating insult with symptoms and signs relating to failure of one or more of the four non-endocrine functions of the kidneys:

- **Waste excretion**: rapid build up of waste products of metabolism (eg urea) is associated with nausea, vomiting and encephalopathic features (confusion, flapping tremor and fits if very severe).
- **Electrolyte balance**: hyperkalaemia may be manifest by bradycardia, with the risk of asystole.
- **Water balance**: oliguria is usual, and is defined as a daily urine output of <400–500 ml; this is the minimum volume to enable excretion of the daily waste products of metabolism. Patients may be overloaded and breathless due to pulmonary oedema. Non-oliguric ARF occurs in 10%; this may be associated with drug toxicity (eg gentamicin) and radio-contrast nephropathy.
- **Acid–base homeostasis**: failure of excretion of acid leads to metabolic acidosis which can result in encephalopathy.

The majority (55%) of cases of ARF result from renal hypoperfusion and ischaemic damage; the resulting renal histopathological lesion is **acute tubular necrosis (ATN)**. Many other patients may have similar ischaemic insults to the kidneys, with an initial period of oliguria, but renal perfusion can then be restored by vigorous haemodynamic management before severe tubular injury ensues; this is termed **pre-renal uraemia** and most cases can be managed without dialysis. In the latter, physiological mechanisms (ie stimulation of the RAA system) are preserved within the kidney, and so the urinary manifestations of sodium and water reabsorption allow differentiation from established ATN. In practice,

the two conditions may be differentiated only by the clinical response to fluid resuscitation – patients with ATN will remain oliguric, whereas those with pre-renal uraemia will usually start diuresing.

Urinary findings	ATN	Pre-renal uraemia
Urine sodium	>40 mmol/l	<20 mmol/l
Urine:plasma osmolality	<1.1:1	>1.5:1
Urine:plasma urea	<7:1	>10:1
Urine volume	Oligo-anuric or polyuria (in the recovery phase)	<1.5 litres

Essential note

Patients with acute tubular necrosis usually remain oliguric following fluid resuscitation, whereas patients with pre-renal uraemia will usually respond with a diuresis

Many patients with pre-existing chronic renal impairment or CRF present with acute deterioration of renal function (**'acute-on-chronic renal failure'**) and require similarly intensive support and clinical management.

The causes of ARF, with approximate relative frequency, are summarised below.

Classification of ARF

- **Pre-renal factors leading to renal hypoperfusion and ATN (55%)**

  - Reduced circulating volume: blood loss; excess GI losses; burns
  - Low cardiac output states: toxic or ischaemic myocardial depression
  - Systemic sepsis
  - Drugs inducing renal perfusion shutdown (eg ACE inhibitors; non-steroidal anti-inflammatory drugs (NSAIDs))

- **Toxic ATN (5%)**

  - Rhabdomyolysis with urinary myoglobin
  - Drugs (eg gentamicin; amphotericin)
  - Radio-contrast nephropathy

- **Structural abnormalities of renal vasculature (5%)**

  - Renal artery occlusion
  - Small vessel occlusion: accelerated-phase hypertension; disseminated intravascular coagulation (DIC); haemolytic–uraemic syndrome (HUS); thrombotic thrombocytopenic purpura (TTP); pre-eclampsia

- **Acute glomerulonephritis and vasculitis (15%)**

  - Idiopathic crescentic glomerulonephritis
  - ANCA-positive vasculitis
  - Goodpasture's syndrome
  - Other proliferative glomerulonephritis (eg systemic lupus erythematosus (SLE); endocarditis; Henoch–Schonlein nephritis)

- **Interstitial nephritis (5%)**
- **Myeloma/tubular cast nephropathy (<5%)**
- **Urinary tract obstruction (10%)**

Investigation of ARF

The history may point to the cause of ARF (eg drugs, skin rash); assessment of the haemodynamic status is imperative, and appropriate fluid resuscitation should be given.

- **Urinary examination**: ATN and pre-renal uraemia can be differentiated by urinary biochemistry (see above); *proteinuria* microscopic haematuria and red cell casts will point to acute glomerulonephritis as the cause.
- A **renal ultrasound** scan will usually show normal sized (or swollen) kidneys, and will identify obstruction (the latter should be urgently treated to reduce irreversible renal injury).
- **Autoantibody profile**: ANF, ANCA, anti-GBM, complement and plasma and urinary electrophoresis should all be routinely performed (unless the cause of ARF is obvious, eg post-myocardial infarction or renal obstruction).
- **Percutaneous renal biopsy** is essential if an intrinsic lesion (eg vasculitis, glomerulonephritis, interstitial nephritis) is suspected, or if no ischaemic cause is apparent.

Management of ARF

The mainstay of treatment involves **optimisation of fluid balance** and avoidance of either hypovolaemia or fluid overload. Patients with single-organ ARF are best managed in a high dependency unit setting. Blood pressure should be controlled, haemoglobin maintained around 10 g/dl and sepsis should be promptly and vigorously treated. 'Renal dose' dopamine and loop diuretics are often given in ATN, although there is no evidence that they alter the outcome of ARF in humans. Some cases of ATN can be managed

without dialysis, with the adoption of careful fluid balance and dietary control; however, many patients with ATN also have multi-organ failure (MOF) and they can only be managed on an ICU.

The most important advances in ARF management have involved attention to **intensive nutritional support** of the sicker patients, and the use of **continuous renal replacement therapies** (eg CVVH: continuous veno-venous haemo-filtration) which are less likely to provoke haemodynamic instability.

Other more specific treatments in ARF depend upon the causative condition and include:

- Specific **immunosuppressive therapy**, and sometimes plasma exchange, may be appropriate for some conditions (eg Goodpasture's syndrome, ANCA +ve vasculitis).
- **Obstruction**: bladder catheterisation for bladder outflow obstruction; nephrostomy drainage for renal obstruction.
- **Other**: eg steroids in acute interstitial nephritis (AIN), plasma exchange in HUS and TTP, chemotherapy in myeloma.

Indications for urgent dialysis in ARF

- Severe uraemia

  - (eg vomiting, encephalopathy, urea > 60 mmol/l)

- Severe acidosis

  - pH <7.1

- Pulmonary oedema
- Hyperkalaemia

  - K >6.5 mmol/l (or less, if ECG changes apparent)

- Uraemic pericarditis

Essential note

Acute renal failure presents with signs and symptoms relating to the failure of one or more of the four non-endocrine functions of the kidney

Prognosis of ARF

The survival prognosis for patients with ARF remains only moderate; 55–60% of patients who require dialytic therapy survive, but this figure partly reflects the very poor outcome of patients who have ATN as a component of MOF who are managed on the ICU. For example, only 10–20% of those with three- or four-organ failure will survive, yet 90% of patients with ARF in isolation survive.

4.2 Rhabdomyolysis

Muscle damage with release of myoglobin can cause severe, hypercatabolic ARF. Serum potassium and phosphate (released from muscle) rapidly rise, calcium is typically low, and the creatine kinase massively elevated; serum creatinine may be disproportionately higher than urea. Sometimes the source of the rhabdomyolytic process requires specific therapy (eg fasciotomy for compartment syndrome, debridement of dead tissue and amputation of non-viable limbs).

Causes of rhabdomyolysis	
Common	*Rare*
Crush injury Trauma; unconsciousness with compression	**Metabolic myopathies** (eg McArdle's syndrome)
Uncontrolled fitting	**Infections** Viral necrotising myositis, infectious mononucleosis
Drugs (eg statins)	**Severe exercise, heat stroke, burns**
Overdose Barbiturates, alcohol, heroin	**Inflammatory myopathies** Polymyositis
	Malignant hyperpyrexia

4.3 Radio-contrast nephropathy

Mild renal dysfunction may complicate up to 10% of angiographic procedures and IVUs. Radio-contrast nephropathy is manifest by non-oliguric ARF, typically occurring 1–5 days after the procedure. The ARF is fully reversible. Recent attention has been directed to prevention of radio-contrast nephropathy with:

- Pre-hydration of patients at greatest risk (eg with N-saline infusion before and during the procedure)
- *N*-Acetyl cysteine (given orally for 2–3 days, from before to 24 h post-procedure).

Risk factors for radio-contrast nephropathy

- High contrast load
- High iodine content of contrast
- Hypovolaemia
- Myeloma
- Age
- Hyperuricaemia
- Diabetes (especially if taking metformin)
- Hypercalcaemia
- Pre-existing CRF

5. CHRONIC RENAL FAILURE (CHRONIC KIDNEY DISEASE) AND RENAL REPLACEMENT THERAPY

5.1 Chronic renal failure (CRF)

A changing nomenclature now sees the term chronic kidney disease (CKD) used interchangeably with CRF. When describing the epidemiology of CRF, distinction has to be made between:

- end-stage renal disease (ESRD), at which stage patients require renal replacement therapy (RRT, ie dialysis or transplantation) and
- less severe, but often progressive, degrees of chronic renal disease (CRF or CKD).

CRF/CKD is very common, and the prevalence is thought to be at least 2000 patients per million (in the elderly, 5–10% of the population have CKD). The incidence of ESRD patients joining RRT programmes in the UK is 80–125/million each year.

There are several recognised stages of **CKD**:

- CKD stage 1: GFR >90 ml/min.*
- CKD stage 2: GFR 60–90 ml/min.*
- CKD stage 3: **moderate CRF** – GFR 30–59 ml/min. Renal anaemia and secondary hyperparathyroidism begin to complicate this level of renal dysfunction. Hypertension should be optimally controlled, ideally with ACE inhibitors or AIIRBs.
- CKD stage 4: **severe CRF** – GFR 15–29 ml/min; patients may have uraemic symptoms (eg anorexia, nausea, sleep disturbance). Patients should receive counselling on the need for future RRT at this stage, and elective commencement of dialysis planned. Dialysis access should be planned; transplant work-up should occur at a GFR of around 20 ml/min with the aim of transplant

listing (for a pre-dialysis ('pre-emptive') transplant) at GFR 15 ml/min.

- CKD stage 5: **ESRD** – GFR <15 ml/min The patient will require RRT, unless conservative treatment is agreed. If RRT is commenced late (eg when GFR <5 ml/min) then there is a risk of developing a life-threatening uraemic syndrome.

* With evidence of renal disease (eg abnormal renal imaging or urinalysis).

CKD 1 and 2 are defined as well-preserved GFR but with urinary (eg microalbuminuria) or structural (eg polycystic change) abnormalities.

Although many cases of CRF progress insidiously, so that very abnormal biochemistry is relatively well tolerated by the patient, about one-third of dialysis patients initially present as uraemic emergencies (which carries a twofold worse prognosis). The key parameters that **differentiate CRF from ARF** are:

- Small kidneys at imaging
- Anaemia
- Renal bone disease
- Clinical tolerance of very severe uraemia.

Essential note

Key parameters differentiating chronic from acute renal failure are: small kidneys, anaemia, renal bone disease and clinical tolerance of severe uraemia

Causes of CRF (approximate relative frequencies)

- **Most common causes of ESRD in UK***
    - Diabetic nephropathy (25%)
    - Chronic glomerulonephritis (15%)
    - Hypertension (15%) – renovascular disease may co-exist in >1/2 of cases
    - Chronic pyelonephritis (12%) – most often due to reflux nephropathy, but also renal calculi (nephrolithiasis) with infection
    - Polycystic kidney disease (8%)
    - Obstructive uropathy (5%)
    - Chronic interstitial nephritis (4%) – eg sarcoidosis, lithium toxicity, myeloma
    - Post-acute renal failure (3%)
    - Amyloidosis (1%)

Causes of CRF (approximate relative frequencies)

- **Some rarer causes of CRF**
    - Analgesic nephropathy
    - Other hereditary disorders, eg Alport's syndrome

* In at least 10% of cases of ESRD, the aetiology remains unknown. These are patients presenting with small kidneys on ultrasound, and in whom renal biopsy will be diagnostically unhelpful. Most likely diagnoses are hypertension, chronic glomerulonephritis or pyelonephritis, or dysplastic kidneys.

Pathogenesis and management of progressive renal dysfunction in CRF

The majority of cases of CRF are slowly progressive towards ESRD, and angiotensin is thought to play a major role in the pathogenesis; this vasoactive mediator not only exacerbates the intraglomerular hypertension seen in remaining nephrons, but it also stimulates fibrosis within the tubulo-interstitium (Figure 2). Proteinuria may also directly damage tubular cells. Hence the **management** of patients with CRF requires attention to:

- **Control of blood pressure**: it is imperative to optimise blood pressure control. Target blood pressures for patients with CRF are equivalent to those required for treatment of diabetic nephropathy (e.g. <125/75 mmHg if significant proteinuria). Hypertension control can slow the progression towards ESRD, and **ACE inhibitors and AIIRB** are logical agents to choose because of their effects upon angiotensin.
- **Reduction of proteinuria**: heavy urinary protein losses (eg >2 g/day) are associated with an increased rate of progression in many cases of CRF. Amelioration of proteinuria by use of ACE inhibitors and AIIRB may also slow progression.
- **Dietary modification**: it is now widely accepted that patients with advanced CRF should maintain a normal protein and high calorie intake to avoid malnutrition in the phase leading up to RRT. However, phosphate restriction and dietary modification of salt and potassium intake should be instituted at an early stage of CRF.
- **Endocrine complications**: anaemia and renal osteodystrophy may begin during CKD stages 2 and 3, and hence early attention should be directed to these endocrine complications (*see* below).

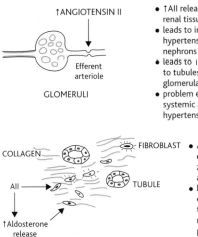

- ↑AII release from damaged renal tissue
- leads to intra-glomerular hypertension in remaining nephrons
- leads to ↑proteinuria (toxic to tubules) and further glomerular injury
- problem exacerbated by systemic and intra-renal hypertension

- AII increases release of aldosterone from zona glomerulosa of adrenal gland
- both have deleterious effects in the renal tubulo-interstitium mediated in part by pro-scarring cytokines (eg TGF-β)

Figure 2 Role of angiotensin II in the pathogenesis of progressive CKD

- **Cardiovascular disease prevention**: CRF creates a pro-atherosclerotic environment due to factors such as hypertension, mixed hyperlipidaemia, anaemia, hyperparathyroidism and, when present, diabetes. Major complications include congestive cardiomyopathy, left ventricular hypertrophy (LVH), vascular calcification, coronary artery disease, stroke and peripheral vascular disease. Patients with CRF therefore have a marked increase in CVS mortality compared to the general population; the importance of early treatment with statins and aspirin is now the subject of a multi-centre trial.

> **Essential note**
>
> Management of CRF centres on: control of blood pressure, reduction of proteinuria, dietary modification, control of endocrine complications, prevention of cardiovascular disease

5.2 Anaemia of CRF

The anaemia of CRF usually first appears when GFR is <50 ml/min; if untreated, it is a major contributor to morbidity in patients with advanced CRF. The major cause is the lack of endogenous erythropoietin (EPO) secretion by the damaged kidneys, but other important contributory factors include:

- Reduced dietary iron intake due to anorexia
- Impaired intestinal absorption of iron
- Reduced red blood cell (RBC) survival (particularly in haemodialysis patients).

> **Essential note**
>
> The main cause of anaemia in CRF is lack of EPO, and management includes replacement EPO and maintenance of iron, ferritin and transferrin status

Recombinant erythropoietin

- Endogenous EPO is normally synthesised by renal peritubular cells; it stimulates proliferation and maturation of erythroid lines within the marrow. Recombinant EPO preparations are now widely available and are used to correct anaemia in patients with CKD (ie pre-dialysis and patients with failing transplants) as well as those receiving dialysis. It is imperative that these patient groups avoid repeated blood transfusion, so that future renal transplantation will not be precluded by allo-sensitisation.

Patients must be iron replete before EPO is commenced. The serum ferritin and the transferrin saturation need monitoring as most patients require supplemental intravenous iron. Target haemoglobin is 11–13 g/dl; haemoglobin correction improves left ventricular hypertrophy (common in dialysis patients), sexual function and other quality of life measures.

> **Causes of resistance to EPO therapy**
>
> - Iron deficiency
> - Sepsis or chronic inflammation
> - Occult GI tract blood loss
> - Hyperparathyroidism
> - Aluminium toxicity (rare)
> - Pure red cell aplasia (PRCA, *see* below)

Main side-effects of EPO therapy: accelerated hypertension with encephalopathy (aim for a monthly Hb increase of <1.5 g/dl), bone aches, flu-like syndrome, fistula thrombosis (rare), and most recently, PRCA (see below).

Pure red cell aplasia (PRCA)

A few cases of unresponsive and progressive severe anaemia have recently been identified in patients treated with EPO. Such patients have antibodies directed at endogenous and exogenous EPO, and they become transfusion dependent. Other marrow functions remain intact.

5.3 Hyperparathyroidism and renal bone disease (renal osteodystrophy)

The regulation of vitamin D and parathyroid hormone (PTH) metabolism is discussed in Chapter 11, Metabolic diseases. Renal bone disease (osteodystrophy) is common in patients with CRF and those receiving dialysis. The pathogenesis is fairly intricate but the most important components are:

- High serum phosphate; phosphate clearance is reduced in renal failure.
- Low plasma ionised calcium: due to several factors. There is lack of 1,25-dihydroxy vitamin D (the 1α-hydroxylation, which markedly increases activity of vitamin D, normally occurs in the kidney). Malnutrition may contribute, but hyperphosphataemia (imbalancing the ionic product of Ca × P) is also very important.
- Stimulation of PTH release: in CRF and ESRD secondary hyperparathyroidism is very common and is the direct response of the glands to hypocalcaemia, hyperphosphataemia and low 1,25-dihydroxy vitamin D levels. Correction of all of these factors (phosphate perhaps the most important) is necessary before the hyperparathyroidism can be optimally controlled. PTH has end-organ effects upon bones (leading to osteoclastic resorption cavities) and also the heart, contributing to LVH, and it is also a major cause of EPO resistance. Tertiary hyperparathyroidism is defined by the presence of elevated PTH and hypercalcaemia; it is due to autonomous PTH secretion from generally hyperplastic parathyroid glands (90%) or an adenoma (10%). Note that primary hyperparathyroidism is only rarely associated with renal failure (due to the nephrotoxic effects of hypercalcaemia or to renal calculus disease).
- Acidosis: increases the severity of bone disease.

Essential note

Abnormal vitamin D and PTH metabolism lead to renal bone disease

---

Histological findings at bone biopsy in osteodystrophy

Several different histological lesions usually co-exist in the same patient:

- Osteomalacia : due to 1,25-dihydroxy vitamin D deficiency.
- Hyperparathyroid bone disease: also termed 'osteitis fibrosa cystica' (von Recklinghausen's disease of bone). Sub-periosteal erosions on the radial border of phalanges are characteristic.

- Osteoporosis: due to relative malnourishment; steroid use.
- Osteosclerosis: a component of the 'rugger jersey' spine appearance at X-ray (bone denser at the vertebral end-plates and thin in the middle of the vertebrae).
- Adynamic bone disease: bone with low turnover; PTH levels (and serum alkaline phosphatase) are usually sub-normal. Although the exact clinical significance is uncertain there is perhaps a greater likelihood of fracturing.
- Aluminium bone disease: now much less common with the use of specially treated water supplies for dialysis and non-aluminium-containing phosphate binders.

Prevention and treatment of renal osteodystrophy

The basic principles are to improve the diet, reduce hyperphosphataemia (eg < 1.7 mmol/l) and acidosis, and to reduce the PTH level. This is brought about by use of phosphate binders (eg calcium carbonate or acetate, sevalemer) oral bicarbonate, dialysis where necessary, and by giving vitamin D in doses that do not provoke hypercalcaemia. Parathyroidectomy may be necessary in resistant cases.

5.4 Maintenance dialysis

Ideally, a patient should be given the opportunity to choose dialysis modality according to lifestyle factors (employment, home environment), their capability and local resources. The two main options are peritoneal dialysis and haemodialysis.

Peritoneal dialysis (CAPD or automated peritoneal dialysis (APD))

A standard CAPD regime would involve four 2-litre exchanges per day. The concentration of dextrose within the dialysate can be altered so that differing ultrafiltration requirements, or patient characteristics, can be addressed. **Automated peritoneal dialysis (APD)** is performed overnight, and can maintain fluid homeostasis in patients with ultrafiltration failure (see below). APD may also be chosen for its convenience by some patients with normal peritoneal membrane characteristics.

The main **complications of CAPD** treatment are:

- Bacterial peritonitis: most cases are treatable. The most common infecting organisms are coagulase-negative staphylococci, Gram-negative bacteria and *Staphylococcus aureus*. Patients who have repeated episodes of peritonitis, and hence several courses of intraperitoneal antibiotics, are prone to develop resistant organisms (eg *Pseudomonas* or fungal peritonitis) and catheter loss, necessitating switch to haemodialysis.
- Ultrafiltration failure: some patients are identified as 'high transporters' of glucose; the osmolar benefit of their CAPD dialysate is rapidly lost and hence these

patients have difficulty with fluid removal (ultrafiltration).

- **Sclerosing peritonitis**: a rare complication of long-term CAPD, perhaps triggered by repeated peritonitis. The peritoneal membrane thickens and encases the bowel. Surgery can be of benefit in some cases.
- **Malnutrition**: renal failure is an anorexic condition; patients often need nutritional supplements.

Essential note

The main complications of peritoneal dialysis are bacterial peritonitis, ultrafiltration failure, sclerosing peritonitis and malnutrition

Haemodialysis

This therapy has been available for several decades; it is an intrinsically more efficient means of RRT than CAPD and so many patients have lived for >20 years whilst being supported by haemodialysis. As this is an intermittent therapy (typically, 4 hours dialysis 3 times each week) water restriction and dietary modification are even more important than for patients receiving CAPD (which gives continuous dialysis). Successful haemodialysis relies upon adequate **vascular access**:

- Arterio-venous fistulae take 4–6 weeks to mature and so vascular access surgery should be planned in timely fashion, when at all possible.
- Patients who present late with severe uraemia, and patients with fistula complications, inevitably require use of temporary or semi-permanent (tunnelled) vascular access catheters. The most frequent complication is line-related sepsis (in particular, *S. aureus* and coagulase-negative staphylococci). Other complications of vascular catheters are venous stenosis or occlusion, reduced if internal jugular or femoral sites are used.

Long-term complications in dialysis patients

Although dialytic therapies will keep patients alive and, with the additional use of EPO, relatively well, many of the metabolic abnormalities of the uraemic condition persist and these patients are at increased risk of:

- **Vascular disease**: dialysis patients have a much greater incidence of cardiovascular events, and higher relative mortality, than the general population. Pathogenetic factors have been discussed earlier in this section. The majority of deaths are due to cardiac disease but this is more often due to arrhythmia or congestive cardiomyopathy (which is exacerbated by fluid overload)

than to overt myocardial infarction. **Vascular calcification** is a major component of the vascular disease affecting patients with renal failure; it is associated with arterial stiffness and LVH.

- **Dialysis-related amyloid**: β_2 microglobulin is a small molecular weight (about 11 000 Daltons) protein normally metabolised and excreted by the kidney. Plasma levels increase greatly in patients on long-term (eg >10 years) haemodialysis, and the protein is deposited as amyloid within carpal tunnels (causing carpal tunnel syndrome), joints and bones (causing bone pains and arthropathy).
- **Arthritis**: pyrophosphate arthropathy (pseudogout) and gout (*see* 'Post-transplantation: non-renal complications' below) are common in patients with renal failure.

5.5 Renal transplantation

About 2000 UK patients benefit from renal transplantation each year, and the vast majority of transplants derive from **cadaveric donors**. There is an overall shortage of organs available for transplantation and so the rate of **live-related transplants** (currently 15% of all grafts) is being increased and non-related live renal donation (often from the spouse) is now occurring. All potential live renal donors have to be screened carefully to ensure that they are clinically fit; absolute contraindications include pre-existing renal disease, a disease of unknown aetiology (eg multiple sclerosis or sarcoidosis), recent malignancy and overt ischaemic heart disease.

Essential note

Absolute contraindications to being a live kidney donor include: pre-existing renal disease, disease of unknown aetiology, recent malignancy and overt ischaemic heart disease

Screening and preparation of potential recipients

All dialysis patients and those with advanced CRF are considered for transplantation. However, less than half will be suitably fit for listing. Exclusion criteria include current or recent malignancy (eg <2 years) and severe co-morbidity (eg debilitating chronic obstructive pulmonary disease (COPD) or stroke, dementia, etc). Advanced age is not an absolute contraindication, but few patients aged >75 years are listed.

- Patients with major risk factors (long-standing diabetes, previous ischaemic heart disease (IHD), heavy smoking) should undergo **CVS screening** prior to referral.

- Patients with obstructed and infected urinary tracts (eg severe reflux, patients with spina bifida) need bilateral native nephrectomy prior to transplantation.

HLA typing

The majority of cadaveric organs are transplanted to the best available tissue match.

- HLA antigens are coded from chromosome 6 (*see also* Chapter 9, Immunology).
- Class 1 antigens are A, B and C; class 2 are the D group antigens.
- Relative importance of HLA matching: DR>B>A>C; most centres accept 1 DR or 1 B mismatch.

Combined kidney–pancreas transplantation

This is now increasingly performed for patients with type I diabetes mellitus. The pancreas is usually transplanted onto the opposite iliac vessels to the kidney, with its duct draining into the bladder. Long-term results are encouraging – normalisation of glycaemic status is expected, and most diabetic microvascular complications (particularly retinopathy and neuropathy) can be stabilised, but not reversed.

Post-transplantation renal function

It is common to see **acute renal transplant dysfunction**, especially in the first few weeks after engraftment. Nevertheless, overall graft survival is >90% at one year and approaching 65% at 10 years. **Chronic graft dysfunction** is common and is responsible for the majority of these renal graft losses beyond 1 year after transplantation. The commoner causes of acute and chronic graft dysfunction are shown in the following table.

Causes of graft dysfunction after transplantation

Acute graft dysfunction

- **Delayed graft function** (ATN of the graft): increased with prolonged cold ischaemia time (seen in 20–50% of all transplants – usually resolves by 2–3 weeks)
- Ureteric leakage (breakdown of anastomosis)
- Vascular thrombosis (arterial or venous thrombosis of the transplant vessels – usually irremediable)
- Urinary tract infection
- Acute ciclosporin or tacrolimus toxicity – resolves rapidly with alteration in dosage
- CMV infection (diagnosed with viral PCR)
- **Acute rejection**: occurs in 25–50% of all transplants (see below)

Causes of graft dysfunction after transplantation

Chronic graft dysfunction

- **Chronic allograft nephropathy**: by far the most common cause of chronic dysfunction of the transplant (see below)
- Recurrent primary disease within the graft (eg glomerulonephritis)
- Calcineurin inhibitor (ciclosporin or tacrolimus) nephrotoxicity. Withdrawal of these agents will often stabilise graft function

---

Acute transplant rejection

This is very common, and should be anticipated in the early weeks after transplantation. Most cases respond rapidly to pulsed i.v. methyl-prednisolone therapy.

Chronic allograft nephropathy (CAN)

This accounts for >90% of graft losses occurring after the first year after transplantation. Proteinuria and slowly progressive graft dysfunction are typical. It is thought to be due to both immunological and non-immunological (hypertension, hypercholesterolaemia, vascular disease within the graft) factors. Management involves:

- optimising hypertension control
- limiting proteinuria (use of ACE inhibitors and AIIRBs)
- **modification of immunosuppressive therapy**: reduction or withdrawal of calcineurin inhibitors (CNI) with introduction of mycophenolate mofetil (MMF), for example, may stabilise the progressive graft dysfunction.

Post-transplantation: non-renal complications

Although the quality of life of most patients is improved after transplantation, patients are still at risk of:

- **Malignancy**: non-Hodgkin's lymphoma (usually EB virus-associated) and **skin cancer** are much commoner in transplant recipients than in age-matched general populations, due to the effects of immunosuppression. All other malignancies are slightly more prevalent.
- **Cardiovascular**: the CVS risk accompanying the patients' previous 'uraemic state' persists after transplantation. Mortality is 2% in the first year after transplantation, half of which is due to CVS disease, and half to infection (*see* below).
- **Infections**: all infections are commoner but patients are also at risk from opportunistic infections such as *Pneumocystis carinii* pneumonia (PCP), and especially cytomegalovirus (CMV), which occurs in up to 30%.

Patients of Asian origin, or those with a previous TB history, are given anti-tuberculous prophylaxis with isoniazid for the first year after transplantation.

- **Gout**: all patients with reduced renal clearance are at increased risk of hyperuricaemia and acute gout. However, prophylaxis with allopurinol is not generally given to all patients, because this agent has many unwanted effects. Treatment of acute gout in patients with renal impairment presents a major problem – there are no truly non-nephrotoxic NSAIDs available, and patients with transplants (or with CRF) are at risk of serious renal dysfunction with their usage.
- **Post-transplantation diabetes mellitus (PTDM)**: the incidence is increased in transplanted patients (3–5% may develop it each year); immunosupressants (particularly tacrolimus) are thought to be responsible.

Essential note

Transplant recipients are at increased risk of: malignancy, cardiovascular disease, infections, gout and diabetes mellitus

Commonly used immunosuppressants for renal transplantation

- Immunosuppressive regimes vary from centre to centre. Historically, a combination of ciclosporin with azathioprine and prednisolone was the favoured regime, but this has changed with the advent of newer agents (particularly tacrolimus, MMF and rapamycin). Most now involve induction with monoclonal antibody (eg basiliximab) followed by a CNI-based regime. Patients who have at least two steroid-responsive acute rejections will usually receive oral corticosteroids for up to 12 months after transplantation.

6. GLOMERULONEPHRITIS AND ASSOCIATED SYNDROMES

6.1 Clinical presentation of glomerulonephritis

The broad definition of glomerulonephritis is inflammatory disease primarily affecting the glomeruli (but note that no inflammation is seen in minimal change disease). Note that other glomerular diseases exist which do not involve glomerulonephritis (eg diabetic nephropathy). Most glomerulonephritis develops as a result of **immune dysregulation**, due to either an inappropriate immune response to a 'self-antigen' (autoimmunity, eg anti-GBM disease, ANCA +ve vasculitis), or to an ineffectual response to a foreign antigen (eg membranous glomerulonephritis secondary to hepatitis B infection).

- This 'immune dysregulation' pathogenesis explains why there is a genetic predisposition to some forms of glomerulonephritis (eg IgA nephropathy).
- Immune complexes are often deposited in the glomeruli (eg SLE nephritis), but in some glomerulonephritides immune complexes form in situ within the glomerulus (eg anti-GBM disease).
- Inflammation often leads to proliferation of cellular structures (mesangial, endothelial or epithelial cells) and/or scarring.
- Glomerulonephritis may be **idiopathic (primary)**, or **secondary** to systemic disease, drugs, etc.
- The long-term clinical outcome often depends more upon the severity of tubulo-interstitial damage rather than on the extent of glomerular injury.
- The type of glomerulonephritis is defined by light microscopic, immunofluorescent and electron microscopic (ultrastructural) characteristics (*see* below).

Essential note

The type of glomerulonephritis is defined by light microscopic, immunofluorescent and electron microscopic (ultrastructural) characteristics

Screening for glomerulonephritis

- Dipstick for proteinuria; 24-h quantification of proteinuria
- Dipstick for haematuria; urine microscopy for red cells and casts
- Hypertension.

Attenuation of progression of glomerulonephritis

- Control blood pressure: for all types of glomerulonephritis
- ACE inhibitors and AIIRB: decrease proteinuria and blood pressure, and may ameliorate progressive scarring (*see* Section 1.3, 'Renin–angiotensin–aldosterone (RAA) system' and Section 5.1 Chronic renal failure (CRF))
- The target blood pressure for patients with chronic renal disease and persistent proteinuria is <125/75 mmHg (*see* Section 5.1 Chronic renal failure (CRF))

Classification of glomerulonephritis

The commoner forms of glomerulonephritis (GN) encountered are:

- Minimal change disease
- Membranous glomerulonephritis
- Focal segmental glomerulosclerosis (FSGS)
- Mesangioproliferative (IgA nephropathy) glomerulonephritis
- Crescentic glomerulonephritis (eg associated with Goodpasture's syndrome or vasculitis)
- Focal segmental proliferative glomerulonephritis (eg associated with vasculitis or endocarditis)
- Mesangiocapillary glomerulonephritis
- Diffuse proliferative glomerulonephritis (eg post-streptococcal).

Renal syndromes and their relationship to glomerulonephritis

There is often confusion regarding the relationship of the various glomerulonephritides to the different renal syndromes. A particular type of glomerulonephritis may manifest several different clinical syndromes (see Table below). For example, membranous glomerulonephritis may be responsible for CRF, persistent proteinuria, nephrotic syndrome and hypertension; any combination of these may be present during the course of the disease. However:

- Certain glomerulonephritides are characteristically associated with typical clinical presentations (eg minimal change disease and nephrotic syndrome, IgA nephropathy and recurrent macroscopic haematuria).
- It should also be borne in mind that a particular syndrome may be due to many conditions other than glomerulonephritis (eg the nephrotic syndrome can be due to accelerated phase hypertension, pre-eclamptic toxaemia or amyloid, as well as various forms of glomerulonephritis, etc).

Definitions of the common renal syndromes

- **Asymptomatic proteinuria**
  - <3 g/day
- **Nephritic syndrome**
  - Characterised by hypertension, oliguria, haematuria and oedema
- **Hypertension**
- **Nephrotic syndrome**
  - >3.5 g proteinuria/day with serum albumin <25 g/l; oedema; hypercholesterolaemia
- **Haematuria**
  - Microscopic or macroscopic
- **Acute and chronic renal failure**
  - (Discussed in previous sections)

Main causes of the nephrotic syndrome

- Primary glomerulonephritis
- Diabetes mellitus
- Infections (eg leprosy, malaria, hepatitis B)
- Myeloma
- Amyloidosis
- Drugs (eg gold, penicillamine)
- Pre-eclampsia

Clinical presentation of glomerulonephritris

	Proteinuria	Nephrotic	Nephritic	Haematuria	ARF	CRF
Minimal change disease	±	+++	−	−	−	−
Membranous GN	+++	++	−	±	−	++
Focal segmental glomerulosclerosis	++	++	±	−	±	++
Mesangial IgA	+	+	+	+++	±	++
Mesangiocapillary GN	++	++	+	+	+	+
Diffuse proliferative GN	+	±	+++	++	++	+
Crescentic nephritis	+	±	+++	++	+++	+
Focal segmental proliferative GN	+	++	++	++	++	+

+++ = Very common presentation; − = never seen/extremely rare

Causes of macroscopic haematuria*

- Urinary infections
- Acute glomerulonephritis
- IgA nephropathy
- Renal calculi
- Urinary tract malignancy
- Renal papillary necrosis
- Loin-pain haematuria syndrome
- Prostatic hypertrophy (dilated prostatic veins)

* It is usually imperative to exclude urinary tract malignancy (urine cytology, cystoscopy, IVU and ultrasound) in patients aged >40 years presenting with macroscopic haematuria.

6.2 Notes on particular glomerulonephritides (*see* Figure 3)

Minimal change disease

The clinical presentation is almost always nephrotic. Although most common in children (causing 80% of nephrotic syndrome due to glomerulonephritis in <15 years), it also accounts for 28% of nephrotic syndrome in adults. It is usually idiopathic, and the majority of cases are steroid-responsive. Other features include:

- Normal renal function and renal histology (by light microscopy – but epithelial cell foot-process fusion on EM)
- May frequently relapse (10%), but renal prognosis is excellent.

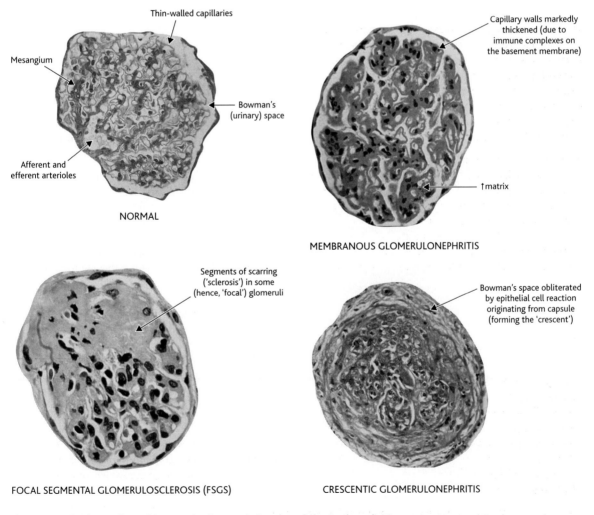

Figure 3 Basic glomerular architecture in characteristic types of glomerulonephritis

Monitoring and treatment: patients with frequently relapsing disease (especially children) are taught to dipstick their urine on a regular basis; three consecutive days of +++ proteinuria is the trigger to commence steroids, which are continued at high dose until urinalysis has remained negative for three consecutive days. The mainstay of treatment is with short courses of high-dose prednisolone. Most relapses are steroid-sensitive; cyclophosphamide (usually orally in children, pulsed i.v. in adults) is used for frequent relapsers or steroid-resistant disease.

Membranous glomerulonephritis (Figure 3)

This is one of the commonest types of glomerulonephritis in the adult; there are two peaks of disease (patients in their mid-20s and those aged 60–70 years). The clinical presentation may be nephrotic syndrome, asymptomatic proteinuria or CRF.

- Renal histology is characterised by granular IgG and complement deposition on the glomerular basement membrane, with immune complexes seen on EM.
- One-third of patients progress through CRF to ESRD, one-third respond to immunosuppressive therapy (eg cytotoxic regimes such as the Ponticelli regime: chlorambucil alternating with corticosteroids), and the disease remits spontaneously in a similar proportion of patients.
- In patients with persistent proteinuria (which can sometimes be in the nephrotic range) the mainstay of treatment is blood pressure control and limitation of proteinuria with ACE inhibitors and/or AIIRBs.
- Renal vein thrombosis may occur in up to 5% of patients.
- Membranous glomerulonephritis may be idiopathic, or secondary to other conditions (*see* below).

Secondary causes of membranous glomerulonephritis

- Malignancy
  - Bronchus, stomach, colon, lymphoma, chronic lymphocytic leukaemia (CLL; high suspicion of these in elderly patients)
- Connective tissue disease
  - eg SLE, rheumatoid arthritis
- Chronic infections
  - eg Hepatitis B or C, malaria
- Drugs
  - eg Gold, penicillamine

Focal segmental glomerulosclerosis (FSGS) (Figure 3)

The **primary** form of FSGS accounts for <10% of nephrotic syndrome in children and the elderly, but up to 20% in young adults. It can also frequently present with proteinuria and/or CRF. There are also familial forms of FSGS. Focal glomerular deposits of IgM are seen at biopsy.

- **Secondary FSGS**: this can be seen in patients with heroin abuse, those with HIV infections and AIDS, and it is frequently seen in patients with obesity.
- **Outcome of FSGS**: 20% of all patients will eventually progress to ESRD.

Mesangioproliferative glomerulonephritis (IgA nephropathy or Berger's disease)

This is a very frequent condition, the commonest primary glomerulonephritis in adults. It typically affects young adults, presenting with microscopic or recurrent macroscopic haematuria. The haematuric episodes are usually 'synpharyngitic' (ie occurring 0–3 days after URTI). Many cases are probably undiagnosed, as most physicians only occasionally biopsy the kidneys of patients with isolated microscopic haematuria. There is a marked increased incidence in the Far East (genetic association). The serum IgA is increased in 50% of patients; the condition is considered to be autoimmune, perhaps due to dysregulation of IgA metabolism. Other features of IgA nephropathy are:

- IgA nephropathy can be associated with cirrhosis, dermatitis herpetiformis and coeliac disease.
- Renal biopsy features show proliferation of mesangial areas of the glomerulus; immunological staining is strongly positive for IgA in these areas. A similar histological picture may be seen in **Henoch–Schönlein nephritis**, and the pathogenesis is thought to be similar in the two conditions.
- **Treatment and outcome of IgA nephropathy**: nephrotic presentations should be treated as for minimal change nephropathy. Otherwise the mainstay of treatment is optimal blood pressure control with ACE inhibitors/AIIRBs, as for other chronic nephropathies. Fifteen to twenty percent of patients will progress to ESRD by 20 years after disease onset; however, the overall prognosis is certain to be better than this as the mildest cases are likely to remain undiagnosed.

Diffuse proliferative glomerulonephritis

This is the histological pattern of the classic post-streptococcal glomerulonephritis which usually presents with the nephritic syndrome or ARF; children and young adults are most often affected. The disorder is typically preceded (by 10–21 days) by a sore throat, or (most often in third world countries) skin disease (impetigo).

- Serum C_3 is low and there is diffuse proliferation within glomeruli at biopsy.
- Post-infective cases usually recover spontaneously with restoration of full renal function.
- The same histological picture may be seen in patients with Goodpasture's syndrome and SLE nephritis.

Rapidly progressive glomerulonephritis (RPGN) – including Goodpasture's syndrome

The term 'rapidly progressive' glomerulonephritis is a clinical description of rapidly deteriorating renal function due to an underlying glomerulonephritis. The histological counterpart is a **crescentic glomerulonephritis**, and so the two terms are (sometimes incorrectly) used interchangeably. They refer to the renal lesions which excite great interest from the nephrologist, not least because patients are often very sick with hypercatabolic ARF and possibly associated systemic disease (eg pulmonary haemorrhage), but also because the underlying disease processes are potentially treatable provided that investigation and therapy are expedient. All age groups may be affected and the presentation is usually ARF or nephritic syndrome.

- Causes of RPGN include Goodpasture's syndrome, ANCA +ve vasculitis and lupus nephritis.
- Crescentic nephritis may be 'idiopathic' but is more often associated with Goodpasture's syndrome, ANCA +ve vasculitis or SLE.

ANCA +ve vasculitis and lupus nephritis are both described in Section 12, Systemic disorders and the kidney, and hence the remainder of this section will concentrate on Goodpasture's syndrome and its treatment, which are similar to that for the former conditions.

Goodpasture's syndrome

This is characterised by the presence of circulating anti-GBM antibodies (the GBM antigen is a component of type 4 collagen), which localise to the glomerular and pulmonary capillary basement membranes. The condition is rare (<1 case/million per year), tends to affect the elderly or patients in their 20–30s and may be triggered by inhaled hydrocarbons.

- **Pulmonary haemorrhage** occurs in 50% of patients with Goodpasture's; the most vulnerable are young male smokers. The occurrence of pulmonary haemorrhage confers a greater mortality and is a definitive indication for plasma exchange.

- Specific biopsy changes are seen in Goodpasture's syndrome, with IgG deposited on the glomerular basement membrane in a linear pattern. Typically there is extensive crescent formation (epithelial cell proliferation arising from Bowman's capsule) (see Figure 3).
- **Prognosis**: Renal functional recovery is rarely seen if the patient presents with advanced ARF (eg creatinine >600 μmol/l) and/or anuria. Overall mortality is >20%. Elderly patients are at particular risk from infective complications after immunosuppression; patients who have pulmonary haemorrhage are at greatest risk of mortality. Transplantation is possible once the patient is rendered autoantibody negative.

Treatment of RPGN and crescentic nephritis

The following is applicable to most diseases causing RPGN and/or crescentic glomerulonephritis. Treatment is with immunosuppressive therapy (high-dose steroids and cyclophosphamide as 3–6 months of induction therapy, followed by 12–18 months of maintenance therapy with lower dose steroid and azathioprine), with or without **plasma exchange** (which effectively removes most plasma proteins, these being replaced by infused human albumin solution). The aim of plasma exchange is to rapidly remove the autoantibodies (eg anti-GBM or ANCA), allowing time for the immunosuppressive drugs to act to reduce their formation.

Essential note

The commoner glomerulonephritides are minimal change disease, membranous glomerulonephritis, focal segmental glomerulosclerosis, IgA nephropathy, diffuse proliferative glomerulonephritis, rapidly progressive glomerulonephritis (RPGN) and Goodpasture's syndrome

---

Plasma exchange in renal disease

- Goodpasture's syndrome
- ANCA +ve diseases: especially with pulmonary–renal presentation (mandatory with severe pulmonary haemorrhage); also for dialysis-requiring ARF
- Myeloma: cases with hyperviscosity
- HUS and TTP

Nephrology

7. INHERITED RENAL DISEASE

The commonest inherited renal diseases are polycystic kidney disease and Alport's syndrome. Rarer disorders include other renal cystic disease, disorders of amino acids and familial glomerulonephritis; the latter conditions are encountered much more often in paediatric nephrology.

Essential note

The commonest inherited renal diseases are polycystic kidney disease and Alport's syndrome

7.1 Autosomal dominant polycystic kidney disease (ADPKD)

Autosomal dominant polycystic kidney disease (ADPKD) is the most common inherited renal condition, and the genes have now been identified:

- **PKD1**: chromosome 16 in 86% of PKD patients
- **PKD2**: chromosome 4 in 10%.

The diagnosis is usually made by ultrasound; cysts usually develop during the teenage years so that first-degree relatives aged >20 years, with a normal scan, can be >90% confident of being disease-free; the confidence level rises to 98% at 30 years of age. The prevalence of ADPKD is 1 in 1000; the condition accounts for about 10% of RRT patients in the UK.

Clinical features

Patients may present with abdominal pain or mass, hypertension, UTI, renal calculi (10%), macroscopic haematuria or CRF.

- The age of onset of CRF varies widely (eg 25–60 years); not all patients develop ESRD.
- **Treatment** of the progressive CRF in ADPKD is as for other chronic nephropathies (ie hypertension control, ACE inhibitors/AIIRB therapy, etc).

Associations of ADPKD

- Liver cysts: 70%
- Berry aneurysms: 8% (leading to sub-arachnoid haemorrhage in some)
- Pancreatic cysts: 10%
- Mitral valve prolapse or aortic incompetence

7.2 Other renal cystic disorders

- **Autosomal recessive PKD**: rare (1/10 000 births). The gene is localised to chromosome 6. ESRF develops early in childhood; 100% have hepatic fibrosis. The prognosis is poor.
- **von Hippel–Lindau (VHL) syndrome**: autosomal dominant, the gene is localised on chromosome 3. Renal cysts are pre-malignant (>50%) and bilateral nephrectomy is often necessary. It is likely that patients previously thought to have renal malignancy in association with ADPKD actually had VHL. Patients are also at risk of spinocerebellar haemangioblastoma, retinal angiomas and phaeochromocytoma.
- **Medullary sponge kidney (MSK)**: sporadic; the cysts develop from ectatic collecting ducts. These may calcify, leading to the classical nephrocalcinosis associated with MSK. Patients have a benign course except that renal calculi and upper urinary tract infections are commonly associated.
- **Simple cysts**: fluid-filled, solitary or multiple, these are usually harmless, incidental findings at ultrasound or IVU. The cysts may grow to considerable size (eg >10 cm). They occasionally require percutaneous drainage because of persistent loin pain. Simple cysts are very common, affecting >20% of the elderly.

Essential note

Renal cystic disorders include: autosomal dominant polycystic kidney disease (PKD), autosomal recessive PKD, von Hippel–Lindau syndrome, medullary sponge kidney and simple cysts

7.3 Alport's syndrome

Eighty-five per cent of patients with Alport's syndrome have X-linked dominant inheritance, but other families may show dominant or recessive inheritance. The primary defect is an abnormal GBM (seen at electron microscopy) with variable thickness and splitting ('basket weave' appearance).

- Clinical presentation is with deafness, persistent microscopic haematuria, proteinuria and CRF; 30% develop nephrotic syndrome.
- Carrier females may have urinary abnormalities (haematuria, proteinuria), and usually do not develop renal failure.
- **Bilateral sensorineural deafness** is characteristic, but the hearing loss may only be mild.

- Ocular abnormalities (**lenticonus** – conical or spherical protrusion of the surface of the lens into the anterior chamber, or cataracts in 40%) may occur.
- The molecular defect involves the gene encoding for the $\alpha 5$-chain of type IV collagen.

7.4 Benign familial haematuria (BFH) and thin membrane nephropathy

Up to 25% of patients referred to a nephrologist for investigation of microscopic haematuria have this condition. It is common in families when it is termed '**benign familial haematuria**'; the inheritance pattern is dominant although the gene has not been identified. Sporadic cases are designated as '**thin membrane nephropathy**'. The normal thickness of the GBM is around 450 nm; patients with BFH/thin membrane nephropathy have an average GBM thickness of <250 nm. Patients usually have normal blood pressure and renal function.

8. RENAL INTERSTITIAL DISORDERS

8.1 Interstitial nephritis

Inflammation of the renal tubulo-interstitium may be acute or chronic; a recognised precipitating cause can be found in the majority of patients.

Acute interstitial nephritis (AIN)

AIN accounts for about 2% of all ARF cases. Most cases are due to an immunologically induced hypersensitivity reaction to an antigen – classically a drug or an infectious agent. The presentation is usually with mild renal impairment and hypertension or, in more severe cases, ARF which is often non-oliguric. Systemic manifestations of hypersensitivity may occur and include fever, arthralgia, rash, eosinophilia and increased IgE.

- **Diagnosis**: urinalysis may be unremarkable (eg minor proteinuria), although urinary eosinophils may be present. If >1% of urinary white cells are eosinophils, then this suggests the diagnosis. Renal biopsy shows oedema of the interstitium with infiltration of plasma cells, lymphocytes and eosinophils; there is often ATN with variable tubular dilatation.
- **Treatment**: cessation of precipitating cause (eg drugs). Most cases will improve without further treatment, but studies show that moderate dose oral steroids (eg 1 mg/kg, tapered over 1 month) can hasten recovery of renal function. Most patients make a near-complete renal functional recovery.

Causes of acute interstitial nephritis

- **Idiopathic** (rare – can be associated with anterior uveitis)
- **Infections**

  - eg viral (eg Hanta virus), bacterial (eg leptospirosis)

- **Drugs**

  - eg allopurinol, penicillin, cephalosporins, sulphonamides, frusemide, thiazide diuretics, aspirin, **NSAIDs**

- **Other**: sarcoidosis.

Chronic tubulo-interstitial nephritis (TIN)

Many diverse systemic and local renal conditions can result in chronic inflammation within the tubulo-interstitium. Patients present with CRF or ESRF; some patients may also manifest RTA (usually type 1), nephrogenic diabetes insipidus or salt-wasting states. Renal biopsy findings involve a chronic inflammatory infiltrate within the interstitium (granulomatous in sarcoid and TB), often with extensive scarring and tubular loss; the latter indicates that renal function can never be fully recovered.

TIN is commonly associated with macroscopically abnormal kidneys (eg scarring in reflux nephropathy). However, **TIN with macroscopically normal kidneys** accounts for about 3% of all ESRD, and the more common causes include sarcoidosis, Sjögren's syndrome and lithium toxicity.

Particular causes of chronic interstitial nephritis

- **Immunological diseases**

  - eg Sjögren's syndrome, rheumatoid arthritis, systemic sclerosis

- **Haematological disorders**

  - Myeloma, light-chain nephropathy

- **Heavy metals (and other toxins)**

  - eg lead, cadmium, Chinese herb nephropathy

- **Metabolic disorders**

  - eg hypercalcaemia, hypokalaemia, hyperuricaemia

- **Granulomatous disease**

  - TB, sarcoidosis

- **Drugs**

Ciclosporin A, cisplatin, lithium, iron, analgesics (*see* 'Analgesic nephropathy and papillary necrosis', below)

Treatment

Treatment is of the underlying condition (or drug/toxin withdrawal); steroids may be beneficial in some auto-immune or inflammatory disorders. The progressive CRF is treated as for other chronic nephropathies.

8.2 Analgesic nephropathy and papillary necrosis

Analgesic nephropathy

In the 1950s to 1970s analgesic nephropathy was the most common cause of both ARF and CRF in parts of Europe and Australia (eg 25% of ESRD in Australia). The condition is now in decline, especially since the withdrawal of phenacetin from the pharmaceutical market; aspirin and NSAIDs are now the most common causative agents. The hallmarks of the condition are the history of chronic analgesic usage (eg for backache, pelvic inflammatory disease, headache) and of addictive or dependent personality traits, renal pain (due to papillary necrosis) and CRF. There is a classical radiological appearance on IVU with features of papillary necrosis and renal scarring.

- Women are affected more often than men (4:1)
- Increased risk of urothelial malignancy (there may be multiple synchronous lesions).

Causes of renal papillary necrosis

- Toxic

    - Classical analgesic nephropathy
    - TB

- Ischaemic

    - Sickle cell disease
    - Acute pyelonephritis
    - Accelerated hypertension
    - Diabetes
    - Urinary tract obstruction
    - Hyperviscosity syndromes
    - NSAID-induced

9. REFLUX NEPHROPATHY AND URINARY TRACT INFECTIONS

9.1 Vesico-ureteric reflux and reflux nephropathy

Reflux nephropathy is the term applied when small and irregularly scarred kidneys (chronic pyelonephritis, CPN) are associated with vesico-ureteric reflux (VUR). It is the commonest cause of CPN, but there are other causes (eg obstructive injury, analgesic nephropathy). Scarring is necessary for the development of reflux nephropathy and this almost only occurs during the first 5 years of life. The end-result of reflux nephropathy is hypertension, protein-uria, CRF and, eventually in some patients, ESRD; reflux nephropathy still accounts for at least 10% of adult patients entering RRT programmes, and is the commonest cause of ESRD in children.

- **Epidemiology**: around 1% of children will have VUR, but this disappears in 40% by the age of 2 years. In young children VUR usually presents with a complicating urinary tract infection (UTI). About 30% of children with UTI will have some degree of VUR and 10% will have evidence of reflux nephropathy. Five per cent of women with symptomatic UTI will have reflux nephropathy.
- **Diagnosis** is by micturating cystography or radionuclide scan; scarring can be demonstrated by ultrasound and DMSA.
- **Genetic predisposition**: first-degree relatives of patients with reflux have a greatly increased chance of VUR; it is recommended that offspring or siblings (if a child) of affected patients undergo screening.

Management of VUR and reflux nephropathy

All children with UTI should be investigated for VUR. The aim of treatment for patients with VUR is to prevent renal scars. As these occur early in life there is no place for anti-reflux surgery to prevent renal scars in adults who have VUR. Children with significant reflux should receive prophylactic antibiotic therapy until puberty in order to minimise UTI. For severe reflux, surgical options include endoscopic injection of collagen behind the intra-vesical ureter, lengthening of the submucosal ureteric tunnel and ureteric re-implantation.

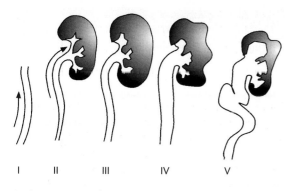

I   II   III   IV   V

Grade I: Ureter only
Grade II: Up to pelvis and calyces, but with no dilatation
Grade III: Mild-moderate dilatation, but with only minimal blunting of fornices
Grade IV: Moderate dilatation, with obliteration of sharp angles of fornices
Grade V: Gross dilatation and tortuosity of ureter and pelvi-calyceal system. Calyces severely clubbed

Figure 4 Classification of vesico-ureteric reflux

9.2 Urinary tract infection (UTI)

Apart from the outer one-third of the female urethra, the urinary tract is normally sterile. UTIs are the commonest bacterial infections managed in general practice; they predominantly affect women (except in infants, patients aged >60 years, and those with co-morbid diseases). Coliforms are by far the most common pathogens. Several important definitions are applied :

- **Acute uncomplicated UTI**: acute cystitis and acute pyelonephritis. The incidence of cystitis is 0.5% per year in sexually active women. It may recur in 40% of healthy women, even when their urinary tracts are normal. Three-day antibiotic treatment regimes are recommended for acute cystitis because of cost, compliance and efficacy. In those with recurrent cystitis, attention to hygiene, post-coital micturition and fluid intake are recommended.
- **Complicated UTI**: these occur in patients with abnormal urinary tracts (eg stones, obstruction, ileal conduits, VUR, neurogenic bladder) and very commonly in patients with urinary catheters (*see* below). The definition also incorporates patients with CRF and renal transplants.
- **Asymptomatic bacteriuria**: two separate urinary specimens showing bacterial colony counts of $>10^5$/ml of the same organism in an **asymptomatic** patient. The prevalence may be 3–5% in adult women (and 0.5% in men); it increases greatly in the elderly (eg 50% of women) and in institutionalised patients. It should always be treated if detected in pregnant women, as 15–20% of patients will otherwise develop acute pyelonephritis.

- **Urinary catheter-associated infection**: up to 5% of all hospital admissions may be due to UTI, and the majority of these occur in patients with long-term in-dwelling catheters. The incidence of bacteriuria is 3–10% per day of catheterisation, and so the duration of catheterisation is the greatest risk factor. Most infections are symptomatic and do not require treatment; if lower urinary tract symptoms occur, a single antibiotic dose may be as effective as a full course of therapy (which predisposes to bacterial resistance); it may also be appropriate to change the catheter (if needed long-term) as organisms are harboured within the bio-film lining of the catheter.

Predispositions to urinary tract infection

- Abnormal urinary tract
  - eg Calculi, VUR, reflux nephropathy, analgesic nephropathy, obstruction, atonic bladder, ileal conduit, in-dwelling catheter, **pregnancy** (where the urinary tract abnormality is temporary)
- Impaired host defences
  - Immunosuppressive therapy (including transplanted patients), diabetes mellitus
- Virulent organisms
  - (eg Urease-producing *Proteus*)

9.3 Tuberculosis of the urinary tract

TB reaches the urinary tract via haematogenous spread. Most patients are 20–40 years of age, with men affected twice as commonly as women. One-quarter of patients are asymptomatic; a further 25% have asymptomatic pyuria or microscopic haematuria, and painless macro-haematuria is common.

- The renal medullary regions are most commonly affected. In the early stages, ulcerating lesions and granulomas are seen in the renal pyramids and collecting systems; renal histology shows chronic interstitial nephritis with granulomas.

- As the disease progresses scarring occurs with ureteric strictures, hydronephrosis, subcapsular collections, perinephric abscesses or renal atrophy. The bladder may be fibrotic and small. The caseating material may eventually calcify.
- **Treatment**: standard anti-tuberculous therapy is recommended. Surgery may be indicated for obstruction and strictures.

10. RENAL CALCULI AND NEPHROCALCINOSIS

10.1 Renal calculi (nephrolithiasis)

Renal stones are common, with an annual incidence of approximately 2 per 1000 and a prevalence of 3% in the UK. Calcium-containing stones are commonest.

Stone composition

- Calcium containing (with oxalate or phosphate): 70%
- Urate: 10% (radiolucent)
- Cystine: 2%
- Staghorns ('struvite' containing magnesium ammonium phosphate and sometimes calcium): 20%; associated with infection with urease-producing bacteria (eg *Proteus* spp.)

Basic investigation

This should include stone analysis, MSU, assessment of renal function, serum calcium and phosphate, and a qualitative test for urinary cystine. The 24-hour urinary excretion of oxalate, calcium (should be <7.5 mmol/day), creatinine and uric acid may also be helpful, and RTA should be excluded (alkaline urinary pH).

Further investigation

Further investigation will involve IVU and/or ultrasound, depending upon clinical presentation.

Commonest predispositions to urolithiasis

- **Metabolic abnormalities**

  - Idiopathic hypercalciuria (most common)
  - Primary hyperparathyroidism (and other causes of hypercalcaemia)
  - Renal tubular acidosis
  - Cystinuria
  - High dietary oxalate intake (eg glutinous rice or leafy vegetables in Thailand)

Commonest predispositions to urolithiasis

- **Renal structural abnormalities**

  - Polycystic kidney disease
  - Medullary sponge kidney
  - Reflux nephropathy

- **Other causes**

  - Chronic dehydration (common, eg chronic diarrhoea, warm climates)

Treatment

General measures: large fluid intake; associated urinary infection should be eradicated where possible (very difficult with staghorn calculi). Treat other underlying causes (eg allopurinol for urate stones, surgery for hyperparathyroidism).

Thiazide diuretics (eg chlorthalidone): increase tubular absorption of calcium in patients with hypercalciuria, and will therefore reduce the likelihood of super-saturation of calcium products within the urine. Citrate may be beneficial for calcium oxalate stones. The specific treatment of patients with **cystinuria** is described in Chapter 11, Metabolic diseases.

Stone removal: ureteric calculi <0.5 cm may be passed spontaneously. Lithotripsy alone may be used for larger ureteric stones and for pelvi-calyceal stones <4 cm; larger calculi can be 'debulked' by this technique before surgical extraction.

10.2 Nephrocalcinosis

This is defined as the deposition of calcium salts within the renal parenchyma; it may be associated with urinary calculi.

Causes

- **Cortical nephrocalcinosis**

  - Cortical necrosis (see 'tram-line' calcification)
  - Chronic glomerulonephritis

- **Medullary nephrocalcinosis**

  - Hypercalcaemia (eg primary hyperparathyroidism, sarcoidosis, hypervitaminosis D, milk-alkali syndrome)
  - Idiopathic hypercalciuria
  - Renal tubular acidosis
  - Primary hyperoxaluria
  - Medullary sponge kidney
  - Tuberculosis

11. URINARY TRACT OBSTRUCTION AND TUMOURS

11.1 Urinary tract obstruction

Chronic urinary tract obstruction (most often due to prostatic disease, calculi and bladder lesions) is a common cause of CRF; obstruction must also be excluded in every case of ARF. The causes of renal tract obstruction are shown in the box below. The term **obstructive nephropathy** refers to pathological renal damage resulting from obstruction.

Acute obstruction

This is often painful due to distension of the bladder, ureter(s) or pelvi-calyceal systems. Complete obstruction will result in anuria and ARF.

- **Diagnosis**: obstruction is one of the few truly reversible causes of renal failure, but diagnosis and treatment need to be expedient in order to allow renal functional recovery. Ultrasound is the chief mode of diagnosis.
- **Treatment and prognosis**: depending upon the site of obstruction, temporary drainage can often be achieved by bladder catheterisation (bladder outflow obstruction), percutaneous nephrostomy or by endoscopic ureteric stenting, pending definitive surgical correction (eg TURP or stone extraction). Relief of obstruction may be followed by massive diuresis (temporary nephrogenic DI); if the obstruction has been relieved within 2 weeks then full renal functional recovery is likely.

Chronic obstructive nephropathy

This is usually associated with CRF or ESRF and it is often complicated by chronic UTI. Obstruction accounts for 5% of all cases of ESRD. There is permanent renal damage that leads to tubular loss, interstitial fibrosis and cortical atrophy. If the obstruction is relieved (eg in <12 weeks), renal functional decline can stabilise and dialysis may be prevented.

Essential note

Urinary tract obstruction may be acute or chronic

Causes of urinary tract obstruction

- **Within the lumen**

  - Tumour (eg urothelial lesions of bladder, ureter or renal pelvis)
  - Renal calculi
  - Papillary necrosis (sloughed papilla)
  - Blood clot

- **External compression**

  - Malignancy: retro-peritoneal neoplasia including para-aortic lymphadenopathy and pelvic cancer (eg cervical or prostatic carcinoma)
  - Other 'tumours': aortic aneurysm; pregnancy (hydronephrosis of pregnancy is very common, is usually asymptomatic, and resolves fully after delivery); haematomas
  - Aberrant arteries (pelvi-ureteric junction (PUJ) obstruction)
  - Retro-peritoneal fibrosis (eg malignant, idiopathic, peri-aortitis, drugs (see below))
  - Prostatic disease: benign hypertrophy or malignancy
  - Inflammatory disorders (eg diverticulitis, Crohn's disease, pancreatitis)
  - Iatrogenic: surgical ligation of ureter

- **Within the wall of urinary tract structures**

  - Neuromuscular dysfunction (eg PUJ obstruction, neuropathic bladder (spina bifida, spinal trauma – see below))
  - Ureteric or vesico-ureteric stricture: eg TB, previous calculi, after surgery, irradiation (eg for seminoma of testis), malignancy
  - Urethral stricture (eg gonococcal) following instrumentation
  - Posterior urethral valves

Neuropathic bladder

In childhood, **spina bifida** with myelomeningocele is by far the commonest cause of a neuropathic bladder. Spina bifida has an incidence of around 1–5 per 1000 births. Urinary tract complications are present at birth in 15%, and will develop in 50%, often over many years. Most of these patients have incomplete bladder emptying due to urethral sphincter dyssynergia.

- The main urinary tract abnormalities are incontinence, infection and reflux with upper tract dilatation, the latter leading to CRF and ESRD.
- Patients usually have associated bowel dysfunction.

- **Treatment**: is with anti-cholinergic drugs, intermittent self-catheterisation, and, in more severe cases, urinary tract diversion into an ileal conduit.

Posterior urethral valves (PUV)

These occur in male infants; the valves are mucosal diaphragms in the posterior urethra at the level of the prostate. PUV can now be detected ante-natally with ultrasound. Urinary diversion should be avoided; self-catheterisation is usually necessary.

11.2 Retroperitoneal fibrosis (RPF)

An uncommon, progressive condition in which the ureters become embedded in dense fibrous tissue (the ureters are drawn medially) often at the junction of the middle and lower thirds of the ureter, leading to obstruction. The majority of cases are thought to result from an immunologically mediated peri-aortitis, and steroids are of benefit in these 'idiopathic' forms of RPF.

- **Other associations**: retroperitoneal malignancy (eg colonic, bladder or prostatic cancer, lymphoma), previous irradiation, inflammatory abdominal aortic aneurysm, other fibrosing conditions (eg sclerosing cholangitis), drugs (eg methysergide and some β-blockers) and granulomatous disease (TB or sarcoidosis).
- **Investigation**: ESR is often very high, IVU shows medial deviation of the ureters and a peri-aortic mass may be seen at CT scan.
- **Treatment**: ureterolysis (with tissue biopsy) with long-term steroid therapy (as relapse is common). Malignant RPF can be palliated with ureteric stenting, or with percutaneous nephrostomy.

11.3 Urinary tract tumours

Benign renal tumours: include adenomata, which are very common (however, just as with thyroid adenoma and carcinoma, their histological differentiation from malignant lesions can be difficult), hamartomas and renin-secreting (juxta-glomerular cell) tumours.

Renal cell carcinoma (hypernephroma): arise from the tubular epithelium; they are more likely in smokers. Other predispositions include von Hippel–Lindau syndrome.

- The hallmark of renal cell carcinoma is its propensity to invade the renal veins, with passage of tumour emboli to lung.
- Other unusual clinical features include pyrexia of unknown origin, left varicocele (renal vein invasion leads to left testicular vein occlusion), and endocrine effects (secretion of erythropoietic factor resulting in polycythaemia, PTH-like substance, renin and ACTH). Five-year survival is about 50%.

Wilm's tumour (nephroblastoma): these are tumours of early childhood, and are derived from embryonic renal tissue. They become enormous and metastasise early. Treatment is with nephrectomy and actinomycin D, providing a three-year survival rate of 65%.

Urothelial tumours: very common and usually derived from transitional epithelium, although squamous carcinoma (far worse prognosis) is recognised. The usual presentation is with bleeding or urinary tract obstruction. Tumours are often multiple, and so investigation of the complete urinary tract is indicated.

- Several carcinogens (eg smoking, rubber and aniline dye exposure, analgesic nephropathy) have been aetiologically linked to this type of malignancy.
- Other risk factors include renal calculi, cystic kidney disease, chronic cystitis (including after cyclophosphamide therapy) and *Schistosoma haematobium* infection
- Nephro-ureterectomy is indicated for lesions of ureter or renal pelvis, and cystectomy with resection of urethral mucosa for advanced bladder cancer; surgery combined with radiotherapy provides a five-year survival of 50%.

Metastatic disease (involving the kidney): most commonly from breast, lung, stomach, lymphoma or melanoma.

Essential note

Malignant tumours of the urinary tract include: renal cell carcinoma, Wilm's nephroblastoma of childhood and urothelial tumours presenting with obstruction and/or bleeding

12. SYSTEMIC DISORDERS AND THE KIDNEY

12.1 Amyloidosis

Amyloidosis is due to over-production of proteinaceous material which deposits in an organised formation within tissues. Kidney involvement leads to presentation with proteinuria, nephrotic syndrome or CRF; biopsy demonstrates characteristic Congo-red-staining extracellular fibrillar material within the mesangium, interstitium and vessel walls. Amyloid is classified according to the amyloid proteins involved, as well as the underlying disease process.

Immunologlobulinic amyloid (AL-amyloidosis)

Free immunoglobulin light chains (hence the 'L') are secreted by a clone of B cells; 25% of patients have an underlying immunoproliferative disease (usually myeloma), but many more probably have a monoclonal gammopathy (MGUS). Median age of presentation is above 60 years.

- AL amyloid may infiltrate any organ other than the brain – eg heart (restrictive cardiomyopathy in 30%, sick-sinus syndrome and arrhythmias), macroglossia, GI tract (motility disturbance, malabsorption, haemorrhage), neuropathy (peripheral and autonomic) and bleeding diathesis.
- **Treatment**: cases associated with myeloma receive conventional therapy. In 'primary amyloid', regimes involving prednisolone with either melphelan or colchicine have been shown to extend survival duration by only 50%. Autologous bone marrow transplantation (after high-dose chemotherapy) provides the only prospect of cure.
- **Prognosis**: is poor, with median survival of 12 months.

AA-amyloidosis

Chronic infections (eg TB, empyema) now account for fewer cases than previously; 70% of cases are due to autoimmune inflammatory conditions. In AA-amyloidosis the kidney is the main target organ – cardiac involvement and neuropathy are uncommon. Prognosis is consequently better than for AL-amyloidosis with median survival of 25 months.

Treatment: the underlying inflammatory or infective disorder should be treated. Colchine has been shown to prevent disease progression in **familial Mediterranean fever** (another form of AA-amyloidosis).

Classification of amyloidosis

- **Primary amyloid**

  AL type, which is serum amyloid protein A coupled with immunoglobulin light chains

- **Hereditary amyloid**

  (eg familial Mediterranean fever)
  The amyloid is of AA type

- **Secondary amyloid**

  This is usually AA type (fibrils composed of acute phase protein)

- **Secondary to chronic suppurative disorders**

  Tuberculosis, osteomyelitis, empyema, bronchiectasis, syphilis, leprosy

- **Secondary to chronic inflammatory disorders**

  Rheumatological conditions

  Rheumatoid arthritis, psoriatic arthritis, ankylosing spondylitis, Still's disease, Reiter's syndrome, Sjögren's syndrome, Behçet's disease

  Gastrointestinal conditions

  Whipple's disease, inflammatory bowel disease

  Para-protein-related conditions

  Myeloma (AL type), benign monoclonal gammopathy (AL type)

- **Other secondary amyloid**

  Heroin abuse, paraplegia, renal cell carcinoma

- **Dialysis-related amyloid**

  This does not deposit in the kidneys, as it is a complication of long-term dialysis. It is due to failure of clearance of β_2-microglobulin (*see* Section 5.4, Maintenance dialysis)

12.2 Renovascular disease

Atherosclerotic renovascular disease (ARVD)

ARVD accounts for >90% of all renovascular disease (Figure 5). It is increased with ageing, is associated with common atherogenic risk factors (ie hypertension, smoking, diabetes, etc) and the presence of generalised vascular disease. As older patients are now readily admitted to RRT programmes, ARVD is found to be increasingly associated with ESRD (15–20%), although it probably only accounts for the renal failure in the minority (*see* below).

Clinical presentation is with hypertension, CRF or ESRD, 'flash' pulmonary oedema (10%), and ARF due to acute arterial occlusion or related to ACE inhibitors. Prognosis is poor (5-year survival <20%) due to co-morbid vascular events. Many cases of ARVD are thought to be incidental, occurring as a result of hypertension and CRF (pro-atherogenic state), rather than being the cause of them.

- **Radiological diagnosis**: **MR angiography** is now the optimum non-invasive screening test for ARVD diagnosis. It is indicated in patients with vascular bruits or asymmetrical kidneys on ultrasound, and in cases of unexplained CRF or severe hypertension. **CT angiography** is also increasingly used, but can be complicated by radio-contrast nephropathy in patients with CRF (N-acetyl cysteine may help prevent this). **Conventional intra-arterial angiography** is now largely reserved for patients with complex anatomy, and when confirming renal arterial anatomy prior to revascularisation. Ninety per cent of RAS lesions are 'ostial' (occurring within the first 1 cm of the renal artery origin).
- **Revascularisation procedures**: renal angioplasty with or without stenting accounts for >95% of all revascularisation (the remainder being surgical reconstructions – especially indicated with complicated lesions, eg related to aortic aneurysm). Improved hypertension control can be anticipated, but cure (ie no need for anti-hypertensive agents) is unusual. Improvement in renal dysfunction is variable. Patients should also receive aspirin and cholesterol-lowering therapy for their general atherosclerotic risk.

Fibromuscular dysplasia (FMD)

FMD accounts for 10% of all renovascular disease; it occurs in the young (20–35 years), and the majority of patients are female. The stenoses tend to be distal in the renal artery; they appear as a 'string of beads' at angiography (Figure 5). Patients usually present with severe hypertension, but renal failure is unusual. As the kidney beyond a fibromuscular stenosis is usually healthy, revascularisation may cure the hypertension, and it often restores renal function completely in the sub-group of patients with renal impairment.

12.3 Connective tissue disorders and the kidney

Most of the connective tissue disorders have the propensity to cause renal disease, and characteristic features are described below (see also Chapter 16, Rheumatology); lupus nephritis and systemic sclerosis merit more detailed coverage.

- **Mixed connective tissue disease**: membranous or proliferative glomerulonephritis (uncommon).
- **Sjögren's syndrome**: renal involvement is most often manifest by renal tubular dysfunction (RTA1 or 2) with interstitial nephritis.
- **Rheumatoid arthritis**: renal disease is common, and usually due to amyloid, or less often the effects of drug therapy (membranous glomerulonephritis with gold or penicillamine therapy).

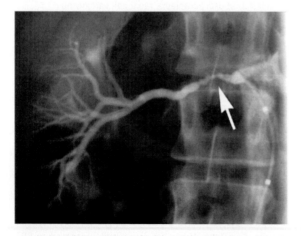

Figure 5a Renal angiogram demonstrating typical 'string of beads' appearance of renovascular narrowing as seen in fibromuscular disease

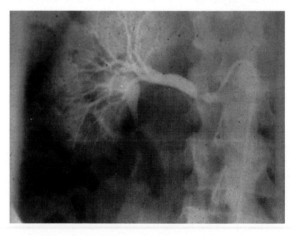

Figure 5b Renal angiogram showing proximal renal artery stenosis of atherosclerotic renovascular disease

SLE nephritis

Over 5% of patients with SLE have renal involvement at presentation, and around 60% of patients will develop overt renal disease at some stage. Lupus nephritis is commoner in black patients and in women (tenfold > than in men), and 90% will have ANF antibodies. Renal disease can be manifest by any syndromal picture (eg proteinuria, nephrotic syndrome, RPGN with ARF, CRF) but proteinuria is present in almost all patients with nephritis. Similarly, many different patterns of glomerular disease are recognised (the histological picture may even change, over time, within the same individual). Note that drug-induced SLE only rarely affects the kidneys. Although lupus nephritis can present with marked patient morbidity, prompt immunosuppressive treatment can be very successful.

Treatment: most patients with significant proteinuria are likely to receive at least prednisolone and ACE inhibitor therapy. Acute SLE with ARF (usually diffuse, crescentic or severe focal proliferative glomerulonephritis) should be treated as for 'RPGN/crescentic nephritis' (*see* Section 6, Glomerulonephritis and associated syndromes), with an intense induction regime (high-dose steroid and usually pulsed i.v. cyclophosphamide) followed by maintenance therapy.

Prognosis of renal lupus: <10% of cases with nephritis now progress to ESRD (historically, renal disease used to be the commonest cause of death in SLE).

Systemic sclerosis

Renal disease is always accompanied by hypertension; the hallmark presentation is 'scleroderma renal crisis' with accelerated hypertension and ARF. Prominent pathological changes are seen in the interlobular arteries (severe intimal proliferation with deposition of mucopolysaccharides – so-called onion skin appearance); fibrinoid necrosis of afferent arterioles and secondary glomerular ischaemia are common. The essential treatment is with ACE inhibitors for hypertension control; many patients progress to ESRD. The overall prognosis is poor because of other organ involvement (especially restrictive cardiomyopathy and pulmonary fibrosis).

12.4 Diabetic nephropathy

Diabetic nephropathy is now the most common cause of ESRD in the UK, accounting for 25% of patients. In recent years there have been advances in the understanding of the natural history, pathogenesis and treatment of diabetic nephropathy, but the mortality of this group remains high, largely because of associated CVS disease.

Epidemiology

Overt nephropathy, defined as persistent proteinuria (>300 mg/24 h), occurs with a cumulative incidence of 30% after 40 years in type I diabetics. In type II diabetics, nephropathy is already prevalent in 10% at the time of diabetes diagnosis (reflecting previous 'sub-clinical' hyperglycaemia), and there is a 25% 20-year cumulative incidence of nephropathy. About one-fifth of these latter patients will develop CRF and be at risk of ESRD (ie 5% of all type II diabetics) – the remainder succumb to other complications of diabetes before they develop significant CRF. As type II diabetes is 10–15 times more common than type I in Western populations, the prevalence of patients with nephropathy in type II diabetes is substantially higher than in those with type I diabetes. In a UK diabetic clinic, the prevalence of nephropathy is about 5% at any time.

- Genetic influence: diabetics in certain racial groups have a far greater risk of developing nephropathy (eg Asians, Pima Indians). In the UK, the likelihood of ESRD is threefold greater in Asian and Afro-Caribbean diabetics than Caucasians.
- Nephropathy is usually associated with retinopathy (common basement membrane pathology); renovascular disease and other arterial pathology are common.

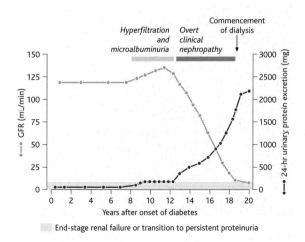

End-stage renal failure or transition to persistent proteinuria

Figure 6 Schematic diagram detailing the natural history of development and progression of diabetic nephropathy

Natural history of nephropathy (Figure 6)

- Microalbuminuria (urinary albumin excretion rate (UAER) 30–300 mg/day, or 20–200 µg/min) develops in 30–50% of patients at 5–10 years after diabetes onset, and 80% of these patients go on to develop overt nephropathy over 10–15 years. The GFR may be elevated at this stage. Blood pressure starts to rise (in 60%).
- 'Established' or 'overt' nephropathy is associated with increasing macro-proteinuria ('persistent proteinuria'), which may become nephrotic in 30%, and declining GFR (eg at 2–10 ml/min per year) in almost all patients. Hypertension is present in most (80%) and is correlated with the rate of decline of GFR. Renal histology typically shows diffuse glomerular sclerosing lesions (all patients) and vascular changes; 10% have Kimmelstiel–Wilson nodules (focal glomerular sclerosis).
- ESRD occurs at an average of 7 years from onset of the overt nephropathy stage.

Screening and prevention

Patients should be **screened** for microalbuminuria in the diabetic clinic; the albumin:creatinine ratio (ACR – *see* Section 2.1 Urinalysis) in an early morning specimen is more practical than obtaining timed urine collections. An ACR of >2.5 is generally taken as the cut-off for microalbuminuria (equivalent to a UAER of >35 µg/min, or 45 mg/24 h).

- Studies in type I diabetics have shown that tight glycaemic control can reduce the likelihood of patients developing microalbuminuria (by 40%), and there is emerging evidence that intensive insulin regimes may prevent some microalbuminuric patients progressing to overt nephropathy.
- However, the latter has been clearly shown with trials using ACE inhibitors in type I diabetes, and with AIIRBs in type II diabetes. These agents also slow the time of doubling of serum creatinine and the time to ESRF in patients with established nephropathy; comparisons with other anti-hypertensive agents suggest that their renoprotective effects are partly independent of hypertension control.
- It is now accepted that blood pressure should be targeted to 125/75 mmHg in patients with overt nephropathy – this will slow, but not prevent, the inexorable decline of GFR.

Outcome

The mortality of these patients is very high (eg patients with insulin-dependent diabetes mellitus have a 20-fold greater mortality than the general population) and this relative risk may be magnified a further 25-fold in those with proteinuria (eg two-year mortality of 30% in patients with ESRD), largely due to co-morbid cardiovascular disease. Many patients with overt nephropathy in type II diabetes will die before they reach ESRD.

> **Essential note**
>
> The mortality of patients with diabetic nephropathy is very high because of the combination of renal and cardiovascular disease

12.5 Thrombotic microangiopathies

Haemolytic–uraemic syndrome (HUS) and **thrombotic thrombocytopenic purpura (TTP)** share similar renal histologic features and pathophysiology (*see also* Chapter 8, Haematology). In both conditions there is a microangiopathic haemolytic anaemia (MAHA), with anaemia, RBC fragments and schistocytes. Platelet clumping occurs within the intra-vascular thrombi, and hence thrombocytopenia is a major feature.

Haemolytic–uraemic syndrome (HUS)

HUS is the commonest cause of ARF in children (because ARF is rare in children), but it is also seen in adults. Children aged <4 years account for 90% of cases. Two main forms of HUS are recognised:

- **Typical or diarrhoea-associated (D$^+$) HUS**: the onset is explosive, with ARF, and epidemics of the disease occur. A third of UK cases are due to verotoxin-producing *E. coli* O157:H7 (VTEC); the toxin damages vascular endothelium, predisposing to the microangiopathy. *Shigella dysenteriae* can also be associated. Ninety per cent of patients with D$^+$HUS make a good recovery, but 5% die during the acute illness.
- **Atypical HUS**: tends to affect older children and adults; most patients have no diarrhoea (D$^-$HUS). Many D$^-$HUS cases are thought to be familial, and there is progressive renal dysfunction with neurologic episodes that can resemble TTP. **Familial forms** of HUS/TTP can be associated with factor H deficiency. These forms have a poorer prognosis.

Treatment: the mainstay of therapy is infusion of fresh frozen plasma (FFP) and plasma exchange.

Thrombotic thrombocytopenic purpura (TTP)

In TTP, explosive ARF is less prominent, but neurological abnormalities are usual (due to formation and release of microthrombi within the brain vasculature).

Secondary cause of HUS and TTP include

- Pregnancy-associated thrombotic microangiopathy
  - TTP
  - HELLP syndrome
  - Post-partum HUS
- HIV-associated thrombotic microangiopathy
- Cancer-associated thrombotic microangiopathy
- Drugs (eg ciclosporin)

12.6 Hypertension and the kidney

A detailed description of hypertension is beyond the scope of this chapter, but see also Chapter 1, Cardiology. The kidney is often damaged by essential hypertension, or it can be central to the pathogenesis of many cases of secondary hypertension.

Primary (essential) hypertension and renal damage

End-organ renal damage is common and is usually manifest with asymptomatic proteinuria and/or CRF (**hypertensive nephrosclerosis**). Microalbuminuria develops in 20–40% of patients with essential hypertension, and persistent proteinuria (occasionally nephrotic) in a smaller proportion. Typical histological lesions include vascular wall thickening and luminal obliteration, with widespread interstitial fibrosis and glomerulosclerosis.

- Elevated creatinine develops in 10–20% of patients; the risk is greater in African-Americans, the elderly and those with higher systolic blood pressure.
- Progression to ESRD occurs in 2–5% over 10–15 years. Hypertension accounts for about 30% of all ESRD in the USA and 15% in the UK.
- It is thought that many patients who present with ESRD of unknown aetiology, especially if having small, smooth kidneys visible at ultrasound, actually have long-standing hypertensive renal disease.

Treatment and targets: all patients should have blood pressure controlled to <140/85 mmHg. In those with proteinuria and/or renal impairment, a target blood pressure of <125/75 mmHg should be sought. ACE inhibitors and AIIRBs are specifically indicated for the reasons described earlier in the chapter.

'Malignant' or accelerated hypertension: this refers to presentation with severe diastolic hypertension (eg DBP > 120 mmHg) with grade 3 (haemorrhages and/or exudates) or 4 (with papilloedema) retinopathy. Patients may have ARF, significant proteinuria and non-renal complications such as encephalopathy or cardiac failure. The condition constitutes a medical emergency. Typical histological lesions include arterial fibrinoid necrosis (which also accounts for the retinal abnormalities) coupled with severe tubular and glomerular ischaemia.

Secondary hypertension

Over 90% of hypertension is idiopathic, approximately 5% is due to renal disease, 2–3% due to primary hyperaldosteronism and <1% has either an alternative rare endocrine or other cause.

Hypertension due to renal disease

Renal disease accounts for the majority of cases of secondary hypertension. The majority of patients with CRF are hypertensive, and it is evident in at least 90% of the dialysis population, and over 60% of transplant patients. It is the chief contributor to the LVH and associated high cardiovascular mortality of these patients.

- **Coarctation of the aorta**: hypertension is seen in the upper limbs only. Rib-notching may be seen on X-ray.
- **Endocrine**: Cushing's syndrome, phaeochromocytoma and acromegaly are all rare causes. It is now believed that **primary hyperaldosteronism** (associated with bilateral or unilateral adrenal hyperplasia) may account for about 3% of all hypertension (see Chapter 1, Cardiology and Chapter 4, Endocrinology).
- **Other secondary hypertension**: alcohol, obesity.

12.7 Myeloma and the kidney

Myeloma occurs with an incidence of 30–40 cases/million, and at a median age of 70–80 years. Renal involvement may present with ARF, CRF and/or proteinuria. Note that Bence–Jones proteinuria is not detected by standard urinary dipsticks.

Renal failure due to myeloma

ARF: some degree of renal impairment is observed in 50% of patients with myeloma; this is reversible in the majority (in those where it is secondary to hypercalcaemia, hypovolaemia, infection or nephrotoxic drugs), but 10% of patients may need dialysis. The latter cases are usually due to **light chain or 'cast' nephropathy**.

CRF: due to amyloidosis (see above), and cast nephropathy associated with chronic interstitial nephritis (see below).

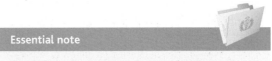

Essential note

Standard urinary dipsticks do not detect Bence–Jones protein

Cast nephropathy

In this, free kappa (the most nephrotoxic) and lambda light chains excreted in the urine damage the tubules by direct nephrotoxicity and by cast formation. The intra-tubular casts are composed of hard, needle-shaped crystals and excite an interstitial infiltrate, often with multi-nucleate giant cells. ATN and tubular atrophy occur, and hence the potential for some recovery from an ARF episode.

- **Treatment and prognosis**: is with rehydration. Hypercalcaemia should be treated with i.v. bisphosphonates. The myeloma should be treated with conventional regimes. Younger patients may be considered for autologous stem cell transplantation. Patients with myeloma and ESRD have poor survival (<50% at 1 year). Those with the greatest tumour mass have the worst prognosis.

12.8 Renal vasculitis

The kidney is often involved in systemic vasculitic illness. Several disorders are recognised, and these are classified and described more fully in Chapter 16, Rheumatology.

> **Essential note**
>
> Types of small vessel vasculitis include: Wegener's granulomatosis, Churg–Strauss syndrome and microscopic polyangiitis (MPA)

Small vessel pauci-immune vasculitis

These conditions affect small vessels (arterioles and veins) and are associated with glomerulonephritis, and pulmonary and skin vasculitis. They are usually associated with +ve serum ANCA (*see* Chapter 9, Immunology). Incidence is 10–20 cases/million each year. The major conditions are defined as :

- **Wegener's granulomatosis**: respiratory tract disease is characteristic and this involves necrotising granulomata within the upper respiratory tract (leading to sinusitis and nasal discharge, as well as damage to the nasal septum) and lungs (with haemoptysis). About 70% of patients are cANCA +ve, and 25% pANCA.
- **Churg–Strauss syndrome**: vasculitis that is associated with asthma, eosinophilia and necrotising inflammation. Sixty per cent have +ve pANCA; 30% are ANCA −ve.
- **Microscopic polyangiitis (MPA)**: vasculitis occurring in the absence of evidence for the above two conditions (ie asthma, eosinophilia or necrotising granulomatous inflammation); 50% are pANCA +ve, and 40% cANCA.

In all conditions, **ARF** is the usual renal presentation; renal histology shows necrotising glomerulitis typically associated with focal proliferative and/or crescentic glomerulonephritis (*see* Section 6.2, Treatment of RPGN and crescentic nephritis). Pulmonary involvement is common. A purpuric vasculitic skin rash is often seen.

- **Treatment**: all of the above three conditions normally merit aggressive immunosuppressive therapy; typical regimes are described in Section 6.2, Treatment of RPGN and crescentic nephritis.
- **Prognosis**: 1-year renal and patient survival is >80%. Poorer renal prognosis is seen in patients with highest creatinine and/or oligo-anuria at presentation. Mortality is increased in patients with pulmonary haemorrhage.

Polyarteritis nodosa (PAN)

PAN is a rare, medium-sized arterial vasculitis which results in microaneurysm formation; hypertension is usually severe, and renal infarcts rather than glomerulonephritis are characteristic. Patients are usually ANCA −ve (unless there is also small vessel involvement, i.e. PAN-MPA overlap). Pulmonary (infiltrates and haemorrhage), GI tract (infarcts), neurological (mononeuritis multiplex) and systemic features (myalgia, PUO) are recognised, but the condition is notoriously difficult to confirm. A few cases are associated with hepatitis B infection. **Treatment** is as for small vessel vasculitis/crescentic nephritis.

Other vasculitides that can affect the kidney

- **Henoch–Schönlein nephritis**: in addition to the typical systemic features of this condition, some patients develop renal disease as a result of small vessel vasculitis.
- **Kawasaki disease**: acute febrile illness, usually in children, associated with a desquamating erythematous rash, and necrotising arteritis in some patients. It is the commonest cause of myocardial infarction in childhood, but significant renal disease is uncommon.
- **Takayasu arteritis**: this can be associated with RAS and renovascular hypertension.

12.9 Sarcoidosis and the kidney

Sarcoidosis (*see* Section 8.1, Interstitial nephritis) can be associated with:

- **ARF**: due to AIN. Ninety per cent of patients have systemic manifestations of sarcoidosis (eg hepato-splenomegaly, hypercalcaemia).
- **CRF**: associated with TIN and hypercalcaemia.

Treatment: most patients respond promptly to oral steroids, which can be tapered at 3–6 months. Relapses occur, but are usually steroid-responsive. Serum ACE may be useful for monitoring disease activity and predicting likelihood of relapses.

13. DRUGS AND THE KIDNEY

(*See also* Chapter 2, Clinical Pharmacology, Toxicology and Poisoning.)

13.1 Renal elimination of drugs
Drugs may be eliminated via the kidneys by two main mechanisms:

- **Glomerular filtration**: a passive process; such drugs will be water-soluble.
- **Active tubular secretion**: drugs act as substrates for secretory processes that are designed to eliminate endogenous molecules, eg penicillin, loop diuretics, thiazide diuretics, cimetidine, metformin, morphine.

13.2 Drug nephrotoxicity
Drugs can lead to renal damage in a number of different ways, and examples are given below.

> **Essential note**
>
> Alterations in renal blood flow, direct tubular toxicity and glomerulonephritis are three ways in which drugs can damage the kidney

Alterations in renal blood flow

- **NSAIDs**: alteration in prostaglandin metabolism can lead to a critical reduction in glomerular perfusion (particularly when there is reduced renal reserve or CRF). Interstitial nephritis may also result from NSAIDs.
- **ACE inhibitors (and angiotensin II receptor blockers)**: ARF or renal impairment occurring in patients who are critically dependent upon the RAA system (those with reduced renal perfusion (eg CCF, loop-diuretics, hypovolaemia and severe renovascular disease)) is well recognised with these agents.
- **Ciclosporin A**: toxicity can be acute (due to renal vasoconstriction) or chronic. The latter is a common cause of transplant dysfunction.

Direct tubular toxicity

- **Aminoglycosides**: disturbance of renal function is seen in up to a third of patients receiving aminoglycosides. Five per cent of filtered gentamicin is actively reabsorbed by proximal tubular cells, within which the drug is concentrated; this can lead to ATN.
- **Cisplatin**: selectively toxic to proximal tubules, by inhibiting nuclear DNA synthesis; ATN results.
- **Amphotericin**: this is toxic to distal tubular cells in a dose-dependent manner; ATN results.

Glomerulonephritis

- **Gold**: proteinuria occurs in about 5% of patients receiving gold, due to an immune-complex glomerulonephritis (usually membranous). It usually resolves within 6 months of discontinuation of the drug.
- **Penicillamine**: the risk of membranous glomerulonephritis is greater than with gold.

Other nephrotoxic effects of drugs
Interstitial nephritis and retro-peritoneal fibrosis are covered in earlier sections, and drug-induced SLE syndromes in Chapter 16, Rheumatology. Nephrogenic DI is the commonest renal complication of *lithium* therapy, but interstitial fibrosis and CRF are also commonly seen.

> **Further revision**
>
> The UK National Kidney Federation at http://www.kidney.org.uk/
>
> Kidney Research UK at http://www.nkrf.org.uk/
>
> Renal disease. In Clinical Medicine (Kumar P, Clark M, eds), Saunders, Edinburgh, 2005
>
> Comprehensive Clinical Nephrology (Johnson RJ, Feehally J eds), Harcourt, London, 2000

Nephrology

You should now know that:

1. The main endocrine functions of the kidney are vitamin D metabolism and the secretion of erythropoietin and renin. The main non-endocrine functions are: waste excretion, electrolyte balance, water balance and acid–base homeostasis.

2. Methods of renal investigation include meaurement of glomerular filtration rate, urinalysis and imaging.

3. Acid–base, water and electrolyte disorders are sequelae of the failure of non-endocrine renal function.

4. Acute renal failure (ARF) presents with signs and symptoms relating to the failure of the kidney's non-endocrine function. Causes include renal hypoperfusion, glomerulonephritis and vasculitis, obstruction, toxicity, structural abnormalities and nephritis. If the renal hypoperfusion and ischaemic damage cause permanent lesions this results in acute tubular necrosis; pre-renal uraemia represents a lesser severity of ischaemic renal injury. The response to fluid resuscitation indicates the pathology: patients with ATN remain oliguric; patients with pre-renal uraemia have a diuresis. ARF is investigated by urinalysis, imaging, autoantibody status and renal biopsy. The mainstay of treatment is optimisation of fluid balance and treatment of the causative condition.

5. Chronic renal failure (CRF) is staged according to GFR and the most common causes are diabetic nephropathy, chronic glomerulonephritis and hypertension. Signs and symptoms relate to the endocrine and non-endocrine functions of the kidney. Most cases progress towards end-stage renal disease (ESRD), requiring dialysis or renal transplant. Management centres on control of blood pressure, reducing the proteinuria, modifying diet, correcting endocrine complications (especially anaemia and bone disease), preventing cardiovascular disease and maintenance dialysis. All dialysis and ESRD patients are considered for renal transplant.

6. The type of glomerulonephritis is defined by light microscopic, immunofluorescent and electron microscopic (ultrastructural) characteristics and include minimal change disease, membranous glomerulonephritis, focal segmental glomerulosclerosis, IgA nephropathy, diffuse proliferative glomerulonephritis, rapidly progressive glomerulonephritis (RPGN) and Goodpasture's syndrome.

7. The commonest inherited renal diseases are polycystic disease and Alport's syndrome. Renal cystic disorders include: autosomal dominant polycystic kidney disease (PKD), autosomal recessive PKD, von Hippel–Lindau syndrome, medullary sponge kidney and simple cysts. Up to 25% of patients referred to a nephrologist for investigation of microscopic haematuria have benign familial haematuria (BFH).

8. Renal interstitial disorders include interstitial nephritis, analgesic nephropathy and papillary necrosis.

9. Reflux nephropathy is the term applied when small and irregularly scarred kidneys (chronic pyelonephritis, CPN) are associated with vesico-ureteric reflux (VUR). The aim of treatment in children is to prevent scarring, which occurs early. Medical treatment includes antibiotic prophylaxis to minimise infection. Urinary tract infections are classified as: acute uncomplicated, complicated, asymptomatic bacterial and urinary-catheter-associated. Susceptibility is increased by structural abnormalities of the urinary tract, immunosuppression and the virulence of the pathogen.

10. Renal stones are common. Basic investigations include: stone analysis, mid-stream and 24-hour urine, assessment of renal function, serum calcium and phosphate and urinary cystine. Further investigations include IVU and/or ultrasound. Treatment includes increased fluid intake, eradication of infection, treatment of underlying cause, diuretics and stone removal.

11. Urinary tract obsruction may be acute or chronic. Diagnosis of acute obstruction is with ultrasound. Treatment must be expedient to avoid permanent damage, and temporary drainage may be achieved by catheterisation. Chronic obstruction is often complicated by UTI.

12. Malignant tumours of the urinary tract include: renal cell carcinoma, Wilm's nephroblastoma of childhood and urothelial tumours presenting with obstruction and/or bleeding.

13. Systemic disorders such as amyloidosis, atherosclerotic renovascular disease, connective tissue disorders, diabetes, thrombotic microangiopathies, hypertension and vasculitis all commonly involve the kidneys and lead to renal impairment.

14. The kidney eliminates drugs by glomerular filtration or active tubular secretion, with the drug excreted in the urine. Drugs can damage the kidney in three main ways: by altering renal blood flow, by a direct toxic effect and through glomerulonephritis.

Neurology

CONTENTS

Revision objectives

You should

1. Be aware of the distinction between neurological signs resulting from central versus peripheral nervous system injury

2. Understand the main types of clinical neurological investigations
3. Know the major categories of neurological disease
4. Have an appreciation of the types of treatment available for neurological disease

1. CEREBRAL CORTEX

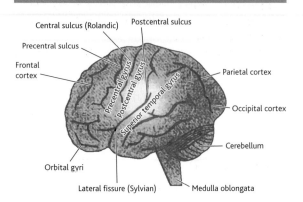

Figure 1 Lateral surface of the human brain

1.1 Cortical localisation

The cortical surface is divided into frontal, parietal, temporal and occipital lobes. Primary motor and sensory cortices are located as follows.

- Motor
  - Frontal lobe (precentral gyrus)
- Auditory
  - Superior temporal lobe (Heschl's gyrus)
- Olfactory
  - Frontal lobe (orbitofrontal cortex)
- Somatosensory
  - Parietal lobe (postcentral gyrus)
- Visual
  - Occipital lobe (calcarine sulcus)

In general, primary sensory cortices receive input from subcortical structures. Signals reach the somatosensory cortex via the posterior limb of the internal capsule (the anterior limb carries descending motor output in the form of the corticospinal tracts). Auditory signals reach the temporal cortex via the medial geniculate nucleus of the thalamus. Visual signals reach the calcarine sulcus (V1) from the lateral geniculate nucleus.

Essential note

Sensory cortices receive input from subcortical structures

After processing in primary sensory areas, corticocortical connections carry signals into secondary association cortices. The pattern of connections of the visual cortex is best understood in the following way. From primary visual cortex (V1), parallel pathways carry signals outward, with different types of processing being carried out in different functionally specialised areas. One way of thinking about visual processing is to contrast a dorsal 'where' stream, passing dorsally into the parietal cortex and concerned with object localisation, with a ventral 'what' stream passing into the temporal cortex and concerned with object identity.

A distributed network of cortical areas in the dominant hemisphere subserves **language function**. Two areas are especially important.

- **Broca's area**: in the dominant (typically left in right-handed individuals) frontal lobe, which is concerned with speech output.
- **Wernicke's area**: in the dominant posterior superior temporal gyrus, which is concerned with word comprehension.

Frontal lobe lesions may cause:

- Anosmia
- Abnormal affective reactions
- Difficulties with planning tasks or those requiring motivation
- Primitive release reflexes (eg grasp, pout, rooting)
- Broca's aphasia ('telegraphic' output aphasia)
- Perseveration
- Personality change (apathetic versus disinhibited).

Parietal lobe lesions tend to cause disorders of spatial representation or apraxias (disorders of learned movement unrelated to muscular weakness) such as those shown below. Parietal lobe lesions may also cause visual field defects, usually a homonymous inferior quadrantanopia, as the upper loop of the optic radiation runs through the parietal lobe.

Essential note

Parietal lobe lesions often cause disorders of spatial representation or apraxia

Parietal lobe lesions may cause:

- Visuospatial neglect or extinction (both usually associated with right parietal lesions)
- Astereognosis (failure to recognise common objects by feeling them)
- Apraxia (dominant)
- Acalculia (inability to perform mental arithmetic; dominant)
- Agraphia (dominant)
- Dressing apraxia (dominant)
- Constructional apraxia (non-dominant)
- Anosognosia (denial of illness; non-dominant).

Occipital lobe lesions may cause:

- Cortical blindness
- Homonymous hemianopia
- Visual agnosia (inability to comprehend the meaning of objects despite intact primary visual perception)
- Specific visual processing defects, eg akinetopsia (impaired perception of visual motion), achromatopsia (impaired perception of colour).

Essential note

Occipital lobe lesions cause visual field defects or more complex visual deficits

Temporal lobe lesions may cause:

- Wernicke's aphasia
- Impaired musical perception
- Auditory agnosia
- Memory impairment (eg bilateral hippocampal pathology)
- Cortical deafness (bilateral lesions of auditory cortex)
- Emotional disturbance with damage to limbic cortex.

Temporal lobe lesions may also cause visual field defects, usually a homonymous superior quadrantanopia, as the lower loop of the optic radiation runs through the temporal lobe.

Essential note

Temporal lobe lesions often result in agnosia, receptive aphasia and memory deficits

1.2 Dementia

Dementia is an acquired, progressive loss of cognitive function associated with an abnormal brain condition. It is not a feature of normal ageing.

Other disorders may masquerade as dementia, including depression, postictal states, acute confusional states (including drug-induced) and psychotic illnesses of old age (*see* below).

By far the commonest cause of dementia is **Alzheimer's disease**. Other important dementias include:

- Lewy body dementia
- Multi-infarct dementia.

Rarer causes of dementia include:

- Fronto-temporal dementia (Pick's disease)
- Creutzfeldt–Jacob disease
- Progressive supranuclear palsy
- AIDS-associated dementia
- Huntington's disease.

Treatable causes of cognitive impairment (which can masquerade as dementia)

- Intracranial tumour
- Normal pressure hydrocephalus
- Thiamine (vitamin B_1) deficiency
- Vitamin B_{12} deficiency
- Hypothyroidism
- Acute confusional state
- Depression
- Chronic drug intoxication

Alzheimer's disease

The earliest symptom of Alzheimer's disease (AD) is typically forgetfulness for newly acquired information. The disease progresses to disorientation, progressive cognitive decline with multiple cognitive impairments and disintegration of personality.

The neuropathology consists of:

- **Macroscopically**: the brain is atrophied with enlarged ventricles. Hippocampal atrophy is particularly prominent and can be one of the first signs of AD.
- **Microscopically**: there is neuronal loss throughout the cortex and two distinctive pathological features; namely, **plaques** (which contain a core of β-amyloid) and **neurofibrillary tangles** (which contain hyperphosphorylated tau protein). Tangles and plaques occur throughout the cortex in overlapping but separate distributions. The density of tangles **can** correlate with dementia severity.

- **Neurotransmitter changes**: there is a loss of cholinergic neurones and a loss of choline acetyl transferase activity throughout the cortex, although other neurotransmitter systems are also affected.

Genetic abnormalities associated with Alzheimer's disease

Fewer than 5% of AD cases are familial (typically autosomal dominant) and three main mutations are described. A point mutation to the presenilin-1 gene (chromosome 14) accounts for up to 50% of familial AD.

- **Down's** syndrome (trisomy 21) is associated with mental retardation and the formation of senile plaques and neurofibrillary tangles in the same brain regions commonly affected by AD. Clinically, Down's syndrome patients develop progressive cognitive impairment from their fifth or sixth decade. The gene coding for amyloid precursor protein is located on chromosome 21 and it is thought that there is overproduction of β-amyloid in these individuals.

- **Apolipoprotein E** (ApoE) is a protein synthesised in the liver that serves as a cholesterol transporter. There are three major forms of ApoE that are specified by different alleles of the ApoE gene on chromosome 19 ($\varepsilon2$, $\varepsilon3$, $\varepsilon4$). The $\varepsilon4$ allele has a greatly increased frequency (around 50%) in patients with AD. The effect of this allele is to decrease the age of onset of AD. After the effect of age, ApoE4 is the most significant risk factor for AD.

Pick's disease

Pick's disease is also known as focal lobar atrophy, and is an example of a focal dementia predominantly affecting frontotemporal function. Atrophy is circumscribed affecting most often the frontal and/or temporal lobes. Pick bodies are seen within the cellular cytoplasm on light microscopy. Clinically, patients present with progressive language disturbance, often affecting output rather than comprehension, and behavioural changes. Frontal lobe features are prominent.

Creutzfeldt–Jakob disease

Creutzfeldt–Jakob disease (CJD) is clinically characterised by:

- Rapidly progressive dementia
- Myoclonus
- Young age of onset.

CSF examination is usually normal, though CSF protein may be mildly elevated. There is a **characteristic EEG** with bi-phasic high-amplitude sharp waves.

The most common cause is sporadic, but there are familial forms. A **new variant CJD** (nvCJD) has recently been reported with a neurobehavioural presentation (often depression) in people aged under 40; this form is thought to be associated with interspecies transmission of the bovine spongiform encephalopathy (BSE) agent.

Invasive brain biopsy is currently the only definitive way of diagnosing CJD ante-mortem, though serological tests show some promise. The disease is rapidly progressive and most patients die within a year of diagnosis.

CJD is a **prion** disease.

- Prion protein is a normal product of a gene found in many organisms
- It is membrane bound
- Infectious agent is resistant to heat, irradiation and autoclaving
- An abnormal isoform accumulates in the spongiform encephalopathies, and this abnormal isoform is thought to be the infectious agent.

See also Chapter 8, Haematology (transfusion transmitted infection).

Normal pressure hydrocephalus

This should be considered in the differential diagnosis of dementia and consists of the triad of dementia, gait abnormality and urinary incontinence. Urinary symptoms are initially of urgency and frequency, and progress to frontal lobe incontinence (patients indifferent to their incontinence). Gait and posture may mimic Parkinson's disease.

The syndrome appears to be due to a defect in absorption of CSF due to thickening of the basal meninges, or in the cortical channels over the convexity and near to the arachnoid villi. The aetiology may be secondary to meningitis, head injury or subarachnoid haemorrhage. The ventricles are dilated and radiologically hydrocephalus is found, but the pressure is only intermittently high.

Headaches are not usually a complaint and papilloedema is **not** found. Treatment with a ventriculoperitoneal shunt may improve symptomatology

1.3 Multiple sclerosis (MS)

Clinical presentation of MS

Multiple sclerosis (MS) is thought to be a cell-mediated autoimmune disease associated with immune activity directed against central nervous system (CNS) antigens, principally myelin. Clinical consensus identifies four different subtypes of MS, which may possibly reflect different immunological subtypes:

- **Relapsing/remitting disease** is the most common form of MS (80–85% of patients). Short-lasting acute attacks (4–8 weeks) are followed by remission and a steady baseline state between relapses. The average number of relapses is around 0.8/year.

- **Secondary progressive disease**: about 30–50% of patients with relapsing/remitting disease will subsequently show progressive deterioration with relapses becoming less prominent within about 10 years of MS disease onset.
- **Primary progressive disease**: 10–15% of patients show progressive deterioration from onset without any superimposed relapses. Age of onset is typically later than for relapsing/remitting disease.
- **Progressive/relapsing disease**: a small number of patients with primary progressive disease also experience superimposed relapses associated with a gradual disease progression.

Good prognostic factors are:

- Relapsing/remitting course
- Female sex
- Early age at onset
- Presence of sensory symptoms.

The aetiology of MS is still unclear but there is undoubtedly a genetic component, with an increased relative risk (20–40%) in siblings compared to the general population. However, as the concordance rate in monozygotic twins is only 25%, there appears to be a substantial environmental component as well.

Optic neuritis is a common presentation of MS:

- Isolated optic neuritis: 40–60% chance of subsequent MS
- A cause of painful visual loss
- Treat with methylprednisolone
- Colour vision is affected early and residual abnormality may persist after recovery.

Diagnosis of MS

This typically requires the demonstration of brain or spinal cord lesions that are disseminated in time and anatomical location. A definitive diagnosis, therefore, is hard to make at the time of the first neurological episode, although if MRI reveals typical lesions this is highly suggestive. Supportive investigations may include:

- T2-weighted MRI showing demyelinating plaques. The presence of gadolinium enhancing lesions is the most predictive MRI parameter, although these are not always present
- Delayed visual evoked response potentials (VEPs)
- Oligoclonal bands in the CSF (but not the serum – *see* below).

Diagnosis of primary progressive disease is often hardest, as clear evidence for lesions disseminated in time and (anatomical) space is often obscured by the progressive course of the disease. Brain MRI may be normal in this form of MS, although multiple lesions may be visible in the spinal cord.

Oligoclonal bands in the CSF

Oligoclonal bands in the CSF indicate intrathecal immunoglobulin synthesis. These are not specific to MS and other causes include neurosarcoidosis, CNS lymphoma, systemic lupus erythematosus (SLE), neurosyphilis, subarachnoid haemorrhage (rare), subacute sclerosing panencephalitis (SSPE) – a rare, late complication of measles – and Guillain–Barré syndrome.

Treatments available for MS

Significant advances have been made in the treatment of MS in recent years, principally in the use of interferon preparations for relapsing/remitting MS.

Steroids

NICE guidelines suggest that individuals suffering an acute relapse should be treated with methylprednisolone, either orally (500 mg to 2 g daily) or intravenously (500 mg to 1 g daily) for three to five days. Steroids have no effect on the incidence of relapses, and are not useful other than for treatment of acute attacks.

Interferon β

Association of British Neurologists guidelines suggest that interferon β should be offered to patients (aged 18 years or older), who have no contraindications to therapy, in the following clinical situations:

Relapsing/remitting MS: patients should be able to walk independently (at least 100 m without assistance) and will have had two clinically significant relapses in the previous two years.

In patients with relapsing **secondary progressive MS**, treatment should only be considered when relapses are the dominant cause of the increasing disability. The following criteria should be fulfilled:

- Able to walk at least 10 m (with or without assistance)
- At least two disabling relapses in the previous two years
- Minimal increase in disability due to slow progression over the previous two years.

Interferons are not currently recommended for primary progressive MS, or in secondary progressive MS without relapses. There are two main forms of interferon (IFN) available:

- IFNβ-1b is produced in a bacterial system and differs slightly from natural human IFNβ
- IFNβ-1a is produced in mammalian cells and is thought to be similar to natural human IFNβ.

All IFNβ preparations reduce the frequency and severity of relapses in relapsing/remitting MS (by about one-third) and delay progression to disability. The accumulation of brain lesions on MRI is reduced. IFNβ also inhibits the progression of disability in secondary progressive MS, but its effect on primary progressive MS is presently unknown.

Treatment with IFNβ is by subcutaneous injection and is generally well tolerated. Common side-effects are 'flu-like' symptoms (fever, chills, myalgia, headache) and local reactions at the injection site. IFNβ is contraindicated in pregnancy. The mechanism of action of IFNβ in MS is not fully understood, but it may act by preventing activated T-lymphocytes from crossing the blood–brain barrier.

The effects of IFNβ are sustained for at least five years after commencement of therapy, but the optimum duration of therapy is not known. Neutralising antibodies can develop to both IFNβ-1b (40% of patients) and IFNβ1a (20% of patients). These antibodies are associated with a reduction in the drug effects on relapse rate and also MRI lesions; in some patients the antibodies disappear subsequently, but in others they persist. It is unclear whether neutralising antibodies influence progression of disability in any way.

1.4 Epilepsy

An epileptic seizure is a paroxysmal discharge of neurones sufficient to cause clinically detectable events apparent either to the subject or an observer. Epilepsy is a disorder where more than one such seizure (not including febrile seizures) has occurred. The prevalence of epilepsy is relatively constant at different ages and is around 0.7%, whereas the incidence follows a U-shaped curve with the highest incidence in the young and elderly.

A simplified classification of epilepsy

- Generalised seizures

  - Tonic–clonic
  - Absences (3 Hz spike-and-wave activity in ictal EEG)
  - Partial seizures secondarily generalised

- Partial seizures

  - Simple partial seizures
  - Complex partial seizures

- Others

  - eg myoclonic or atoni

- A typical **tonic–clonic** seizure begins without warning. After loss of consciousness and a short tonic phase, the patient falls to the ground with generalised clonic movements. There may be incontinence and there is post-ictal confusion.
- **Simple partial seizures** may affect any area of the brain, but consciousness is not impaired and the ictal EEG shows a local discharge starting over the corresponding cortical area. Any simple seizure may progress (for example, motor seizures may show a Jacksonian march) and become secondarily generalised with a supervening tonic–clonic seizure.
- Consciousness is impaired by **complex partial seizures** that typically have a medial temporal (often hippocampal) focus. An aura (sense of déjà vu, strong smell or rising sensation in the abdomen) may precede the seizure, followed by loss of consciousness. There may be automatisms (repetitive stereotyped semi-purposeful movements).

Neuroimaging is usually carried out in most if not all patients with seizures; focal seizures usually imply a focal pathology and imaging is mandatory in such circumstances.

Anticonvulsant agents are discussed in Chapter 2, Clinical Pharmacology, Toxicology and Poisoning.

Treatment of epilepsy

Patients presenting with a first seizure have an overall risk of recurrence of about 35% at two years. Most neurologists do not therefore advocate routine treatment for a first seizure. However, some groups have a higher recurrence risk (eg 65% at two years for patients with a remote neurological insult and an EEG with epileptiform features) and in these sub-groups treatment may be considered.

- After the second or subsequent seizures, drug treatment is routinely advised as the recurrence risk is much higher.
- Carbamazepine and sodium valproate are widely accepted as drugs of first choice for partial and generalised seizures, respectively.
- Note that 40% of patients with epilepsy will be women of child-bearing age. As valproate is associated with a higher incidence of neural tube defects than other agents, the choice of monotherapy may need to be reviewed (*see* Chapter 2, Clinical Pharmacology, Toxicology and Poisoning).

Any anti-epileptic should be introduced at a low dose and the clinician must be vigilant for idiosyncratic reactions. The dosage can then be escalated until either control is achieved or the maximum allowed dose is reached. If control is not achieved with monotherapy, then at least one additional trial of monotherapy is recommended before combination therapy is considered.

Epilepsy and driving

Current regulations are such that following a first seizure (whether diagnosed as epilepsy or not), driving is not permitted for one year, with a medical review before restarting driving. Loss of consciousness in which investigations have not revealed a cause is treated in the same way as for a solitary fit.

Patients with epilepsy may be allowed to drive if they have been free from any epileptic attack for one year, or if they have had an epileptic attack whilst asleep more than three years ago and attacks subsequently only when asleep.

To obtain a vocational (HGV, etc) driving licence patients should have been free of epileptic attacks AND off all anti-epileptic medication AND free from a continuing liability to epileptic seizures (eg structural intracranial lesion) for 10 years.

Epilepsy and pregnancy

Seizure rate in pregnancy is predicted by seizure rate prior to pregnancy. All anti-epileptic drugs have teratogenic effects including:

- Cleft-lip/palate
- Congenital heart defects
- Urogenital defects
- Neural tube defects (especially with valproate).

Teratogenic effects are more likely if more than one drug is used. Nevertheless, anti-epileptic drugs are not contraindicated in pregnancy, as the effects of uncontrolled epilepsy may be more risky.

There is no increase in infant mortality for epileptic mothers. Folic acid supplementation decreases the incidence of malformations.

2. MOVEMENT DISORDERS

2.1 Tremors, myoclonus, dystonia and chorea

Essential tremor is a postural tremor of the hands in the absence of any identifiable cause such as drugs.

- Autosomal dominant with incomplete penetrance (35% will have no family history)
- Propranolol is the most effective medication
- Stress will worsen the tremor
- Alcohol will improve the tremor.

Resting tremor is seen when the limbs are completely supported and relaxed, and is typical of Parkinsonism ('pill-rolling').

An **action (intention) tremor** is typically caused by an ipsilateral cerebellar hemisphere lesion. **Myoclonus** is characterised by the occurrence of sudden involuntary jerks ('fragmentary epilepsy').

Causes of myoclonus

- Physiological (normal) hypnic jerks whilst falling asleep
- Drug-induced (eg amitriptyline)
- Alzheimer's disease
- Juvenile (and inherited) myoclonic epilepsy
- Metabolic (liver or renal failure)
- Creutzfeldt–Jakob disease
- Following anoxic cerebral injury (eg cardiac arrest)
- As part of a progressive myoclonic encephalopathy (eg Gaucher's disease)

Dystonia is characterised by prolonged spasms of muscle contraction; focal dystonias include spasmodic torticollis, writer's cramp and blepharospasm. Myotonic dystrophy is discussed in Section 9.1.

Chorea is a continuous flow of small, jerky movements from limb to limb.

Causes of chorea

- Huntington's disease
- Rheumatic (Sydenham's) chorea
- SLE
- Polycythaemia rubra vera
- Chorea gravidarum (during pregnancy)
- Thyrotoxicosis
- Drug-induced (eg oral contraceptives, phenytoin, neuroleptics, L-dopa)
- Wilson's disease (*see also* Chapter 5, Gastroenterology)
- Antiphospholipid syndrome

Athetosis is a slow sinuous movement of the limbs, and is often seen after severe perinatal brain injury. In the past, athetosis was also used to describe movements that would now be called dystonic.

2.2 Parkinson's disease

Parkinsonism refers to a triad of symptoms:

- Resting tremor
- Bradykinesia
- Rigidity.

This pattern of symptoms comprises an akinetic-rigid syndrome.

The diagnosis of idiopathic Parkinson's disease is often inaccurate and there is no single diagnostic test.

Pointers include:

- An asymmetric onset
- Persistent asymmetry
- Good therapeutic response to L-dopa initially (over 90% will improve symptomatically).

Treatment of Parkinson's disease

Levodopa has been the mainstay of symptomatic treatment of Parkinson's disease since the 1970s. However, in recent years levodopa has been used less frequently as a first-line treatment, particularly for young patients, because of its involvement in the generation of long-term motor complications (eg end of dose wearing-off effect, unpredictable on/off switching). Such complications affect 10% of patients for every year of levodopa treatment.

- Modified-released levodopa has a similar rate of long-term motor complications.
- **Selegiline** was commonly added to levodopa in later disease as initial studies suggest that it might have neuroprotective effects. However, this was not confirmed in subsequent trials and indeed one trial found increased mortality with selegiline (although this has not been confirmed by follow-up of other treated patients).
- **Anticholinergics** (eg benzhexol) are frequently used for the control of tremor, but they are probably less efficacious than levodopa in respective of other motor symptoms (and they have a worse side-effect profile).

More recently, modern **dopamine agonists** (eg ropinirole, pramipexole, cabergoline and pergolide) have been introduced. Initial trial results suggest that monotherapy with these agents may be marginally less efficacious than with levodopa, but these agents generate fewer long-term motor complications. Many neurologists would now recommend that Parkinson's disease is initially treated with such dopamine agonist monotherapy, particularly for young patients, with small amounts of levodopa added as the disease progresses.

However, there is no absolute consensus on treatment of Parkinson's disease and the outcome of several therapeutic trials, which are in progress, is awaited.

2.3 Huntington's disease (Huntington's chorea)

Huntington's chorea is inherited as an autosomal dominant disorder that normally begins in the third or fourth decade and which is clinically characterised by the triad of:

- Chorea (which patients can temporarily suppress)
- Cognitive decline
- Positive family history.

Other motor symptoms include dysarthria, dysphagia, ataxia, myoclonus and dystonia. Childhood onset is atypical and may be associated with rigidity.

Genetics of Huntington's chorea

- Autosomal dominant with complete penetrance
- There is expansion of the CAG trinucleotide repeat within this gene (leading to 'anticipation' – *see* Chapter 6, Genetics)
- Gene is on chromosome 4 and codes for a protein, huntingtin
- Genetic testing in asymptomatic individuals is now available

Neuropathologically the disease causes neuronal loss in cortex and striatum, especially the caudate. Treatment is unsatisfactory and relies on neuroleptics, which partially relieve chorea through interfering with dopaminergic transmission.

3. NEURO-OPHTHALMOLOGY

3.1 Visual field defects

This section should be read in conjunction with Chapter 14, Ophthalmology.

The optic pathways and the visual defects resulting from various lesions at different sites are illustrated in the following figure.

Optic nerve fibres leave the retina, and travel in the optic nerve to the optic chiasm. Lesions of the retina and optic nerve produce field defects in the **ipsilateral eye alone**. Lesions at the optic chiasm typically produce **bitemporal hemianopia**. Causes include:

- Pituitary tumour (compression from below)
- Craniopharyngioma
- Intracranial aneurysm
- Meningioma
- Dilated third ventricle.

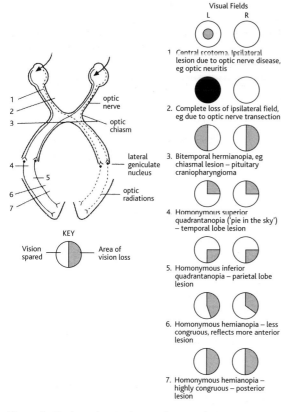

Figure 2 Optic pathway abnormalities and associated defects

From the optic chiasm fibres run in the optic tract to the lateral geniculate nucleus (thalamus). **Retrochiasmal** lesions produce congruous (**homonymous**) field defects; the degree of congruity increases with more posterior lesions. From the lateral geniculate fibres pass in the optic radiation to the primary visual cortex, located in the occipital cortex. The fibres from the lower and upper quadrants of the retina diverge, the upper fibres (lower half of the visual field) passing though the parietal lobes, the lower fibres (upper half of the visual field) through the temporal lobes. Hence:

- Temporal lobe lesions may cause superior quadrant homonymous hemianopia
- Parietal lobe lesions may cause inferior quadrant homonymous hemianopia.

Note that the decussation of fibres at the optic chiasm means that the right visual field is represented in the left occipital cortex and vice versa.

- At the very tip of the occipital lobe, the representation of the fovea (macula) is a vascular watershed, supplied by the posterior and middle cerebral arteries. Sparing of this area ('foveal sparing') may therefore occur with a posterior cerebral artery cerebrovascular accident (CVA).

3.2 Pupillary abnormalities

Pupil size depends on both pupillodilator (sympathetic) and pupilloconstrictor (parasympathetic) fibres. Pupilloconstrictor fibres travel from the Edinger–Westphal nucleus in the midbrain to the orbit on the third nerve. The path of sympathetic fibres is described below.

The pupillary light reflex pathway has two parts:

- **Afferent**: retina, optic nerve, lateral geniculate body, midbrain
- **Efferent**: Edinger–Westphal nucleus (midbrain) to third nerve.

Afferent pupillary defect

This is detected by the 'swinging flashlight' test. If the amount of light information carried by one eye is less than that from the contralateral side when the light is swung from the normal to the abnormal side, pupil dilatation is observed. This is also known as a Marcus Gunn pupil.

Essential note

The 'swinging flashlight test' is used to detect the afferent pupillary defect

An afferent pupillary defect is a sign of **asymmetrical disease anterior to the chiasm**.

Causes:

- Retinal disease (eg vascular occlusion, detachment)
- Optic nerve disease (eg optic neuritis, glaucoma) with asymmetric nerve damage.

Causes of a small pupil (miosis)

Miosis can be caused by:

- **Senile miosis**
- **Pontine haemorrhage**
- **Horner's syndrome**: see below
- **Argyll Robertson pupil**: bilateral (may be asymmetrical) small irregular pupils which do not react to light but accommodate normally. They dilate poorly in the dark and in response to mydriatics. Characteristically seen in neuro-syphilis
- **Drugs**: systemic (opiates); topical (pilocarpine)
- **Myotonic dystrophy**.

Horner's syndrome

Horner's syndrome is caused by interruption of sympathetic pupillomotor fibres, and is one of the causes of a small pupil (miosis), accompanied by enophthalmos, ptosis and anhidrosis.

Causes of a large pupil (mydriasis)

Mydriasis can be due to:

- **Adie's (tonic) pupil**: idiopathic dilated pupil with poor reaction to light and slow constriction to prolonged near effort. Seventy per cent female, 80% initially unilateral, 4% per year becoming bilateral. Associated with decreased deep tendon reflexes (Holmes Adie syndrome)
- **Third nerve palsy**: *see* below
- **Drugs**: systemic (eg antidepressants, amphetamines); mydriatrics (eg tropicamide, atropine)
- **Trauma**: sphincter pupillae rupture.

3.3 Oculomotor disorders

Essential note

A mnemonic to remember oculomotor innervation is:
$LR_6(SO_4)_3$

The sixth nerve supplies lateral rectus, the fourth supplies superior oblique and the third nerve innervates the others.

Causes of oculomotor disorders

- Ischaemic infarction of a nerve
- Intracerebral aneurysm
- Head trauma
- Neurosarcoidosis
- Myasthenia gravis
- Tumours at the base of the brain (eg glioma, metastasis, carcinomatous meningitis)
- Ophthalmoplegic migraine
- Arteritis
- Meningitides (eg syphilitic or tuberculous)
- Orbital lymphoma
- Orbital cellulitis
- Thyroid eye disease

The effects of paresis on diplopia are predicted by three rules.

1. Paresis of horizontally acting muscles tends to cause horizontal diplopia, and vertical paresis leads to vertical diplopia.

2. The direction of gaze in which the separation of the images is maximum is the direction of action of the paretic muscles.
3. The image seen furthest from the centre of gaze (the **false** image) usually belongs to the paretic eye, so when covering the paretic eye, this image will disappear.

Third nerve

The third nerve nucleus is a large nucleus located in the midbrain at the level of the superior colliculus. Fibres pass through the red nucleus and the pyramidal tract in the cerebral peduncle. The nerve then passes between the posterior cerebral and superior cerebellar arteries, through the cavernous sinus and into the orbit via the superior orbital fissure. The large nuclear size of the third nerve means that it is rarely entirely damaged by lesions and complete third nerve palsies tend to be caused by **peripheral lesions**.

Complete third nerve palsy causes:

- Ptosis
- Inability to move the eye superiorly, inferiorly or medially
- Eye deviated down (preserved superior oblique) and out (preserved lateral rectus)
- Pupil fixed and dilated.

Lateral gaze is intact and attempted downward gaze causes intorsion (inwards rotation of the eye); normal down gaze requires not only superior oblique but also inferior rectus.

The pupil may be normal (pupil-sparing or 'medical' third) or dilated and fixed to light (so-called surgical third). This is because parasympathetic pupilloconstrictor fibres run on the surface of the nerve; these are fed by the pial vessels and are therefore spared in palsies of vascular aetiology. However, they are affected early by a compressive lesion (when the pupil is involved in 95% of cases).

Causes of a third nerve palsy

- Posterior communicating artery aneurysm (usually but not always painful)
- Diabetes, usually pupil-sparing (75%)
- Arteriosclerotic
- Cavernous sinus pathology (eg thrombosis, aneurysm, fistula, pituitary mass). Frequently associated with lesions of cranial nerves IV, V and VI
- Orbital apex disease, such as tumours, thyroid disease, orbital cellulitis, granulomatous disease; often associated with palsies of cranial nerves IV–VI and optic nerve dysfunction

Causes of a third nerve palsy

- Trauma
- Uncal herniation; the third nerve travels anteriorly on the edge of the cerebellar tentorium and may be compressed by the uncal portion of the temporal lobe with increased intracranial pressure due to a supratentorial cause

Causes of a sixth nerve palsy

- Vascular
- Trauma
- Cavernous sinus syndrome
- Orbital apex syndrome
- Increased intracranial pressure (false localising sign due to stretching of the nerve)

Fourth nerve

The fourth nerve nucleus lies in the midbrain at the level of the inferior colliculus. The fourth nerve has the longest intracranial course, passing between the posterior cerebral and superior cerebellar arteries, lateral to the third nerve and into the orbit through the cavernous sinus and superior orbital fissure. It is the only nerve to exit the dorsal aspect of the brainstem. A fourth nerve lesion is the commonest cause of vertical diplopia. Looking down and in is most difficult and classically the patient notices diplopia descending stairs or reading.

Disorders of conjugate gaze

Symmetrical and synchronous movements of the two eyes together are known as **conjugate eye movements**. The commonest cause of horizontal disconjugate eye movements is **internuclear ophthalmoplegia**. This is due to a lesion in the medial longitudinal fasciculus that connects the IIIrd and IVth cranial nerve nuclei in the pons (see Figure 3), and causes impaired adduction of the ipsilateral eye with contralateral nystagmus on abduction. It is most commonly secondary to multiple sclerosis.

Causes of **impaired vertical conjugate gaze** include Graves' ophthalmopathy and thalamic or midbrain pathology.

Causes of a fourth nerve palsy

- Vascular (20%)
- Diabetes
- Vasculitis
- Cavernous sinus syndrome
- Congenital (decompensation causes symptoms) (30%)
- Trauma (susceptible to contrecoup injury, for example whiplash because of dorsal brainstem exit) (30%)
- Orbital apex syndrome

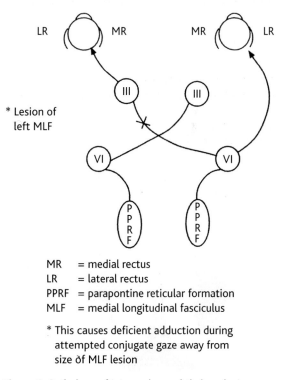

* Lesion of left MLF

MR = medial rectus
LR = lateral rectus
PPRF = parapontine reticular formation
MLF = medial longitudinal fasciculus

* This causes deficient adduction during attempted conjugate gaze away from size of MLF lesion

Figure 3 Pathology of internuclear ophthalmoplegia

Sixth nerve

The sixth nerve nucleus lies in the mid-pons inferior to the IVth ventricle, and is motor to the lateral rectus. A sixth nerve palsy causes convergence of the eyes in primary position and diplopia maximal on lateral gaze towards the side of the lesion. The affected eye **deviates medially** due to the unopposed action of medial rectus.

3.4 Nystagmus

Nystagmus is a defect of control of ocular position that leads to a rhythmic involuntary to-and-fro oscillation of the eyes.

> **Essential note**
>
> There are three types of nystagmus: pendular, jerk and rotatory

Causes of acquired nystagmus

- **Vestibular lesions**: the lesion may be in the VIIIth nerve, inner ear, brainstem or vestibular pathway. Jerky nystagmus with fast phase away from the side of the lesion and made worse by gaze in that direction; typically improves with visual fixation.
- **Cerebellar lesions**: fast phase towards the side of the lesion.
- **Drug-induced** (eg alcohol, barbiturates, phenytoin).

Downbeat nystagmus (where the fast phase is down) is associated with foramen magnum lesions (eg Arnold–Chiari malformation, spinocerebellar degeneration, syringobulbia, platybasia), whereas upbeat nystagmus is typically due to intrinsic brainstem disease, or rarely cerebellar vermis lesions.

4. OTHER BRAINSTEM AND CRANIAL NERVE DISORDERS

4.1 Facial and trigeminal nerves

The brainstem and locations of the principal cranial nerve nuclei are illustrated in Figure 4.

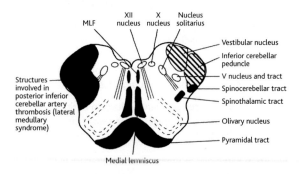

Figure 4 Locations of the principal cranial nerve nuclei within the brainstem

The facial nerve has the following functions:

- Motor to the muscles of facial expression
- Taste fibres from the anterior two-thirds of the tongue (in the chorda tympani)
- Taste from the palate (nerve of the pterygoid canal)
- Secretomotor parasympathetic fibres to parotid, submandibular and sublingual glands
- Nerve to stapedius.

Taste fibres, nerve to stapedius and to the facial muscles leave the nerve **below** the geniculate ganglion.

> **Causes of facial nerve palsy**
>
> - Brainstem tumour
> - Neurosarcoidosis
> - Cerebello-pontine angle lesions (eg acoustic neuroma)
> - Cholesteatoma
> - Lyme disease
> - Stroke
> - Multiple sclerosis
> - Otitis media
> - Ramsay–Hunt syndrome
> - Diabetes
> - Guillain–Barré syndrome

If the palsy is bilateral, exclude myasthenia gravis, facial myopathy (look for ptosis) and neurosarcoidosis. Weakness of frontalis (forehead) muscle(s) indicates a nuclear or infra-nuclear (LMN) lesion.

Bell's palsy

An isolated facial nerve palsy of acute onset, thought secondary to viral infection.

- Unilateral facial weakness
- Pain behind ear
- Absent taste sensation on anterior two-thirds of tongue

Usually recovery begins by two weeks but the palsy may be prolonged and 10% have residual weakness. Electrophysiological tests can help predict the outcome and tapering dose of steroids (given from onset) improves the outcome. Tarsorrhaphy may be needed to prevent corneal damage

Ramsay–Hunt syndrome

Features include Herpes zoster, affecting the geniculate ganglion, and facial palsy with herpetic vesicles in the auditory meatus. Deafness is a complication.

> **Essential note**
>
> Facial nerve lesions lead to facial nerve palsy, Bell's palsy and Ramsay–Hunt syndrome

Trigeminal neuralgia

This is characterised by brief lancinating pain in the distribution of one of the divisions of the trigeminal nerve. It is more common in patients over the age of 50 and in women. Maxillary and mandibular divisions are most often affected, it is almost always unilateral and trigger points are common. It may be a presenting symptom of MS in younger patients. Treatment includes:

- Carbamazepine/phenytoin
- Clonazepam
- Baclofen
- Thermocoagulation of trigeminal ganglion
- Surgical section of nerve root.

4.2 Vestibulocochlear nerve and deafness

Damage to the eighth cranial nerve may result in deafness or vertigo (see below). At the bedside, sensorineural and conductive deafness are distinguished by Rinne's and Weber's tests.

Rinne's test

- Involves tuning fork testing each ear
- Air>bone conduction normally
- Hearing decrease and bone<air conduction in conduction deafness
- Hearing decreased and air>bone conduction in sensorineural deafness.

Weber's test

- Involves tuning fork applied to front of forehead
- Central normally
- Lateralises to normal side in sensorineural deafness
- Lateralises to deaf side in conduction deafness.

Causes of deafness

Conduction	Sensorineural
Ear wax	Acoustic neuroma
Otosclerosis	Paget's disease
Middle ear infection	Central lesions (MS/CVA/glioma)
	Congenital (maternal infections, congenital syndromes)
	Ménière's disease
	Head trauma
	Drugs and toxins (aminoglycoside antibiotics, frusemide, lead)

Several drugs may cause tinnitus, including aspirin, frusemide and aminoglycosides.

> **Essential note**
>
> Rinne's and Weber's tests are used to distinguish between sensorineural and conductive deafness

Vertigo

Neurological disorders causing vertigo are typically due to pathology of the labyrinthine structures of the middle ear, the brainstem vestibular nuclei, or the vestibulocochlear nerve that connects the two.

Common causes of vertigo

Labyrinthine (peripheral)	Brainstem (central)
Trauma (including barotrauma)	Acute vestibular neuronitis
Ménière's disease	Vascular disease
Acute viral infections	MS
Chronic bacterial otitis media	Space-occupying lesions (eg brainstem glioma)
Occlusion of the internal auditory artery	Toxic causes (eg alcohol, drugs)
	Hypoglycaemia

Acoustic neuroma

Acoustic neuroma is a benign tumour arising on the eighth cranial nerve as it emerges from the brainstem in the cerebellopontine angle. It is a common cause of a **cerebellopontine angle syndrome**:

- Cranial nerve VIII is affected early, but the patient may not report hearing loss, tinnitus and vertigo
- Corneal reflex (cranial nerve V) is absent
- Facial sensation is abnormal (V nerve)
- The facial nerve is affected late

Investigation is by use of MRI or high-resolution CT scanning, and treatment is surgical removal.

5. SPINAL CORD DISORDERS

5.1 Neuroanatomy

The spinal cord ends at the lower border of L2. There is one principal descending pathway, the corticospinal tract, which crosses in the midbrain. The two principal ascending sensory pathways are the dorsal columns and spinothalamic tracts (see below).

Ascending sensory pathways	
Dorsal (posterior) columns	Spinothalamic tracts
Joint position sense and vibration	Pain and temperature
Carry sensation from the same side of the body (ipsilateral – uncrossed)	Incoming fibres cross immediately or within a few segments
Synapse in the brainstem at the cuneate and gracilis nuclei, then decussate	Crossed tract results in **lamination** with fibres from legs outside fibres from the arms

5.2 Brown–Séquard syndrome

This clinical syndrome is caused by lateral hemisection of the spinal cord resulting in:

- Ipsilateral upper motor neurone (UMN) weakness below the lesion (severed descending corticospinal tract fibres)
- Ipsilateral loss of joint position sense and vibration (severed ascending dorsal column fibres)

- Contralateral loss of pain and temperature sensation (severed crossed ascending spinothalamic tract fibres).

Light touch sensation is often clinically normal below the lesion, and the clinical syndrome is most commonly (but not exclusively) caused by multiple sclerosis.

5.3 Motor neurone disease

Motor neurone disease (MND) is a degenerative disorder affecting both lower motor neurones (LMN) and upper motor neurones (UMN) supplying limb and bulbar muscles. There is no involvement of sensory nerves, and the aetiology is unknown. There are three principal types.

- **Progressive muscular atrophy**: typically presents with LMN signs affecting a single limb that then progresses. Best prognosis (still poor).
- **Amyotrophic lateral sclerosis**: both LMN and UMN are involved; typical clinical picture would be LMN signs in the arms and bilateral UMN signs in the legs. Intermediate prognosis.
- **Progressive bulbar palsy**: bulbar musculature affected with poor prognosis.

Examination may initially show only fasciculation but progresses to widespread wasting and weakness, spastic dysarthria and exaggerated reflexes.

Diagnosis of MND

Diagnosis is largely clinical but confirmatory investigations include nerve conduction studies and EMG, which show evidence of chronic partial denervation and widespread fasciculation with normal sensory nerves and preserved motor nerve conduction velocity (these latter features distinguish the disorder from peripheral neuropathies). CSF protein concentration may be slightly increased. Prognosis is poor with death within five years typical.

Treatment of motor neurone disease

Riluzole is a drug that affects glutamate neurotransmission in a complex fashion. It is usually well tolerated, is associated with a modest improvement in survival (about 2–3 months at 18 months) and is NICE-approved for treatment of probable or definite MND. However, its effects upon quality of life remain unknown and it should be emphasised that the mainstay of treatment of MND remains symptomatic, with a multidisciplinary approach to problems such as nutrition and ventilation.

6. VASCULAR DISORDERS, CEREBRAL TUMOURS AND OTHER CNS PATHOLOGIES

6.1 Transient Ischaemic attacks, stroke and subarachnoid haemorrhage

A transient ischaemic attack (TIA) is a focal CNS disturbance developing and fading over minutes or hours to give full recovery within 24 hours. Most TIAs are caused by embolism.

Differential diagnosis of TIA

- Migraine
- Malignant hypertension
- MS (unusual)
- Epilepsy
- Hypoglycaemia

Modifiable risk factors for TIA include hypertension, diabetes mellitus, cigarette smoking, drug use (drugs of abuse, oral contraceptive pill, alcohol), elevated haematocrit and carotid stenosis. Medical management with oral aspirin significantly decreases the chance of subsequent TIA or stroke.

Carotid arterial stenosis

If a severe (70–99%) carotid stenosis is present then the existing evidence suggests that carotid endarterectomy (by an experienced surgeon) should be undertaken. Carotid endarterectomy carries a relatively high (about 8%) risk of perioperative stroke, so the patient trades a short-term increased risk of stroke for a significant long-term reduction in subsequent risk.

Stroke

A completed stroke is a focal CNS disturbance due to a vascular cause where the deficit persists. The aetiology may be embolic, thrombotic or haemorrhagic. The presenting symptoms depend on the vascular territory involved.

Lacunar strokes

Lacunar infarctions occur where small intracerebral arteries are occluded by atheroma or thrombosis. Typically small low-density subcortical lesions are seen in the area of the internal capsule.

- Lacunar syndromes cause a pure motor, sensorimotor or pure sensory stroke, with no involvement of higher cortical functions.
- Lacunar infarcts have a low mortality and relatively good prognosis for recovery; they are primarily associated with hypertension.

Other types of stroke involve either the anterior or posterior cerebral circulation. **Intracerebral haemorrhage** is primarily associated with the rupture of micro-aneurysms situated in the basal ganglion or brainstem.

Risk factors for stroke

- Diabetes
- Hypertension
- Smoking
- Cocaine abuse
- Previous TIA or stroke
- Male sex
- Increased Hb, haemoglobinopathy
- Family history
- Atrial fibrillation

Diagnosis of stroke is on clinical grounds supported by neuroimaging. (CT is commonly used initially in order to distinguish between haemorrhage and ischaemic causes; however, note that up to 50% of early CT scans will be normal in acute ischaemic stroke.) Management of stroke is initially conservative, though patients with expanding cerebellar or cerebral haematoma may need surgical treatment. Aspirin is effective in secondary prevention. Mortality from stroke is between 20 and 30%, with poorer prognosis in old patients with depressed level of consciousness.

Factors associated with a poor prognosis in stroke

- Complete paralysis of a limb (MRC grade 0 or 1)
- Loss of consciousness at onset of stroke
- Higher cerebral dysfunction
- Coma or drowsiness at 24 hours
- Old age

Subarachnoid haemorrhage

Around 5–10% of all strokes are due to subarachnoid haemorrhage (SAH). Causes include:

- Ruptured arterial aneurysm
- Trauma
- Ruptured arteriovenous malformation
- Cocaine or amphetamine abuse
- Hypertension.

Eighty per cent of intracranial aneurysms are located in the anterior circulation, most on the anterior communicating artery, and 15% are bilateral.

Investigation of subarachnoid haemorrhage

SAH is typically investigated with CT and lumbar puncture (LP).

- CT may be negative in up to 20% of suspected SAH, so a normal CT does not exclude the diagnosis
- LP shows xanthochromia (due to red cell breakdown products, only visible >4 hours after haemorrhage)
- Other recognised findings include transient glycosuria, low CSF glucose or lengthening of the QT interval (leading to tachyarrhythmias or torsades des pointes).

Treatment of SAH

The management of SAH depends upon making the diagnosis, locating the underlying aneurysm and occluding it. About a quarter of patients will die within a day of presentation, and a third of those that survive the first day will subsequently die of complications or rebleeding. At presentation, several factors have prognostic value for poor outcome, the most important of which are decreased level of consciousness, increasing age and amount of blood visible on CT scan.

- All patients are typically treated with oral nimodipine, which reduces intracranial vasospasm and so can prevent delayed cerebral ischaemia. It probably reduces the risk of poor outcome by about a third.
- Early operative intervention to occlude the causative aneurysm is now usual practice for most patients in reasonable condition, but this is not supported by randomised controlled trial evidence.

Complications of subarachnoid haemorrhage

Neurological	Systemic
- Rebleeding	- Fever
- Hydrocephalus	- Tachyarrhythmias secondary to catecholamine release
- Focal ischaemic injury from cerebral vasospasm	- Neurogenic pulmonary oedema (rarely)
	- Hyponatraemia secondary to syndrome of inappropriate antidiuretic hormone

Intracranial aneurysms are associated with:

- Polycystic kidney disease
- Ehlers–Danlos syndrome
- Fibromuscular dysplasia causing renal artery stenosis
- Medium vessel arteritides (eg polyarteritis nodosa)
- Coarctation of the aorta.

6.2 Headache

Headache is an extremely common symptom that has a multiplicity of causes. Leaving aside acute unexpected headaches caused by, for example, subarachnoid haemorrhage, important causes of chronic recurrent headache include:

- Tension headache
- Classical (accompanied by focal neurological symptoms) or common migraine
- Cluster headache
- Headaches in association with raised intracranial pressure.

Migraine

Migraine is classically preceded by a visual aura followed by a unilateral throbbing headache with photophobia and nausea.

Features of migraine

- EEG and neurovascular abnormalities associated with the headache
- Rarely may result in stroke
- May have unilateral lacrimation
- Can be associated with (reversible) neurological signs (eg hemiplegic migraine)

The neurological symptoms suggest a vascular origin, and a popular hypothesis is that of 'spreading depression' of cortical blood flow. However, whilst changes in cerebral perfusion undoubtedly occur, it is presently not clear whether these are primary or whether brainstem neuroregulatory abnormalities of serotonergic or noradrenergic neurotransmitters are more important. Therapy is aimed at stopping an attack (abortive) or if the frequency of attacks is high enough, regular medication is given as a prophylactic agent.

Migraine therapy

Abortive	Prophylactic
Paracetamol	Propranolol
Codeine ± antiemetic	Pizotifen
Ergotamine*	Amitriptyline
Sumatriptan (5HT$_1$ agonist)	Methysergide

* Ergotamine is contraindicated with cardiovascular/ peripheral vascular disease as it is a vasoconstrictor; also in pregnancy, Raynaud's or with renal impairment.

Cluster headache

Cluster headache has a distinct pattern, with attacks occurring in clusters lasting days or weeks and remissions lasting months. Males are more often affected than females, and onset of attacks is typically between 25 and 50 years.

Typical features of cluster headache

- Unilateral severe headache lasting up to an hour
- Lacrimation
- Partial Horner's may occur
- Pain may be retro-orbital
- Redness of ipsilateral eye
- Nasal stuffiness

The aetiology is not known and treatment is difficult. Management of the acute attack includes inhaled oxygen (face mask), ergotamine and sumatriptan. Steroids may be helpful. Lithium treatment is used for prophylaxis.

Benign intracranial hypertension (BIH)

Patients (often overweight young women) present with headaches and profound papilloedema, yet have no focal neurological signs or intracranial lesion on imaging. Clinical features include:

- Headache
- Blurred vision
- Dizziness
- Transient visual obscurations
- Horizontal diplopia.

Papilloedema is found on examination, with peripheral constriction of the visual fields and enlarged blind spot. The CSF pressure is elevated.

Iatrogenic (drug-induced) causes include:

- Oral contraceptive pill
- Steroids
- Tetracycline
- Vitamin A
- Nitrofurantoin
- Nalidixic acid.

Treatment of BIH
This consists of weight loss, acetazolamide and repeated lumbar puncture to reduce the CSF pressure. In more resistant cases or those associated with regular recurrence, **ventriculoperitoneal shunt** may be necessary. **Optic nerve sheath fenestration** can be performed in patients whose sight is threatened.

6.3 Cerebral tumours

Primary and secondary intracranial neoplasms have an approximately equal incidence. Both produce presenting symptoms through local neural damage giving rise to focal neurological symptoms, epilepsy or symptoms of raised intracranial pressure, such as headache. The most common presenting symptoms of a glioma are epilepsy and headache.

Gliomas

Gliomas are the most common primary intracranial neoplasm. Most commonly gliomas are derived from the astrocyte cell line, though less commonly oligodendrogliomas, ependymomas and gangliogliomas may occur.

- **Treatment**: confirmation of diagnosis necessary by brain biopsy. If possible, surgical removal should be undertaken followed by radiotherapy. Adjuvant chemotherapy for high-grade gliomas is under evaluation.
- **Prognosis**: this is relatively poor. Even grades I and II astrocytomas have survival rates of 10–30% at five years, whereas glioblastoma multiforme (grade IV astrocytoma) is usually rapidly fatal within a year.

6.4 Wernicke's encephalopathy

This is an acute ophthalmoplegia characterised by:

- Ataxia
- Ophthalmoplegia
- Nystagmus
- Global confusional state
- Polyneuropathy (in some cases).

It may evolve into Korsakoff's syndrome, with a dense amnesia and confabulation. The syndrome is commonly associated with alcoholism and may be precipitated by a sudden glucose load, but may also be caused by prolonged vomiting (eg hyperemesis gravidarum), dialysis or gastro-intestinal cancer.

Red cell transketolase activity is reduced. Neuro-pathogically it is characterised by periaqueductal punctate haemorrhage. Treatment with thiamine should lead to rapid reversal of the neurological symptoms, though the memory disorder may endure.

7. CNS INFECTIONS

CSF abnormalities in bacterial and viral meningitis are dis-cussed in Section 10 of this chapter and causative organ-isms are listed in Chapter 10, Infectious Diseases and Tropical Medicine. For HIV-related neurological disease see Chapter 7, Genito-urinary Medicine and AIDS.

7.1 Encephalitis

Acute viral encephalitis involves not simply the meninges (a viral meningitis) but also the cerebral substance. Confusion and altered consciousness are thus prominent, and seizures and focal neurological signs may occur. Viral encephalitis is often secondary to herpes simplex, but may also be second-ary to infection with mumps, zoster, EBV or Coxsackie and echoviruses. See also Chapter 10, Infectious Diseases and Tropical Medicine.

Clinical features of herpes simplex encephalitis

- Fever
- Focal symptoms (eg musical hallucinations)
- Confusion
- Focal signs (eg right-sided weakness and aphasia)

Focal signs in herpes simplex encephalitis are related to anterior temporal lobe pathology, which may be visible on CT or MRI. Normal CSF findings are occasionally seen, but typically there is a lymphocytosis with red cells also present. In a minority (20%) of cases the CSF sugar may be low. Investigation with imaging or with EEG may confirm focal temporal lobe involvement, and definitive diagnosis can be made with polymerase chain reaction (PCR) to detect viral DNA in the CSF. Treatment with aciclovir should be started on suspicion of the diagnosis.

7.2 Lyme disease

Lyme disease is caused by a spirochaete, *Borrelia burgdorferi*, which is transmitted by ticks. The illness can be subacute or chronic and evolves in poorly defined stages. A ring-like erythematous lesion (erythema migrans) at the site of the tick bite is accompanied by influenza-like symptoms, with neurologic (or cardiac) symptoms appearing weeks to months later. Usually, neurological involvement appears as 'viral-like' meningitis with or without cranial mono-neuropathies. Treatment is with oral doxycycline in the initial stages but the meningitis is usually treated with intra-venous ceftriaxone.

Neurological abnormalities in Lyme disease

- Cranial neuropathies
- Bell's palsy
- Low-grade encephalitis
- Meningitis
- Cerebellar ataxia
- Mononeuritis multiplex

8. PERIPHERAL NERVE LESIONS

8.1 Mononeuropathies

A peripheral lesion of a single nerve is known as a mononeu-ropathy. Commonly mononeuropathies are associated with compressive lesions or have a vascular aetiology. Two of the most important mononeuropathies (other than oculomotor palsies) are carpal tunnel syndrome and common peroneal nerve palsy.

Essential note

Mononeuropathies include carpal tunnel syndrome, common peroneal nerve palsy and wasting of small muscles of the hand

Carpal tunnel syndrome

The most common peripheral nerve entrapment syndrome. Symptoms are of numbness and dysaesthesia affecting median nerve (lateral three-and-a-half fingers), and weak-ness of median nerve innervated muscles (see below). Conditions associated with carpal tunnel syndrome:

- Pregnancy
- Obesity
- Hypothyroidism
- Acromegaly
- Amyloidosis
- Rheumatoid arthritis.

Treatment is with wrist splints, occasionally diuretics or surgical decompression.

Common peroneal nerve palsy

This nerve is motor to tibialis anterior and the peronei muscles. Patients usually present with foot drop and weakness of:

- Inversion (L4) of the foot
- Dorsiflexion (L5; tibialis anterior)
- Eversion (S1; peronei).

Sensory loss over the dorsum of the foot is usually present, but not prominent. Distinction from L5 root lesion is made by demonstrating that foot eversion is intact (for a root lesion).

Causes of common peroneal palsy

- Compression at the fibula neck, where the nerve winds round the bone (eg below-knee plasters)
- Connective tissue disease/vasculitis
- Weight loss
- Diabetes mellitus
- Polyarteritis nodosa
- Leprosy

Unilateral foot drop can also be caused by prolapsed invertebral disc, or from lesions to the central nervous system such as stroke or multiple sclerosis.

Other mononeuropathies affecting the hand and arm

The **median nerve** supplies some of the muscles of the thenar eminence (abductor pollicis, flexor pollicis brevis and opponens pollicis) and the lateral two lumbricals.

The **ulnar nerve** supplies the muscles of the hypothenar eminence (abductor digiti minimi), the medial two lumbricals and all the interossei (remember dorsal abduct, palmar adduct – 'dab and pad').

The **radial nerve** does not supply muscles in the hand. It supplies primarily the extensor compartment of the forearm.

Causes of wasting of the small muscles of the hand

- Arthritis
- Motor neurone disease
- Other cervical cord pathology
- Syringomyelia
- Polyneuropathies
- Brachial plexus injury (eg trauma, Pancoast's tumour)

8.2 Polyneuropathies

Polyneuropathies have a heterogeneous set of causes. Typically peripheral nerves are affected in a diffuse symmetrical fashion; symptoms and signs are most prominent in the extremities. Different aetiologies may be associated with involvement of mainly motor, mainly sensory or mainly autonomic fibres.

Causes of polyneuropathy

Mainly sensory neuropathies	Mainly motor neuropathies
Diabetes mellitus	Guillain–Barré syndrome (*see* below)
Leprosy	
Amyloidosis	Porphyria
Vitamin B_{12} deficiency	Lead poisonin
Carcinomatous neuropathy	Diphtheria
Uraemic neuropathy	Hereditary sensory and motor neuropathy (HSMN) types I and II
	Chronic inflammatory demyelinating polyneuropathy (CIDP)

Motor neuropathies cause partial denervation of muscle. An important sign of denervation is fasciculation, which is particularly prominent in disorders of the anterior horn cell in addition to the motor neuropathies described above.

Causes of fasciculation

- Motor neurone disease
- Thyrotoxicosis
- Cervical spondylosis
- Syringomyelia
- Acute poliomyelitis
- Metabolic – severe hyponatraemia, hypomagnesaemia
- Drugs (clofibrate, lithium, anticholinesterase, salbutamol)

Autonomic neuropathies

Autonomic neuropathy may present with:

- Postural hypotension
- Abnormal sweating
- Diarrhoea or constipation
- Urinary incontinence
- Absence of cardiovascular responses (eg to Valsalva's manoeuvre)
- Impotence

Principal causes of autonomic neuropathy

- Diabetes mellitus
- Amyloidosis
- Chronic hepatic failure
- Guillain–Barré syndrome
- Renal failure
- Multiple system atrophies (eg Shy–Drager syndrome and olivopontocerebellar atrophy)

Guillain–Barré syndrome

Guillain–Barré syndrome (GBS) is an uncommon acute post-infective polyneuropathy. A progressive ascending symmetric muscle weakness (ascending polyradiculopathy) leads to paralysis, maximal by one week in more than half of patients. Symptoms frequently begin after a respiratory or gastrointestinal infection; *Campylobacter jejuni* infection is associated with a worse prognosis.

Sensory symptoms may be present but are typically not associated with objective sensory signs. Papilloedema may occur. The condition may be associated with urinary retention or cardiac arrhythmia (autonomic involvement). Some patients will require intubation and artificial ventilation.

Investigation typically reveals:

- Elevated CSF protein (often very high)
- Normal CSF white cell count

- Slowing of nerve conduction velocity and denervation on EMG.

Poor prognostic features include:

- Rapid onset of symptoms
- Age
- Axonal neuropathy on nerve conduction studies
- Prior infection with *Campylobacter jejuni*.

Treatments include plasma exchange and intravenous immunoglobulin.

9. DISORDERS OF MUSCLE AND NEUROMUSCULAR JUNCTION

9.1 Myopathies

Disorders of muscle are known as myopathies. The most important feature is muscle weakness, variably accompanied by wasting, hypertrophy, pseudohypertrophy or other symptoms, such as myotonia. Signs are invariably symmetrical. Myopathies are usually painless (with the exception of inflammatory myopathies).

Note that fasciculations are signs of muscle denervation, and they indicate a disorder of motor nerves or the neuromuscular junction. They are not a feature of myopathy.

There are a number of different types of myopathies.

Classification of myopathies

- **Inflammatory** (eg polymyositis; *see* Chapter 16, Rheumatology)
- **Metabolic** (eg mitochondrial)
- **Drug-induced** (alcohol, chloroquine, corticosteroids, HMG-CoA reductase inhibitors (eg simvastatin), penicillamine and zidovudine)
- **Inherited – dominant** (eg dystrophia myotonica; *see* below); **recessive** (eg Duchenne; *see* below)
- **Secondary to endocrine disease** (principally thyrotoxicosis or hypothyroidism)

Muscular dystrophy

Duchenne muscular dystrophy is an X-linked disorder affecting about 1 in 3500 male births, though occasionally females may be affected (due to translocation of the short arm of the X chromosome, Xp21).

- The gene has now been isolated in this Xp21 region, and produces a protein named dystrophin that is normally present on the muscle sarcolemmal membrane. The function of this protein unknown.

- In Duchenne dystrophy, the dystrophin protein is absent.
- Serum creatine kinase is elevated.
- There is no effective treatment at present and death usually occurs in the second or third decade of life

In the milder **Becker dystrophy**, the dystrophic protein is seen but it is dysfunctional and present at a lower level than normal (see Table in Section 9.2, Chapter 6, Genetics).

Dystrophia myotonica

An inherited myopathy (autosomal dominant) with onset in the third decade.

Features of dystrophia myotonica

- Myotonic facies
- Myotonia (delayed muscular relaxation after contraction)
- Wasting and weakness of the arms and legs
- Frontal baldness
- Testicular/ovarian atrophy
- Diabetes mellitus
- Cataract
- Cardiomyopathy
- Mild cognitive impairment

Diagnosis depends on the characteristic myotonic discharge on EMG in association with the clinical features listed above. Usually severe disability results within 10–20 years, and there is no treatment available though phenytoin may be used for symptomatic relief of myotonia.

9.2 Neuromuscular junction

Neuromuscular transmission is dependent on cholinergic transmission between the terminals of motor nerves and the motor end plate.

Myasthenia gravis

This is an antibody-mediated autoimmune disease affecting the neuromuscular junction; antibodies are produced to the acetylcholine receptors. It is a relatively rare disorder with a prevalence of about 1 in 20 000.

Most (but not all) patients have ptosis. Many have ophthalmoplegia, dysarthria and dysphagia, but any muscle may be affected. The pupil is never affected, but weakness of eye closure and ptosis is common.

Myasthenia gravis may mimic MND, mitochondrial myopathies, polymyositis, cranial nerve palsies or brainstem dysfunction.

Diagnosis of myasthenia gravis

- Tensilon test
- ACh receptor antibodies (present in 85–90%)
- Electrophysiology (repetitive stimulation gives rise to diminution in the amplitude of the evoked EMG response)
- Thyroid function tests (up to 10% have co-existent thyrotoxicosis)
- CT mediastinum

Treatment of myasthenia gravis

Primary treatment is with cholinesterase (ChE) inhibitors (eg pyridostigmine), and some patients will achieve control with these agents alone. The cause of the disease is usually modified with treatments directed at the **immune system**:

- **Immunosuppression**: steroids, azathioprine, cyclophosphamide, ciclosporin A
- Plasmapheresis
- Intravenous immune globulin infusion.

In those with thymoma or hyperplasia of the thymus, up to 60% will improve or achieve remission after **thymectomy**. The benefits of surgery are greatest in patients aged less than 40 years.

10. NEUROLOGICAL INVESTIGATIONS

10.1 Cerebrospinal fluid

Normal CSF findings

- Pressure
    - 60–150 mmH$_2$O of CSF (patient recumbent)
- Protein
    - 0.2–0.4 g/l
- Cell count
    - Red cells 0, White cells <5/mm^3 (few monocytes or lymphocytes)
- Glucose
    - More than 2/3 blood glucose

Abnormal CSF findings

Elevated protein

- Very high; >2 g/l

  - Guillain–Barré syndrome
  - Spinal block
  - TB meningitis
  - Fungal meningitis

- High

  - Bacterial meningitis
  - Viral encephalitis
  - Cerebral abscess
  - Neurosyphilis
  - Subdural haematoma
  - Cerebral malignancy

Low CSF glucose

- Bacterial meningitis
- TB meningitis
- Fungal meningitis
- Mumps meningitis (20%)
- Herpes simplex encephalitis (20%)
- Subarachnoid haemorrhage (occasionally)

Polymorphs

- Bacterial meningitis

Lymphocytes

- Viral encephalitis/meningitis
- Partially treated bacterial meningitis
- Behçet's syndrome
- CNS vasculitidies
- HIV-associated
- Lymphoma
- Leukaemia
- Lyme disease
- Systemic lupus erythematosus

Oligoclonal bands in CSF

- Multiple sclerosis
- Neurosarcoidosis
- CNS lymphoma
- Systemic lupus erythematosus
- Subacute sclerosing panencephalitis (SSPE)
- Subarachnoid haemorrhage (unusual)
- Neurosyphilis
- Guillain–Barré syndrome

10.2 Neuroradiology

CT and MR scanning of the brain and spinal cord are the mainstays of imaging investigations in neurological diseases. A comprehensive account is beyond the remit of this section.

Essential note

Major neurological investigations include analysis of CSF, neuroradiology and electrophysiology

10.3 Electrophysiological investigations

EEG

The EEG is characteristically abnormal in the following conditions:

- **Absence seizures**: 3 Hz spike-and-wave complexes
- **Creutzfeldt–Jakob**: periodic bursts of high-amplitude sharp waves.

Nerve conduction tests

Nerve conduction tests are used to investigate peripheral neuropathies. The technique involves stimulating a peripheral nerve (sensory or motor) and recording the action potential latency and amplitude further along the same nerve. This allows calculation of the conduction velocity of the nerve. These measures can be used to distinguish (amongst other things) between axonal and demyelinating neuropathies.

- **Axonal**: reduced amplitude (loss of axons) but **preserved** conduction velocity
- **Demyelinating**: preserved amplitude but **reduced** conduction velocity (loss of myelin).

Electromyography (EMG)

EMG is useful in disorders of the neuromuscular junction or investigation of myopathic processes. The technique involves stimulating the motor nerves while recording the compound action potential from muscles.

Characteristic abnormalities:

- **Myasthenia gravis**: diminished response to repetitive stimulation
- **Lambert–Eaton syndrome**: enhanced response to repetitive stimulation
- **Polymyositis**: fibrillation due to denervation hypersensitivity, reduced amplitude and duration of motor units
- **Myotonic syndromes**: 'dive bomber' discharge (high-frequency action potentials).

Further revision

Basic neuroscience tutorial (very good) at
http://thalamus.wustl.edu/course/

Eye movement simulator at
http://cim.ucdavis.edu/Eyes/eyesim.htm

Neurology/Neuropathology MCQs at
http://www.medlib.med.utah.edu/WebPath/EXAM/
MULTORG/EXAMIDX.html

Textbook of neuromuscular disease at
http://www.neuro.wustl.edu/neuromuscular/

Searchable database of neuroscience resources on the
internet at http://www.neuroguide.com/index.html

Neuroradiology whole brain atlas at
http://www.med.harvard.edu/AANLIB/home.html

Stroke syndromes (and other teaching material on
stroke) at http://www.strokecenter.org/prof/
syndromes/index.htm

The National Institute of Neurological Disorders and
Stroke at http://www.ninds.nih.gov/index.htm

The American Association of Neurology at
http://www.aan.com/professionals/

Donaghy M. *Neurology: an Oxford core text*. 2005.
Oxford: Oxford University Press.

Revision summary

You should now know that:

1. Neurological syndromes affecting the central nervous system (brain and spinal cord) cause upper motor neurone signs in affected limbs. Cortical involvement can lead to disorders of higher cognitive function and behaviour. In contrast, syndromes affecting the peripheral nervous system (motor, sensory and autonomic nerves) tend to result in lower motor neurone signs affecting the limbs, and do not give rise to disorders of higher cognitive function.
2. Major neurological investigations include: analysis of cerebrospinal fluid, neuroradiology, nerve conduction studies and electromyography (EMG).

3. The major categories of neurological disorder include: dementia, MS, epilepsy, movement disorders, Parkinson's disease, Huntingdon's disease, motor neurone disease, sequelae of cerebrovascular accidents, headache, tumours and CNS infections.
4. Cholinesterase inhibitors, steroids, interferons, antiepileptic agents, modulators of dopaminergic neurotransmission, aspirin, analgesics, triptans and antibiotics are among the pharmacological agents used in the treatment of the major categories of neurological disease described above.

Ophthalmology

CONTENTS

Pupillary and eye movement disorders, nystagmus and visual field defects are all covered in the neuro-ophthalmology section of Chapter 13, Neurology.

Revision objectives

1. To understand the basic anatomy of the eye and the adnexal structures and their function
2. To perform basic assessment of ocular function
3. To understand the common causes of acute and chronic visual disturbance

Ophthalmology

1. ANATOMY, HISTORY AND EXAMINATION

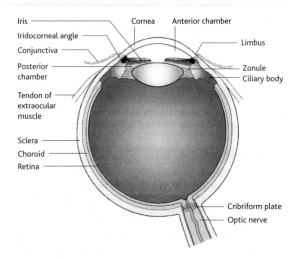

Figure 1 The basic anatomy of the eye
Source *Lecture Notes on Ophthalmology* 8th edition, by B James *et al.* (1997), published by Blackwell Science. ISBN 086542 723 2

1.1 Orbit
The orbit houses the globe, extraocular muscles, lacrimal gland, orbital fat and attendant arteries, veins and nerves.

1.2 Extraocular muscles
The extraocular muscles are responsible for movement of the eye. The four rectus muscles and the superior oblique arise at the orbital apex and pass forward to insert into the globe. The inferior oblique arises from the anteromedial orbital floor and runs along the lower surface of the globe to insert into its posterolateral aspect. The innervation and primary action of each muscle are shown in the following table – other movements are due to the action of two muscles acting together.

Muscle	Nerve Supply	Primary action
Superior rectus	III	Elevation in abduction
Inferior rectus	III	Depression in abduction
Medial rectus	III	Adduction
Lateral rectus	VI	Abduction
Inferior oblique	III	Elevation in adduction
Superior oblique	IV	Depression in adduction

1.3 The globe
Key features of the constituent parts are:

- **Cornea**: clear structure.
- **Conjunctiva**: thin mucous membrane covering anterior sclera and lining eyelids.
- **Sclera**: tough fibroelastic coat.
- **Uveal tract**: iris, ciliary body and choroid.
- **Retinal pigment epithelium**: the outermost layer of the retina.
- **Retina**: light-sensitive innermost layer of the globe. It comprises: (1) rods – more plentiful in the peripheral retina, sensitive to low light and movement detection; and (2) cones – concentrated within the macular region, particularly at the fovea, important for acuity and colour vision. Vascular supply is from the central retinal artery.
- **Lens**: positioned posterior to the iris and anterior to the vitreous.

Essential note

Rods are sensitive to low light and movement detection; cones are important for acuity and colour detection

1.4 Ophthalmic history
Key questions to be addressed include:

- Subjective visual acuity and how this affects the patient's function
- Perceived changes in visual field
- Presence of symptoms such as ocular pain, irritation, redness, lacrimation and photophobia
- Past ocular history
- Systemic enquiry, including past medical history and drug history.

1.5 Ophthalmic examination
Visual acuity is critical in the ophthalmic assessment of patients. Standard Snellen acuity is measured using a chart at a distance of 6 m. The patient reads down the chart and the acuity is recorded in relation to the line of letters they achieve. If the patient can see none of the letters they move closer to the chart in 1 m intervals until they are able to read the top letter. Visual acuity less than this is measured as counting fingers, hand movements or perception of light. Visual fields should be examined by confrontation, comparing the patient's field of vision to that of the examiner.

Pupil reactions, direct and consensual and the presence of an afferent pupillary defect, to a bright light stimulus, and an accommodative target should be assessed. A relative afferent pupillary defect occurs due to an abnormality affecting the retina or optic nerve anterior to the chiasm. This is further discussed in the neuro ophthalmology sub-section of the Neurology chapter.

Extraocular movements should be tested to a light target in the cardinal positions of gaze, looking for under actions and the presence of diplopia.

Red colour vision is important in the assessment of optic nerve function – however it is important to be aware that 10% Caucasian males are red–green colour blind.

Essential note

Distance acuity is measured using Snellen charts. At the bedside visual fields are assessed by confrontation

2. CAUSES OF A RED EYE

2.1 Conjunctivitis

Typically presents with irritation, watery or purulent discharge and diffuse injection. It is usually bilateral. The main infective agents are bacteria, viruses and Chlamydia. It may also be allergic. Vision is normal or only mildly reduced. The pre-auricular lymph node may be enlarged in viral disease.

2.2 Corneal abrasions and ulceration

History of trauma or foreign body usually associated with corneal abrasion. Associated with pain, which may be severe. Variable reduction in vision. Defect stains with fluorescein. Secondary bacterial infection may occur – contact lenses are major risk factor.

- **Herpes simplex**: 'dendritic', corneal ulceration may be seen when lesions appear like the branches of a tree, or 'geographic' when they become much larger with an amoeboid shape. The corneal stroma may subsequently become involved. Treatment is with topical antiviral agents.

Essential note

Causes of red eye include conjunctivitis, corneal abrasions and ulceration, uveitis, scleritis and acute glaucoma

2.3 Uveitis

Uveitis is inflammation of the uveal tract, which may be anterior and/or posterior.

- **Anterior uveitis** typically presents with pain, photophobia, a red eye, lacrimation and decreased vision.
- **Posterior uveitis** is frequently asymptomatic or presents with floaters (due to inflammatory debris in the vitreous) or impaired vision, as macular oedema may occur.

Uveitis of any cause may be complicated by cataract or glaucoma. Anterior uveitis is most commonly idiopathic but there are also associations with systemic diseases.

Systemic associations with uveitis

- HLA-B27-associated uveitis
- Ankylosing spondylitis
- Sarcoidosis
- Inflammatory bowel disease
- Juvenile idiopathic arthritis

  - (Previously termed juvenile chronic arthritis)

- Reiter's syndrome
- Infections

  - TB, syphilis, herpes simplex, herpes zoster, toxoplasmosis, toxocariasis, AIDS, leprosy

- Behçet's disease
- Malignancy

  - Non-Hodgkin's lymphoma
  - Leukaemia
  - Retinoblastoma
  - Ocular melanoma

2.4 Scleritis

Presents as a diffuse red eye associated with lacrimation, photophobia and severe, deep, boring pain.

Inflammation of the sclera may be caused by

- Herpes zoster
- Ankylosing spondylitis
- Sarcoidosis
- Inflammatory bowel disease
- Gout
- Vasculitis: polyarteritis nodosa (PAN), systemic lupus erythematosus (SLE), Wegener's, relapsing polychondritis, dermatomyositis, Behçet's

2.5 Acute glaucoma

- Rapid decrease in visual acuity associated with severe ocular and periocular pain often with vomiting.
- More common in hypermetropes (long-sightedness).
- It is due to closure of the drainage angle resulting in a massive rapid elevation in intraocular pressure.
- Corneal oedema results in a cloudy appearance.
- The pupil is oval, mid-dilated and non reacting.
- Failure to treat pressure rapidly results in permanent visual loss.

3. CAUSES OF ACUTE LOSS OF VISION

3.1 Retinal venous occlusion

Retinal vein occlusion may affect the central retinal vein (CRVO) or one of its branches (BRVO).

Aetiology

- Systemic hypertension (most common)
- Increased intraocular pressure (central occlusion only)
- Diabetes mellitus
- Hyperviscosity states

Clinical signs of retinal venous occlusion

- **Painless loss of vision**

  - Variable extent depending on macular involvement and degree of retinal ischaemia

- **Relative afferent pupillary defect**

  - With retinal ischaemia

Clinical signs of retinal venous occlusion

- **Multiple retinal haemorrhages**

  - Mainly superficial, in nerve fibre layer

- **Retinal venous dilatation**
- **Cotton wool spots**
- **Vascular sheathing**
- **Neovascularisation**

  - May occur in 20% of CRVO and 1% BRVO due to ischaemia, ie similar pathogenesis to diabetic retinopathy. In the anterior segment this may produce neovascular glaucoma, or in the retina it can cause vitreous haemorrhage or retinal traction. Treatment is by retinal laser to abolish the ischaemic stimulus

3.2 Retinal arterial occlusion

Occlusion of the central artery or one of its branches produces retinal infarction and painless visual loss corresponding to the area supplied.

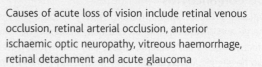

Essential note

Causes of acute loss of vision include retinal venous occlusion, retinal arterial occlusion, anterior ischaemic optic neuropathy, vitreous haemorrhage, retinal detachment and acute glaucoma

Aetiology

- **Embolic**
- **Sudden rapid increase in intraocular pressure**

  - To more than central retinal arterial pressure

- **Arteritic**

  - Most commonly giant cell arteritis (GCA). However, visual loss in GCA is only due to central retinal artery occlusion in 10% of cases; it usually affects vision by producing anterior ischaemic optic neuropathy, which damages the optic nerve head

Clinical signs of retinal arterial occlusion

- Sudden, profound, painless loss of vision
- Pale oedematous retina with cherry red spot at fovea (only lasts around 48 hours)

  - This is due to the choroidal reflex showing through at the fovea as the retina is thinner here

- Relative afferent pupillary defect
- Neovascular complications (occur later)

  - Much rarer than with venous occlusions, probably because the retina is too severely damaged to produce angiogenic factor

Treatment, by lowering the intraocular pressure rapidly, either surgically or pharmacologically, may sometimes dislodge the embolus if presentation occurs within a few hours of onset.

3.3 Anterior ischaemic optic neuropathy

Infarction of the anterior portion of the optic nerve results in acute severe painless visual loss, which generally does not improve. This is the usual method by which **giant cell arteritis** affects vision (90%), retinal artery occlusion occurring in the other 10% of cases. A history of temporal headache with jaw claudication is classical. The erythrocyte sedimentation rate (ESR) is usually markedly elevated associated with a raised C-reactive protein (CRP) and thrombocytosis. It is essential to exclude this condition as it rapidly becomes bilateral. Giant cells and loss of the internal elastic lamina are evident histologically on temporal artery biopsy.

Ischaemic optic neuropathy is not always due to inflammatory arteritis; other causes include arteriosclerosis and hypotensive events. If visual loss is incomplete an altitudinal (ie horizontal) field defect results.

3.4 Vitreous haemorrhage

Intraocular bleeding may occur secondary to neovascularisation, eg diabetic retinopathy, or when the vitreous detaches from the retina, which is a physiological event. Frequently occurring in middle age due to liquefaction of the vitreous.

The patient experiences a variable reduction in vision and floaters corresponding to the density of haemorrhage.

The red reflex is normal but retinal details may be obscured on fundoscopy.

3.5 Retinal detachment

More common in myopes. Patient complains of floaters, photopsia (flashing lights) and painless loss of vision that varies in severity. Surgical intervention is required.

3.6 Acute glaucoma

See Section 2.5 above.

4. CAUSES OF CHRONIC VISUAL LOSS

Any longstanding visual loss may only be noted acutely by the patient.

4.1 Cataract

Cataract, an opacity of the lens, is the commonest cause of blindness worldwide. Surgery is indicated:

- When decreased vision affects the patient's life
- If the view of the fundus is impaired when monitoring or treating another condition (eg diabetes).

Essential note

Causes of chronic visual loss include cataract, chronic glaucoma and age-related macular degeneration

Causes of cataracts

- Congenital

  - Autosomal dominant (25%)
  - Maternal infection – rubella, toxoplasmosis, CMV, herpes simplex, varicella zoster
  - Maternal drug ingestion – corticosteroids, thalidomide
  - Metabolic – galactosaemia, hypocalcaemia, hypoglycaemia
  - Chromosomal abnormalities (eg Down's syndrome, Turner's syndrome)

- Drug-induced

  - eg steroids

- Secondary to ocular disease

  - (eg uveitis)

Continued over

Causes of cataracts

Continued

- **Metabolic**
  - Diabetes
- **Traumatic**
  - Penetrating or blunt injury, radiotherapy
- **Miscellaneous**
  - Myotonic dystrophy, atopic dermatitis
- **Senile**

4.2 Chronic glaucoma

Glaucoma describes a group of conditions in which elevated intraocular pressure causes visual damage with characteristic optic disc cupping. The normal intraocular pressure is <22 mmHg.

- Chronic glaucoma is an insidious asymptomatic disease.
- Intraocular pressure is elevated (usually not as markedly as in acute glaucoma), resulting in cupping of the optic nerve head and loss of the visual field.
- Classically an arcuate scotoma develops, which progresses to generalised field constriction.
- Familial tendency but no strict inheritance pattern.
- More common in women and myopes (those who are short-sighted).

4.3 Age-related macular degeneration

Usually a bilateral, gradual decline in vision with classically central visual loss and a preserved peripheral field; navigational ability is therefore maintained.

An acute loss of central vision may occur due to the development of 'wet' macular disease, which may be amenable to treatment with laser or photodynamic therapy.

4.4 Retinitis pigmentosa

Retinitis pigmentosa (RP) is a term describing a group of progressive inherited diseases affecting the photoreceptors and the retinal pigment epithelium. It is characterised by the triad of:

- **Night blindness**: due to loss of rod function
- **Tunnel vision**: loss of peripheral field also due to rod dysfunction; central visual acuity loss due to cone disease may also occur but tends to be a later feature
- **Pigmented bony spicule**: the classical fundal appearance with associated disc pallor and blood vessel attenuation.

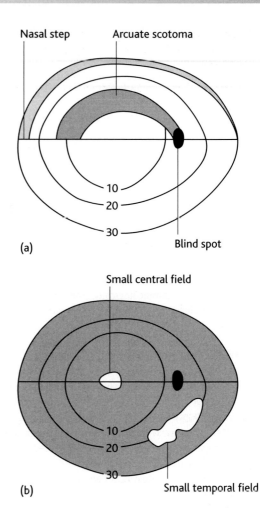

(a)

(b)

Figure 2 The characteristic pattern of visual field loss in chronic open angle glaucoma: (a) an upper arcuate scotoma, reflecting damage to a cohort of nerve fibres entering the lower pole of the disc (remember – the optics of the eye determine that damage to the lower retina creates an upper field defect; (b) the field loss has progressed, a small central island is left (tunnel vision), sometimes this may be associated with a sparing of an island of vision in the temporal field.
Source *Lecture Notes on Ophthalmology* 8th edition, by B James *et al.* (1997), published by Blackwell Science. ISBN 086542 723 2

5. OPTIC NERVE DISORDERS

5.1 Optic neuritis

Inflammation of the optic nerve may affect the:

- **Nerve head** – producing **papillitis** with optic disc swelling, hyperaemia and haemorrhages

- **Retrobulbar portion of the nerve** – in which the nerve appears normal ('the patient sees nothing, the doctor sees nothing').

It is the presenting feature of 25% of patients with multiple sclerosis (MS): up to 70% of patients who have an attack of optic neuritis will develop MS (20% in the first two years).

Clinical signs of optic neuritis

1. **Reduced visual acuity**
   Usually monocular (90%), progresses rapidly over a few days; improves over four to six weeks, achieving virtually normal vision in 90%, although relative afferent pupillary defect (RAPD) usually persists
2. **Pain**
   Precedes visual loss by a few days, worsened by eye movements
3. **Red colour desaturation**
4. **Relative afferent pupillary defect**
5. **Paracentral or central scotoma**
6. **Visual evoked potential prolonged**
   Reflecting delayed conduction in optic pathway

Causes of optic neuritis/papillitis

- **Demyelination** (also post-viral syndromes)
- **Infections**: viral encephalitis (measles, mumps, chicken-pox), infectious mononucleosis, herpes zoster
- **Inflammatory**: contiguous with orbital inflammation, sinusitis or meningitis secondary to granulomatous disease (eg TB, sarcoid, syphilis)
- **Other systemic disease**: (eg diabetes)

5.2 Causes of optic atrophy

Optic disc pallor may be associated with a variable degree of reduced visual acuity, visual field defects or it may be asymptomatic. Depending on the cause, it may be unilateral or bilateral.

Causes of optic atrophy

- **Congenital**
  - Dominant or recessive

Causes of optic atrophy

- **Secondary to optic nerve compression**
  - (eg pituitary mass, meningioma, orbital cellulitis)
- **Drugs**
  - Ethambutol, isoniazid, chloramphenicol, digoxin
- **Radiation neuropathy**
- **Carcinomatous**
  - Due to microscopic infiltrates of the nerve and its sheath
- **Post-papilloedema**
- **Post-optic neuritis**
  - See above
- **Post-trauma**
- **Toxic neuropathy**
  - (eg tobacco (cyanide), arsenic, lead, methanol)
- **Nutritional**
  - Vitamins B_1, B_2, B_6, B_{12}, folic acid and niacin deficiencies
  - Tobacco–alcohol amblyopia may be toxic or nutritional with a good prognosis for recovery
- **Infiltrative neuropathy**
  - (eg sarcoid, lymphoma, leukaemia)

5.3 The swollen optic nerve head

Papilloedema

Papilloedema means optic nerve head swelling **secondary to increased intracranial pressure**. This may be due to:

- Space-occupying lesion
- Hydrocephalus
- CO_2 retention
- Idiopathic intracranial hypertension.

Papilloedema is usually bilateral. Features include:

- Hyperaemia of the disc
- Peripapillary splinter haemorrhages
- Blurring of the disc margins
- Exudates and cotton wool spots
- Loss of spontaneous venous pulsation: absent in 20% of normal people
- Loss of the cup is a late feature.

On clinical examination papilloedema produces an enlarged blind spot. **Transient visual obscurations** – with blacking out of vision lasting a few seconds, often due to positional change – also occur. Visual loss occurs late.

Papillitis

This refers to inflammation of the optic nerve head (as distinct from retrobulbar neuritis) and is most frequently due to a demyelinating episode (*see* Section 4.1).

Other causes of swelling of the optic nerve head

- Central retinal vein occlusion
- Orbital mass (eg optic nerve glioma, nerve sheath meningioma, thyroid eye disease and metastases)
- Accelerated phase hypertension (see above)
- Infiltrative neuropathy (eg lymphoma)
- Toxic neuropathy.

Ophthalmic features of HIV/AIDS are covered in Chapter 7, Genito-urinary medicine and AIDS.

6. MISCELLANEOUS DISORDERS

6.1 Diabetic retinopathy

Diabetic retinopathy is the commonest cause of blindness in patients aged 30–60 years. It is related to disease duration and control. It is unusual in type I diabetes until 10 years after diagnosis, but eventually occurs in nearly all patients. It is present in 10% of type II patients at diagnosis (reflecting that diabetes has previously been undetected in many patients), in 50% after 10 years' disease and in 80% after 20 years' disease.

Essential note

Diabetic retinopathy is the commonest cause of blindness in the working population. Age-related macular degeneration is the commonest cause of blindness over the age of 65

Diabetic retinopathy is a **microvascular** disease. Pathological changes include:

- **Loss of vascular pericytes**: thought to be responsible for the structural integrity of the vessel wall. A decrease therefore results in disruption of the blood–retinal barrier and leakage of plasma constituents into the retina.
- **Capillary endothelial cell damage**.
- **Basement membrane thickening** with carbohydrate and glycogen deposition.

- Changes in red cell oxygen-carrying capabilities and increased platelet aggregation are also thought to contribute. The production of an angiogenic factor by ischaemic retina is the likely cause of neovascularisation. At all stages, good control of diabetes, any coexisting hypertension and stopping smoking have been shown to reduce serious sequelae.

Classification of diabetic retinopathy

- **Background retinopathy**
  - Does not affect visual acuity
  - Microaneurysms – first clinical change, saccular pouch, either leaks or resolves due to thrombosis
  - Haemorrhages – dot, blot and flame-shaped
  - Exudates – leakage of lipid and lipoprotein intoretina
  - No local treatment required; adequate control of diabetes only

- **Diabetic maculopathy**
  - Most common cause of visual loss
  - More common in type II diabetes
  - Retinopathy within the macular region
  - Oedematous retina may require laser treatment

- **Preproliferative retinopathy**
  - Cotton wool spots – represent areas of axonal disruption secondary to ischaemia
  - Venous dilatation, loops, beading and reduplication
  - Large deep haemorrhages
  - Treatment controversial: some advocate prophylactic laser treatment, others recommend improving disease control and more frequent monitoring

- **Proliferative retinopathy**
  - More common in type I diabetes
  - Retinal neovascularisation: new vessels occur in thin-walled friable clumps on the venous side of the retinal circulation. Initially flat, they then grow into the vitreous leading to haemorrhage, fibrosis and tractional retinal detachment
  - Iris neovascularisation (rubeosis): may be complicated by glaucoma
  - Treatment with retinal laser photocoagulation abolishes the production of angiogenic factor from ischaemic retina

Rapid progression of diabetic retinopathy may occur in:

- Pregnancy – 5% of patients with background changes develop proliferative retinopathy
- Sudden improvement in control in previously poorly managed disease.

Other ophthalmic changes occurring in diabetes

- Diabetic papillopathy

  - Is typically a bilateral process in young type I diabetic patients
  - Is associated with mild to moderate visual loss
  - Fundal examination reveals disc swelling, macular oedema with exudates and macular star
  - Management is good control of the diabetes
  - Spontaneous recovery is usual within 6 months

- Fluctuating vision secondary to osmotic changes with varying glucose levels (very common)
- Cataract
- Mononeuropathies affecting the IIIrd, IVth and VIth cranial nerves causing diplopia.

6.2 Hypertensive retinopathy

Retinal abnormalities can reflect the severity of hypertension and are characterised by:

- Vascular constriction causing focal retinal ischaemia
- Leakage leading to retinal oedema, haemorrhage and lipid deposition.

Arteriosclerotic changes reflect the duration of the hypertension. These include vessel wall thickening secondary to intimal hyalinisation, medial hypertrophy and endothelial hyperplasia.

Classification of hypertensive retinopathy

- Grade 1

  - Arteriolar attenuation

- Grade 2

  - Focal arteriolar attenuation (with 'arteriovenous nipping')

- Grade 3

  - Haemorrhages, cotton wool spots (due to infarction of nerve fibre layer of retina)

- Grade 4

  - Disc swelling – 'malignant' or 'accelerated' phase

Grades 3 and 4 are associated with severe target organ hypertensive damage (eg renal disease) and high mortality (accelerated phase hypertension). Treatment is aimed purely towards the hypertension and any underlying cause.

6.3 Thyroid eye disease

Thyroid eye disease may pre-date, coincide with or follow the systemic disease. The classic triad of Graves' disease is ocular changes, thyroid acropachy and pretibial myxoedema. Signs and symptoms range in severity and include:

- Lid lag and retraction: latter is adrenergic and more likely with active hyperthyroidism
- Corneal exposure: secondary to lid changes or proptosis
- Soft tissue swelling
- Proptosis and diplopia – secondary to orbital fat proliferation and muscle infiltration
- Optic nerve compression – sight threatening.

Management of ocular manifestations may be divided into:

- **Surface abnormalities**: ocular lubricants, tarsorrhaphy
- **Muscle changes**: prisms or patches to control diplopia; surgery after defect stable
- **Optic nerve compression**: systemic steroids, radiotherapy, surgical decompression
- **Cosmetic**: improve lid position, remove redundant tissue.

6.4 Ocular tumours

Primary tumours

- **Choroidal melanoma**: this is the commonest primary intraocular tumour. It presents as a unilateral lesion with variable pigmentation (amelanotic to dark brown). Symptoms include reduced vision or field loss depending on the site of the lesion.

Secondary tumours

The eye may be affected by metastases to the choroid or orbit. Cerebral metastases may also affect the visual pathway or cause oculomotility disorders.

- **Choroidal metastases** occur most frequently from breast, bronchial and renal primary tumours and are usually multiple and bilateral. Lesions appear pale and are minimally elevated and are associated with metastatic disease elsewhere. The effect upon vision depends on the site; macular lesions are most common and can cause marked visual loss. Palliative radiotherapy is usually successful in improving vision.

6.5 Syphilitic disease

The ophthalmic abnormalities are related to the particular stage of syphilis:

- **Congenital**: interstitial keratitis (leads to clouding of the corneas in the second decade of life), iritis, chorioretinitis and optic atrophy
- **Primary**: chancre may occur on the eyelid
- **Secondary**: iritis occurs in 4% of patients with secondary syphilis and is usually bilateral; optic neuritis, chorioretinitis and scleritis are all associated
- **Tertiary**: associated with optic atrophy, chorioretinitis, iritis, interstitial keratitis and the **Argyll Robertson pupil** (accommodates but does not react to a light stimulus).

6.6 Blind registration

Blind registration is completed by ophthalmologists and can facilitate rehabilitation and Social Services support. Monocular vision is not a criterion for registration. Two levels for blind registration exist:

- **Partial sight registration** – visual acuity is < or =6/24 in both eyes, or when there is constriction of visual fields, including hemianopia
- **Blind registration** – visual acuity is < or =3/60 in both eyes.

Further revision

Royal National Institute for the Blind at www.rnib.org.uk

www.mrcophth.com is a very extensive site with a student and GP section and many photos, clinical quizzes and videos of eye movement abnormalities

An eye movement simulator can be found at http://cim.ucdavis.edu

Journals: *Current Opinion in Ophthalmology* and *Survey of Ophthalmology*

Revision summary

1. The optic nerve (IInd cranial nerve) transmits visual information from the eye. Pupil dilatation is sympathetic and constriction parasympathetic. Ocular movement is mediated by the four recti and two oblique muscles, supplied by the IIIrd, IVth and VIth cranial nerves.

2. In assessing ocular function, corrected acuity, visual fields, pupil reactions, dilated fundal examination and ocular movements should be performed.

3. Acute visual loss is caused by acute glaucoma, retinal detachment and vascular events. Chronic visual loss is caused by cataract, chronic glaucoma and age-related macular degeneration.

Respiratory medicine

CONTENTS

Revision objectives

1. Develop a thorough understanding of lung anatomy and physiology

2. Be able to identify common diseases of the respiratory system

Continued over

Revision objectives (*continued*)

3. Diagnose airways disease and differentiate asthma from COPD
4. Understand the spectrum of lung infections
5. Have a basic understanding of cystic fibrosis
6. Develop an overview of occupational lung disease
7. Understand the presentation of lung cancer and clinical management
8. Develop a working knowledge of pleural disease, particularly the causes of pleural effusion and pneumothorax management
9. Have an overview of rare lung disorders
10. Be aware of guidelines pertaining to the management of respiratory problems

1. LUNG ANATOMY AND PHYSIOLOGY

The human lung is made up of approximately 300 million alveoli each around 0.3 mm in diameter. Gas exchange takes place in the alveoli, and air is transported to these via a series of conducting airways. It is warmed and humidified in the upper airways and transported through the trachea, main bronchi, lobar and segmental bronchi to the terminal bronchioles, the smallest of the conducting tubes. These airways take no part in gas exchange and constitute the anatomical dead space (approximately 150 ml). The terminal bronchioles lead to the respiratory bronchioles, which have alveoli budding from their walls. Lung tissue distal to the terminal bronchiole forms the primary lobule.

1.1 Ventilation

The most important muscle of inspiration is the diaphragm, a muscular dome that moves downwards on inspiration. The external intercostal muscles assist inspiration by moving the ribs upwards and forwards in a 'bucket-handle' movement.

- The accessory muscles of respiration include the scalene muscles, which elevate the first two ribs, and the sternocleidomastoids, which elevate the sternum; these are not used during quiet breathing.
- Expiration is passive during quiet breathing.
- During exercise, expiration becomes active and the internal intercostal muscles and the muscles of the anterior abdominal wall are utilised.
- The greatest ventilation is achieved at the lung bases and this is matched by increased perfusion in these areas.

Essential note

Ventilation of alveoli is greatest at the lung base

Normal lung is very compliant. **Compliance** is reduced by pulmonary venous engorgement and alveolar oedema and in areas of atelectasis. Surfactant, secreted by type 2 alveolar epithelial cells, substantially lowers the surface tension of the alveolar lining fluid, increasing lung compliance and promoting alveolar stability. Lack of surfactant leads to respiratory distress syndrome.

Essential note

Surfactant increases lung compliance and stability by reducing alveolar surface tension

Resistance to airflow is related to the radius of the airway, but the greatest overall resistance to flow occurs in medium-sized bronchi. Airway calibre is influenced by lung volume; at low lung volumes small airways may close completely leading to areas of atelectasis, particularly at the lung bases.

1.2 Perfusion

The pulmonary vessels form a low-pressure system conducting deoxygenated blood from the pulmonary arteries to the alveoli where they form a dense capillary network. The pulmonary arteries have thin walls with very little smooth muscle; the mean pulmonary artery pressure is 15 mmHg (2.00 kPa) and the upper limit of normal pressure is 30 mmHg (4.00 kPa).

- Pulmonary vascular resistance is one-tenth systemic vascular resistance.
- Hypoxic vasoconstriction refers to contraction of smooth muscle in the walls of the small arterioles in a hypoxic region of lung; this helps to divert blood away from areas with poor ventilation so maintaining ventilation and perfusion matching.

1.3 Control of respiration

The respiratory centre is made up of a poorly defined collection of neurones in the pons and medulla; to a certain extent, the cortex can override the function of the respiratory centre. Chemoreceptors are crucial to the control of respiration, and these may be **central** or **peripheral**:

- **Central chemoreceptors** are located on the ventral surface of the medulla. They respond to increased hydrogen ion concentration in the cerebrospinal fluid (CSF), generated by increased carbon dioxide tension (pCO_2) in the blood.
- **Peripheral chemoreceptors** are located in the carotid bodies (at the bifurcation of the common carotid arteries) and the aortic bodies (near the aortic arch); they respond to hypoxaemia, hypercapnia and pH changes.

In people with normal respiratory function the most important factor for control of ventilation is the pCO_2, which is maintained to within 3 mmHg (0.4 kPa) of baseline (normal range 35–45 mmHg (4.67–6.00 kPa). However, in patients with severe lung disease, chronic CO_2 retention develops and the hypoxic drive to ventilation becomes very important.

- Ventilation may increase by 15 times the resting level during severe exercise.
- Cheyne–Stokes respiration is characterised by periods of apnoea separated by periods of hyperventilation; it occurs in severe heart failure or brain damage, and at altitude.

1.4 Pulmonary function tests (PFTs)

Peak flow

- Tables of normal values depending on age, sex and height are published for both peak flow and spirometry.
- Is measured in litres per minute and is a useful guide to airways obstruction.

- Is most useful in asthma, as it reflects central airways obstruction, but may underestimate disease severity in chronic obstructive pulmonary disease (COPD).
- Attention to technique is important.

Spirometry

- FEV_1 refers to the volume of gas expired in the first second of a forced expiration.
- Forced vital capacity (FVC) refers to the total volume of gas expired on forced expiration from maximal inspiration.
- The normal ratio of FEV_1/FVC is 0.7–0.8.
- Reduction in FEV_1 with a preserved FVC occurs in airways obstruction (eg asthma or COPD); in patients with severe COPD a slow vital capacity is a more accurate measurement, as it allows time for the lungs to empty fully and a true FEV_1/FVC ratio to be determined.
- Restriction refers to a reduction in FVC with a preserved FEV_1/FVC ratio and occurs in conditions such as pulmonary fibrosis, neuromuscular disorders, obesity and pleural disease.

Flow volume loops

A flow volume loop is produced by plotting flow on the *y* axis against volume on the *x* axis.

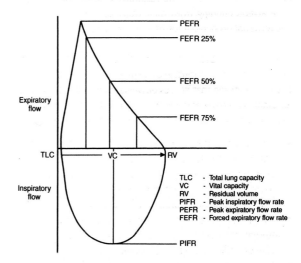

Figure 1 Typical flow volume loop

If a subject inspires rapidly from residual volume (RV) to total lung capacity (TLC) and then exhales as hard as possible back to RV, then a record can be made of the maximum flow volume loop. This loop shows that expiratory flow rises very rapidly to a maximum value, but then declines over the rest of expiration. During the early part of a forced expiration the maximum effort-dependent flow

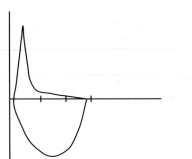

Pressure-dependent collapse
If intrathoracic airways collapse immediately expiration begins there is an abrupt early fall from peak flow, ie pressure-dependent collapse typical in emphysema

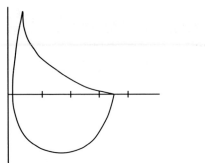

Volume-dependent collapse
If the airways collapse progressively with expiration, the scooping out of the expiration limb is more gradual, ie volume-dependent collapse. This is seen in chronic pulmonary disease

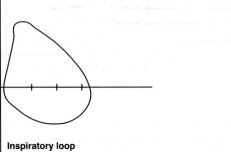

Inspiratory loop
If the lungs are abnormally stiff or springy, airway closure is delayed, as in children and young women, producing a descending portion which is convex. Inspiration is opposed slightly, producing a flatter inspiratory loop

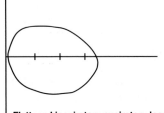

Flattened inspiratory expiratory loops
If extrathoracic obstruction exists both the inspiratory and expiratory loops will be flattened, eg tracheal compression by goitre, nodes

Figure 2 Flow volume loops in different disorders

rate is achieved within 0.1 s, but the rise in transmural pressure leads to the airways being compressed and therefore to the flow rate being reduced. The flow rate is then said to be effort-independent.

Lung volumes

- Tidal volume, inspiratory and expiratory reserve volumes and vital capacity can all be measured by use of a spirometer.
- Total lung capacity, residual volume and functional residual capacity can be measured using a helium dilution method, nitrogen washout or body box.

1.5 Gas transfer

Transfer of carbon monoxide is limited solely by diffusion and is used to measure gas transfer. Either a single breath hold or a steady-state method can be used. Results are expressed both as total gas transfer (DLCO) or gas transfer corrected for lung volume (KCO, i.e. KCO = DLCO/VA where VA is alveolar volume).

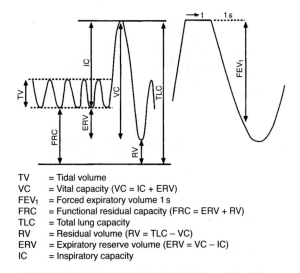

TV	= Tidal volume
VC	= Vital capacity (VC = IC + ERV)
FEV$_1$	= Forced expiratory volume 1 s
FRC	= Functional residual capacity (FRC = ERV + RV)
TLC	= Total lung capacity
RV	= Residual volume (RV = TLC − VC)
ERV	= Expiratory reserve volume (ERV = VC − IC)
IC	= Inspiratory capacity

Figure 3 Subdivision of lung volume

- Hypoventilation

  - (eg opiate overdose, paralysis of respiratory muscles)

- Ventilation/perfusion (*V/Q*) mismatch

  - (eg pulmonary embolus)

- Low inspired partial pressure of oxygen (pO_2)

  - (eg high altitude, breathing a hypoxic mixture)

- Diffusion impairment

  - (eg pulmonary oedema, fibrosing alveolitis, bronchiolar–alveolar cell carcinoma)

- Shunt*

  - (eg pulmonary arteriovenous (A–V) malformations, cardiac right to left shunts)

*Hypoxaemia caused by shunt cannot be abolished by administering 100% oxygen

Oxygen and carbon dioxide transport

Oxygen is transported in the blood by combination with haemoglobin (Hb) in the red cells. A tiny amount is dissolved (0.3 ml/100 ml blood, assuming pO_2 of 100 mmHg, 13.3 kPa). The oxyhaemoglobin dissociation curve is sigmoidal in shape. Once oxygen saturation falls below 90% the amount of oxygen carried to the tissues falls rapidly. The $p50$ (the partial pressure at which haemoglobin is 50% saturated) is 26 mmHg (3.47 kPa).

- The curve is shifted to the right by high temperature, acidosis, increased pCO_2, and increased levels of 2,3-diphosphoglycerate (2,3-DPG); this encourages offloading of oxygen to the tissues.
- The curve is **shifted to the left** by changes opposite to those above, and by carboxyhaemoglobin and fetal haemoglobin.

Carbon dioxide (CO_2) is transported in the blood as bicarbonate, in combination with proteins as carbamino compounds, and it is also dissolved in plasma. CO_2 is 20 times more soluble than oxygen and about 10% of all CO_2 is dissolved. CO_2 diffuses into red blood cells where carbonic anhydrase facilitates the formation of carbonic acid, which dissociates into bicarbonate and hydrogen ions. Bicarbonate diffuses out of the cell and chloride moves in to maintain electrical neutrality.

Acid–base control

The normal pH of arterial blood is 7.35–7.45. Blood pH is closely regulated and variation outside this pH range results in compensation by the lung or the kidney to return pH to normal. Failure to excrete CO_2 normally results in a respiratory acidosis; this is usually due to hypoventilation. Hyperventilation causes lowering of the pCO_2 and alkalosis.

pH can also be altered by metabolic disturbance. Metabolic acidosis and alkalosis are considered in Chapter 11, Metabolic diseases.

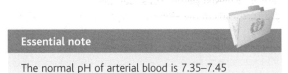

Essential note

The normal pH of arterial blood is 7.35–7.45

1.6 Adaptation to high altitude

The barometric pressure decreases with altitude; at 18 000 feet (5486 m) it is half the normal 760 mmHg (101 kPa). Hyperventilation, due to hypoxic stimulation of peripheral chemoreceptors, is an early response to altitude. The respiratory alkalosis produced is corrected by renal excretion of bicarbonate.

- Hypoxaemia stimulates the release of erythropoietin from the kidney, and the resultant polycythaemia allows increased carriage of oxygen by arterial blood.
- There is an increased production of 2,3-DPG, which shifts the oxygen dissociation curve to the right, allowing better offloading of oxygen to the tissues.

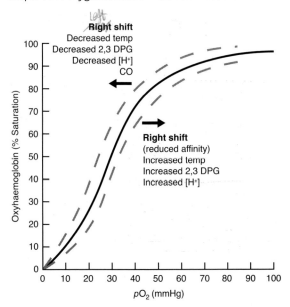

Right shift
Decreased temp
Decreased 2,3 DPG
Decreased [H⁺]
CO

Right shift
(reduced affinity)
Increased temp
Increased 2,3 DPG
Increased [H⁺]

Oxyhaemoglobin (% Saturation) vs pO_2 (mmHg)

Figure 4 Oxygen dissociation curve

● Hypoxic vasoconstriction increases pulmonary artery pressure causing right ventricular hypertrophy. Pulmonary hypertension is sometimes associated with pulmonary oedema – altitude sickness. In some individuals, hypoxic vasoconstriction is abnormally pronounced. High transmural pressures cause the pulmonary capillaries to tear and fluid leaks into the alveoli.

2. DISEASES OF LARGE AIRWAYS

2.1 Asthma

Asthma is a chronic inflammatory disorder of the airways. In susceptible individuals this inflammation causes symptoms associated with widespread but variable airflow obstruction that is reversible either spontaneously or with treatment. There is an increase in airway sensitivity to a variety of stimuli.

The prevalence of asthma has been increasing in recent years, principally among children. Approximately 5.1 million people suffer from asthma in the UK – 1.4 million of these are children. Around 1500 asthma deaths occur annually in the UK.

The development of asthma is almost certainly due to a combination of genetic predisposition and environmental factors. Atopy is strongly associated with asthma. The most important allergens are the house dust mite (*Dermatophagoides pteronyssinus*), dog allergen (found in pelt, dander and saliva), cat allergen (predominantly in sebaceous glands), pollen, grasses and moulds.

Essential note

The incidence of asthma in the UK is increasing – 5.1 million sufferers in the UK

Asthma attacks may be provoked by the following

● Exposure to sensitising agents
● Infection
● Drugs, including aspirin, non-steroidal anti-inflammatory agents (NSAIDs), β-blockers
● Exercise
● Gastro-oesophageal reflux
● Cigarette smoke, fumes, sprays, perfumes, etc
● Failure to comply with medication

In patients with asthma the airways are narrowed by a combination of contraction of bronchiolar smooth muscle, mucosal oedema and mucus plugging. In the early stages changes are reversible; however, in chronic asthma, structural changes (including thickening of the basement membrane, goblet cell hyperplasia and hypertrophy of smooth muscle) develop and ultimately lead to irreversible fibrosis of the airways. Asthma is regarded as a complex inflammatory condition and mast cells, eosinophils, macrophages, T-lymphocytes and neutrophils are all involved in the pathogenesis. A variety of inflammatory mediators are released, including histamine, leukotrienes, prostaglandins, bradykinin and platelet activating factor (PAF).

Chronic asthma

The hallmark of chronic asthma is variable and reversible airflow obstruction. This causes:

● Shortness of breath
● Chest tightness
● Wheeze
● Cough.

At times the cough may be productive of sputum, which may be clear, or yellow/green, due to the presence of eosinophils. The normal diurnal variation in airway calibre is accentuated in asthmatics and symptoms may be worse at night.

Physical signs of asthma

● Tachypnoea
● Hyperinflation of the chest
● Nasal polyps (particularly in aspirin-sensitive asthmatics)
● Wheezing, most marked in expiration
● Atopic eczema

Lung function tests may show

● Significant (>20%) diurnal peak expiratory flow rate (PEFR) variability on at least 3 days per week for a minimum of 2 weeks
● Significant improvement in PEFR and FEV_1 (>15% improvement and at least 400 ml) after a bronchodilator or trial of oral or inhaled steroids
● Increased lung volumes
● Reduced FEV_1
● FEV_1/FVC ratio <0.7

Diagnosis of asthma

The diagnosis of asthma is clinical and is often confirmed by diary recordings of PEFR. Challenge tests with histamine or methacholine, or with exercise, can be used to assess airway responsiveness where the diagnosis is unclear. Responsiveness is expressed as the concentration of provoking agent required to decrease the FEV_1 by 20%.

Helpful additional information

- History of asthma in childhood or a family history of asthma
- Symptoms of perennial rhinitis, nasal polyps or chronic sinusitis
- History of eczema or hay fever
- History of wheezing associated with aspirin, NSAIDs or β-blockers

---

Skin prick tests

Skin prick tests can be use to assess atopy. Many asthmatic subjects make immunoglobulin E (IgE) in response to common allergens. A tiny quantity of allergen is introduced into the superficial layers of the dermis and tests are read at 20 min. The diameter of the weal is measured in millimetres, the size of the weal correlating well with bronchial challenge testing. Serum total IgE is commonly raised in asthmatics. Specific IgE may be measured by radio-allergo-sorbent testing (RAST).

Treatment

The mainstay of treatment is inhaled corticosteroid with short acting β-agonists to relieve symptoms. Treatment is altered in a stepwise fashion as recommended in the British Thoracic Society (BTS) and Scottish Intercollegiate Guidelines Network (SIGN) National Guidelines. The dose of inhaled steroid should be low to moderate initially and subsequently reduced once adequate control has been achieved. Long-acting β-agonists (eg salmeterol or formoterol) should be added in patients inadequately controlled on doses of 200 µg/day of beclomethasone diproprionate or equivalent. Oral theophylline preparations or $β_2$-agonist tablets are of benefit in some patients. Leukotriene receptor antagonists (*see also* Chapter 2, Clinical pharmacology, toxicology and poisoning) may be particularly useful for exercise-induced asthma, and in patients with aspirin sensitivity. Long-term oral corticosteroids are reserved for patients with very severe asthma.

It is very important to check that patients are able to use their inhalers correctly and are compliant with therapy.

Allergen avoidance may be helpful in reducing the severity of existing disease in patients sensitised and exposed.

All inhalers are now required to be CFC-free.

Acute severe asthma

Asthma symptoms may worsen acutely, necessitating prompt treatment to relieve the attack. An immediate assessment is essential, looking for signs of severity which include the following:

- Speech impairment
- Tachycardia (pulse >110 beats/min)
- Respiratory rate >25 breaths/min
- PEFR 33–50% predicted

Life-threatening asthma is associated with any one of the following

- Hypoxaemia
- PEFR <33% predicted
- Exhaustion
- Bradycardia (pulse <60 beats/min), hypotension
- Silent chest
- Normal or raised pCO_2

Arterial blood gases should be performed if the patient is hypoxic on air (saturations <92%) and a chest radiograph is necessary to exclude pneumothorax.

Management consists of high-flow oxygen therapy, nebulised bronchodilators (β-agonists ± ipratropium), steroids and, if infection is considered likely, antibiotics. PEFR should be measured regularly to assess the response to treatment. If there is no improvement with nebulisers, then intravenous infusions of either salbutamol or aminophylline should be used. A single dose of intravenous magnesium can be given to patients who have not had a good response to bronchodilators or patients with life-threatening asthma.

If the patient is severely ill, or not improving with treatment, they should be promptly transferred to an Intensive Care Unit.

Further revision

The British Thoracic Society at http://www.brit-thoracic.org.uk/

National Asthma Campaign at http://www.asthma.org.uk/

NICE Guidelines at http://www.nice.org.uk/

Continued over

Further revision (*continued*)

Scottish Intercollegiate Guidelines Network (SIGN) at http://www.sign.ac.uk/guidelines/index.html

Allergic bronchopulmonary aspergillosis

Most patients with allergic bronchopulmonary aspergillosis are asthmatics but the condition may occur in non-asthmatics.

The disease is due to sensitivity to *Aspergillus fumigatus* spores mediated by specific IgE and IgG antibodies. The allergic response results in airways becoming obstructed by rubbery mucus plugs containing *Aspergillus* hyphae, mucus and eosinophils; plugs may be expectorated. See also section 3.6.

Characteristics of allergic bronchopulmonary aspergillosis

- Lobar or segmental collapse of airways occurs
- Fleeting chest radiograph shadows due to intermittent obstruction of airways
- Positive skin-prick tests and RAST to *Aspergillus*
- Positive precipitins to *A. fumigatus*
- Raised serum IgE >1000 ng/ml
- Peripheral blood and pulmonary eosinophilia
- May result in proximal bronchiectasis
- Treatment is with oral corticosteroids which may be required long-term; itraconazole is also useful and may allow the dose of steroid to be reduced

2.2 Chronic obstructive pulmonary disease (COPD)

COPD is defined as a chronic, slowly progressive disease characterised by airflow obstruction that does not markedly change over several months. Most of the lung function impairment is fixed although some reversibility can be produced by bronchodilator therapy. Long-term prognosis is determined by post-bronchodilator FEV_1.

The diagnosis is made by:

- History of cough with sputum production, wheeze and shortness of breath
- History of frequent winter bronchitis and delayed recovery from viral infections
- Reduced FEV_1/FVC ratio.

Causes of COPD

- Smoking (usually a history of at least 20 pack-years; 1 pack year is 20 cigarettes per day for 1 year)
- Dust exposure
- α_1-antitrypsin deficiency
- Air pollution
- Low birth weight and low socioeconomic status

COPD is due to a combination of chronic bronchitis and emphysema.

Chronic bronchitis is defined as chronic cough and sputum production for at least 3 months of 2 years consecutively in the absence of other diseases recognised to cause sputum production.

Emphysema is characterised by abnormal, permanent enlargement of the air spaces distal to the terminal bronchioles, accompanied by destruction of their walls without obvious fibrosis. Emphysema may be centriacinar (predominantly affecting the upper lobes and associated with smoking), panacinar, paraseptal or predominantly localised around scars (scar emphysema). Panacinar predominantly affects the lung bases. Paraseptal is adjacent to the septae in the periphery of the lung.

COPD accounts for 6–7% of all UK deaths at present, however the incidence of COPD is increasing; it is set to rise from the fourth commonest cause of death worldwide currently to the third by 2020.

Signs of COPD

- Hyperinflation
- Weight loss
- Flapping tremor (CO_2 retention)
- Pursed-lip breathing
- Wheeze
- Central cyanosis
- Cor pulmonale: raised jugular venous pressure (JVP), right ventricular heave, loud P2, tricuspid regurgitation, peripheral oedema, hepatomegaly

Investigations

- **PFTs**: FEV_1 <80% predicted, FEV_1/FVC <0.7; patients have large lung volumes and reduced gas transfer factor (KCO) in emphysema. COPD may be graded by the pattern of FEV_1:

  - **Mild COPD**: FEV_1 50–80% of predicted

- **Moderate COPD**: FEV_1 30–50% of predicted
- **Severe COPD**: FEV_1 <30% of predicted.

- **Chest radiograph**: may be normal or show evidence of hyperinflation, bullae or prominent vasculature due to pulmonary hypertension.
- **Arterial blood gases**: may indicate type 1 or type 2 respiratory failure.
- **Full blood count (FBC)**: possible polycythaemia.
- **ECG**: may show p pulmonale, right axis deviation, right bundle branch block.
- **Sputum culture**: *Haemophilus influenzae*, *Streptococcus pneumoniae* or less commonly *Staphylococcus*, *Moraxella catarrhalis* or Gram-negative organisms.

Treatment of COPD

Several recent clinical trials have shown no impact of inhaled steroids on disease progression in COPD. Pulmonary rehabilitation is increasingly recognised as an important part of disease management.

Treatments available for COPD

- Smoking cessation
- Inhaled anti-cholinergic drugs
- Inhaled short- or long-acting β_2-agonists
- Inhaled or systemic steroids
- Long-term oxygen therapy (LTOT)
- Lung volume reduction surgery (for patients with severe emphysema) or bullectomy
- Theophyllines
- Diuretics
- Pulmonary rehabilitation
- Transplantation

Treatment of acute exacerbations

Antibiotics are indicated for acute exacerbations if two of the following are present:

- Increased breathlessness
- Increased sputum volume
- Increased sputum purulence.

Regular bronchodilators, either nebulised or inhaled, are given, in addition to short courses of oral steroids and controlled oxygen therapy. Non-invasive positive pressure ventilation (NIPPV) via facemask may also be useful for patients with type 2 respiratory failure. Patients should be treated along conventional lines for an hour and arterial blood gases (ABGs) repeated. If significant acidosis (pH <7.35) with hypercapnia persists then NIPPV should be instituted.

Further revision

COPD: NICE Guideline, First Consultation at http://www.nice.org.uk/page.aspx?o=84988. Published in *Thorax* 2004; **59** (Suppl 1)

2.3 Long-term oxygen therapy (LTOT)

Patients are eligible for LTOT if they **exhibit all of the following**:

- pO_2 on air <7.3 kPa (55 mmHg)
- Normal or elevated pCO_2
- FEV_1 <1.5 litres
- pO_2 7.3–8 kPa (55–60 mmHg) with evidence of pulmonary hypertension, peripheral oedema or nocturnal hypoxaemia or secondary polycythemia.

Arterial blood gases must be measured when the patient is clinically stable, and on two occasions which are at least 3 weeks apart. pO_2 on oxygen should be >8 kPa (60 mmHg) without an unacceptable rise in pCO_2. Oxygen should be given via a concentrator for at least 15 hours per day. The patient must have stopped smoking before LTOT is considered.

α_1-Antitrypsin deficiency

A cause of emphysema in patients younger than typical of COPD; it is thought to result from an imbalance between neutrophil elastase in the lung, which destroy elastin, and the elastase inhibitor α_1-antitrypsin, which protects against the proteolytic degradation of elastin. The decline in lung function is accelerated in smokers.

Characteristics

- PFTs show airflow obstruction, large lung volumes and reduced KCO
- Cirrhosis of the liver is associated
- Smoking cessation is imperative
- Replacement of α_1-antitrypsin is not routinely given
- Lung transplantation may be an option for some patients
- Genetic counselling should be offered and siblings of index cases should be genetically tested

2.4 Respiratory failure

Respiratory failure is an inability to maintain adequate oxygenation and carbon dioxide excretion. There are two recognised types of respiratory failure.

- **Type 1** respiratory failure is present when there is hypoxaemia with normal or low levels of carbon dioxide

  - **Type 1 respiratory failure** may be corrected by increasing the inspired oxygen concentration.
  - **Type 2** respiratory failure is hypoxaemia with high pCO_2
  - **Type 2 respiratory failure** may require mechanical ventilatory support; respiratory stimulants such as doxapram may be useful for those with reduced respiratory drive.

Arterial blood gases

- Normal values: pH 7.37–7.43, pO_2 >10.3 kPa (77 mmHg) whilst breathing room air, pCO_2 4.7–6.0 kPa (35–45 mmHg), HCO_3 22–28 mmol/l
- Always state the percentage of inspired oxygen when recording blood gases
- To convert from kPa to mmHg multiply by 7.5.

Essential note

Normal ABG values: pO_2 >10.3 kPa on air, pCO_2 4.7–6.0 kPa, HCO_3 22–28 mmol/l

---

Causes of respiratory failure

- **Reduced ventilatory drive**

  - Opiate over dosage, brainstem injury

- **Mechanical problems**

  - Chest trauma causing flail chest
  - Severe kyphoscoliosis
  - Obesity

- **Alveolar problems**

  - Barriers to diffusion

    - Pulmonary oedema
    - Pulmonary fibrosis

Causes of respiratory failure

- *V/Q* mismatch

  - Pulmonary embolus
  - Shunt (cardiac or pulmonary)

- Reduced inspired partial pressure of oxygen

  - High altitude

- **Neurological conditions (affecting chest wall muscles)**

  - Guillain–Barré syndrome
  - Polio

- **Upper airway obstruction**

  - Laryngeal tumour
  - Obstructive sleep apnoea

- **Lower airway obstruction**

  - Bronchospasm
  - Sputum retention

2.5 Ventilatory support

This may be invasive or non-invasive.

Non-invasive positive pressure ventilation (NIPPV)

This involves the use of a securely fitting nasal or full face-mask. The technique has been used to provide long-term respiratory support in the community for patients with respiratory failure due to conditions such as severe chest wall deformity or old polio. It is used increasingly to manage episodes of acute respiratory failure due, for example, to exacerbations of COPD as an alternative to (and often more appropriate than) ventilation on the Intensive Care Unit (ICU). The technique can be carried out on general wards using portable, bi-level pressure support ventilators. Regular monitoring of blood gases is necessary and the ventilator settings are altered in response. As the patient improves, time spent off the ventilator is lengthened until the patient is weaned. A decision as to whether ICU referral is appropriate if the patient deteriorates further should be clearly stated in the notes when treatment is instituted.

Positive pressure ventilation (PPV)

Conventional ventilation requires access to the airway, by means of either an endotracheal tube or tracheostomy.

Indications for positive pressure ventilation

- Type 2 respiratory failure from any cause
- Paralysis of respiratory muscles (eg Guillain–Barré syndrome)
- Multiple organ failure
- Trauma cases, including injury to the chest or cervical spine
- Inability to maintain a clear airway
- Reduced conscious level – Glasgow coma scale <5
- During and after certain surgical procedures

Ventilation should be considered when there is failure to maintain oxygenation (pO_2 <8 kPa or 60 mmHg) despite high inspired oxygen concentrations (usually associated with hypercapnia and acidosis). It is often necessary in patients with multiple organ dysfunction associated with sepsis or trauma.

Continuous positive airways pressure (CPAP)

CPAP is delivered through a tightly fitting facemask or it may be used in conjunction with conventional ventilation. It provides a pneumatic splint to the airway and is the treatment of choice for obstructive sleep apnoea. CPAP improves oxygenation in patients requiring high concentrations of oxygen by the recruitment of collapsed airways. It may, however, cause hypotension, the rise in mean intrathoracic pressure inhibiting venous return and reducing cardiac output.

3. LUNG INFECTIONS

HIV/AIDS-associated respiratory disease is covered in Chapter 7, Genito-urinary medicine and AIDS.

3.1 Pneumonia

Pneumonia is an acute inflammatory condition of the lung usually caused by bacteria, viruses or, rarely, fungi.

The chest radiograph will show consolidation, the hallmark of which is air bronchograms.

Community acquired pneumonia

The incidence is 5–11 per 1000 of the adult population per year, being much more common in the elderly.

Causal organisms

- *Streptococcus pneumoniae* (60–70%)
- Atypical organisms, including *Mycoplasma pneumoniae* (5–15%), *Legionella pneumophila*, *Chlamydia psittaci*, *Chlamydia pneumoniae* and *Coxiella burnetii* (Q fever)
- *Haemophilus influenzae*
- *Staphylococcus aureus*
- Gram-negative organisms
- Viruses, including influenza, varicella zoster, cytomegalovirus (CMV)

General investigations for patients admitted to hospital

- Full blood count
- Urea and electrolytes (U&Es)/liver function test
- C-reactive protein (CRP)
- ABGs
- Blood and sputum cultures
- Chest radiograph
- Paired serological tests for atypical organisms and viruses (selected cases)

Signs of severity (CURB-65 criteria)

- Confusion (<8/10 score on abbreviated mental test (AMT))
- Urea >7 mmol/l
- Respiratory rate >30 breaths/min
- BP systolic <90 mmHg and/or diastolic <60 mmHg
- Age >65

Patients with three or more CURB criteria are at high risk of death and are regarded as having severe community acquired pneumonia. Hypoxaemia (pO_2 <8 kPa despite oxygen therapy) and multilobe involvement also confer a worse prognosis. Age >50 years and the presence of co-existing disease are 'pre-existing' bad prognostic factors.

Specific pneumonias

Streptococcus pneumoniae

There is an abrupt onset of illness, with high fever and rigors. Examination reveals crackles or bronchial breathing, and herpetic cold sores may be present in more than one-third of cases.

- Elderly patients may present with general deterioration or confusion.
- Capsular polysaccharide antigen may be detected in serum, sputum, pleural fluid or urine.
- Increasing incidence of penicillin resistance, particularly in countries such as Spain.
- Vaccine available.

Mycoplasma pneumoniae

Mycoplasma tends to affect young adults; it occurs in epidemics every 3–4 years. There is typically a longer prodrome, usually of 2 weeks or more, and the white cell count may be normal. Cold agglutinins occur in 50%; the mortality is low.

- Extrapulmonary complications include: peri/myocarditis, erythema multiforme, erythema nodosum and Stevens–Johnson syndrome.

Legionella pneumophila

Outbreaks are usually related to contaminated water cooling systems, showers, or air conditioning systems, but sporadic cases do occur. Legionnaires' disease usually affects the middle-aged and elderly, patients often having underlying lung disease. Males are affected more than females (3:1). Diagnosis is by direct fluorescent antibody staining or serological tests; antigen may be detected in the urine. Atypical pneumonias are treated with macrolide antibiotics or the newer fluoroguinolones.

Clinical and laboratory features

- Gastrointestinal upset common; diarrhoea, jaundice, ileus and pancreatitis may occur
- White cell count (WCC) often not elevated with lymphopenia; thrombocytopenia/pancytopenia may occur
- Hyponatraemia due to syndrome of inappropriate antidiuretic hormone (SIADH)
- Headache, confusion and delirium are prominent, and focal neurological signs may develop
- Abnormal liver and renal function in approximately 50%
- Acute renal failure, interstitial nephritis and glomerulonephritis may develop

---

Staphylococcus aureus

Staphylococcus aureus pneumonia may follow a viral illness (often influenza); it has a high mortality (30–70%). The disease is more common in intravenous drug addicts.
Specific features include:

- Toxin production with extensive tissue necrosis

- Staphylococcal skin lesions may develop
- Chest radiograph shows patchy infiltrates with abscess formation in 25% and empyema in 10%
- >25% of patients have positive blood cultures.

Treatment of pneumonia

All patients should be given appropriate concentrations of oxygen and may require intravenous fluids if volume depleted.

- Treatment is with oral amoxicillin and erythromycin for non-severe cases requiring hospitalisation and with
- a third-generation cephalosporin and clarithromycin intravenously in severe cases using the CURB criteria.
- A single antibiotic can be used for community patients or those admitted to hospital for non-medical reason.
- Newer fluoroquinolones provide an alternative for patients who are allergic to penicillin or macrolides.

Intravenous treatment should be stepped down to oral treatment after 48 hours provided the patient is improving. If a specific organism is isolated the appropriate antibiotic is given. Treatment should continue for 7–10 days depending on response. Up to 21 days treatment is recommended for *Legionella*.

Nosocomial (hospital-acquired) pneumonia

This is defined as pneumonia that develops 2 days or more after admission to hospital (0.5–5% of hospitalised patients). The organisms usually involved include:

- *Staphylococcus aureus*
- Gram-negative bacteria: *Klebsiella*, *Pseudomonas*, *Escherichia coli*, *Proteus* spp, *Serratia* spp, *Acinetobacter* spp
- Anaerobes
- Fungi
- *Streptococcus pneumoniae* (and other streptococci) are less common.

Treatment is with broad-spectrum agents (eg third-generation cephalosporins).

Aspiration pneumonia

Aspiration pneumonia may complicate impaired consciousness and dysphagia. Particulate matter may obstruct the airway, but also chemical pneumonitis may develop from aspiration of acid gastric contents, leading to pulmonary oedema.

- Anaerobes are the principal pathogens, arising from the oropharynx.
- There are typically two to three separate isolates in each case.
- Multiple pulmonary abscesses or empyema may result.

- Treat with metronidazole in combination with broad-spectrum agent (eg third-generation cephalosporin).

Cavitation may develop with the following infections

- *Staphylococcus aureus*
- *Klebsiella pneumoniae*
- *Legionella pneumophila* (rare)
- Anaerobic infections
- *Pseudomonas aeruginosa*
- *Mycobacterium tuberculosis* and atypical mycobacterial infections

3.2 Empyema

A collection of pus in the pleural space may complicate up to 15% of community acquired pneumonias and is more common when there is a history of excess alcohol consumption, poor dentition, aspiration or general anaesthesia.

- A diagnosis of empyema is suspected if a patient is slow to improve, has a persistent fever or elevation of the WCC or CRP and has radiological evidence of a pleural fluid collection. The pH of pleural fluid is <7.2.
- Untreated, extensive fibrosis occurs in the pleural cavity, weight loss and clubbing develop and the mortality rate is high.
- The mainstay of treatment is drainage of the pleural space combined with continuous high-dose intravenous antibiotic treatment. Daily intra-pleural administration of streptokinase has been shown to liquefy the pus and facilitate percutaneous drainage with improved resolution rates.
- For those who fail to resolve with medical therapy, thoracotomy and decortication of the lung may be necessary.

Lung abscess

This maybe suspected when the patient is slow to improve. A chest radiograph will show single or multiple fluid-filled cavities. Prolonged courses of antibiotics are needed sometimes with percutaneous drainage.

3.3 Tuberculosis

The number of new cases of tuberculosis (TB) declined in the UK throughout the 20th century mainly due to the improvement in living standards. In recent years, however, the incidence of TB has begun to increase again. Those at risk include:

- Those on low incomes
- Homeless people
- Alcoholics
- HIV-positive individuals
- Immigrants from countries with a high incidence of TB.

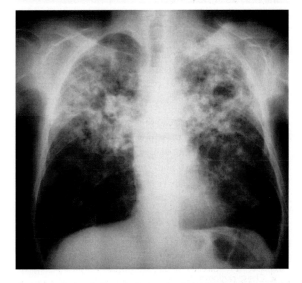

Figure 5 Frontal chest radiograph of the lungs of a patient with pulmonary tuberculosis (TB)

Credit SCIENCE PHOTO LIBRARY

The most commonly involved site is the lung – with lymph node, bone, renal tract and gastrointestinal (GI) tract being less common. Tuberculous meningitis is the most serious complication.

Primary TB

Primary infection occurs in those without immunity. A small lung lesion known as the Ghon focus develops in the mid or lower zones of the lung and is composed of tubercle-laden macrophages. Bacilli are transported through the lymphatics to the draining lymph nodes, which enlarge considerably and caseate. Infection is often arrested at this stage and the bacteria may remain dormant for many years. The peripheral lung lesion and the nodes heal and may calcify. The entire process is often asymptomatic; however, specific immunity begins to develop and tuberculin skin tests become positive.

Post-primary TB

Organisms disseminated by the blood at the time of primary infection may reactivate many years later. The most common site for post-primary TB is the lungs, with bone and lymph node sites being less common. Reactivation may be precipitated by a waning of host immunity, for example due to malignancy or immunosuppressive drugs including steroids.

Clinical picture

Primary infection is often asymptomatic, but may cause mild cough and wheeze or erythema nodosum.

Reactivation or reinfection may cause

- Persistent cough
- Night sweats
- Pleural effusion
- Meningitis
- Weight loss
- Haemoptysis
- Pneumonia
- Lymphadenopathy

Miliary TB

This is caused by widespread dissemination of infection via the bloodstream. It may present with non-specific symptoms of malaise, pyrexia and weight loss. Eventually hepato-splenomegaly develops and choroidal tubercles may be visible on fundoscopy. The chest radiograph shows multiple rounded shadows a few millimetres in diameter, 'millet seeds'. It is universally fatal if left untreated.

Diagnosis of TB

- Chest radiograph

  - May show patchy shadowing in the upper zones with volume loss and cavitation, and ultimately fibrosis

- Pleural fluid aspiration and biopsy
- Lymph node biopsy
- Bone marrow aspirate
- Morning sputum collections

  - For acid-alcohol fast bacilli smear

- Bronchoscopy and lavage

  - Used for those unable to expectorate; transbronchial biopsy if miliary disease is a possibility

- Early morning urine specimens

  - For renal tract disease

- CSF culture

Specimens are examined for Acid alcohol fast bacilli (AAFB) using Ziehl-Neelsen or auramine stains and then cultured on Löwenstein-Jensen medium. Cultures are continued for at least 6 weeks, as the organism is slow growing. Polymerase chain reaction (PCR) for tuberculous DNA can be used to provide a rapid diagnosis.

Essential note

TB is a notifiable disease

Treatment

This is with a combination of four drugs:

- Rifampicin
- Isoniazid
- Pyrazinamide
- Ethambutol.

Short courses of treatment for 6 months are now standard. All drugs are given for 2 months and isoniazid and rifampicin are continued for a further 4 months. Sensitivity testing will identify drug resistance and all four drugs are continued until sensitivities are known. If pyrazinamide has to be discontinued due to side-effects, a 9-month regime is necessary. Second-line agents (eg ethionamide, propionamide, streptomycin, cycloserine) may be needed. Compliance can pose major problems and directly observed therapy (DOT – larger doses of drugs administered 3 times per week) is used when poor compliance is anticipated.

- Side-effects are common, rifampicin, isoniazid and pyrazinamide all causing hepatitis, whereas ethambutol may cause optic neuritis – visual acuity should be checked before treatment is initiated. Isoniazid may cause peripheral neuropathy, 10 mg pyridoxine daily being given in those at particular risk of this complication (eg alcoholics, diabetics and in patients with renal failure). If hepatid toxicity develops (ACT/AST >5 × normal) all drugs should be stopped until the LFTs normalise. They should then be re-introduced individually with the least lively culprit first, initially at half the recommended dose. The LFTs should be monitored as the dosage and drugs are increased.
- Multi-drug resistant TB (MDR-TB) signifies resistance to rifampicin and isoniazid; it currently accounts for 2% of tuberculous infections nationally and is mainly concentrated in London.

Prevention

BCG vaccination is given to most children aged 13 years provided that a Heaf test shows grade 0–1 reactivity. BCG provides approximately 70% protection against TB and prevents disseminated disease developing. In infants at particular risk, vaccination is given at birth. Chemoprophylaxis (isoniazid for 6 months or rifampicin and isoniazid for 3 months) is given to those with evidence of recent infection (Heaf conversion) but no clinical or radiological disease.

Patients with pulmonary TB, particularly those who are sputum smear positive for AAFB, are potentially infectious and close contacts should be screened for disease. Once 2 weeks of antituberculous chemotherapy has been completed, the patient is rendered non-infectious. TB is a notifiable disease.

Opportunistic mycobacterial infections
These account for 10% of all mycobacterial infections.

Causative organisms

- *Mycobacterium kansasii*
- *Mycobacterium xenopi*
- *Mycobacterium malmoense*
- *Mycobacterium avium intracellulare*

These organisms cause disease that is clinically and radiologically identical to TB. Pulmonary disease, lymphadenitis (in children) and disseminated infection are the commonest clinical problems. They are ubiquitous in the environment and are low-grade pathogens. Opportunistic mycobacterial infections constitute a relatively higher proportion of mycobacterial infections in AIDS patients. The onset of symptoms is usually gradual. Treatment programmes are generally longer than for TB, and are often continued for 18 months to 2 years. Rifampicin and ethambutol are the main agents used, but for those not responding streptomycin, clarithromycin or ciprofloxacin may be added. Atypical infections do not need to be notified. Contact tracing is unnecessary as person-to-person infection is very rare.

3.4 Bronchiectasis
This is the permanent dilatation of sub-segmental airways which are inflamed, tortuous, flabby and partially/totally obstructed by secretions. Bronchiectasis may be cystic, cylindrical or varicose. The obstruction often leads to post-obstructive pneumonitis so that the lung parenchyma may be temporarily or permanently damaged.

Causes

- Congenital
- Post-infective (eg following episodes of childhood measles, pneumonia or pertussis)
- Immune deficiency
- Post-tuberculosis
- Allergic bronchopulmonary aspergillosis (ABPA) – proximal

Causes

- Complicating sarcoidosis or pulmonary fibrosis
- Idiopathic – 60%
- Distal to an obstructed bronchus or one severely compressed from encroaching lymph nodes
- Secondary to bronchial damage resulting from a chemical pneumonitis (eg inhalation of caustic chemicals)
- Mucociliary clearance defects: primary ciliary dyskinesis or associated with situs inversus (Kartagener's syndrome) or associated with azoospermia and sinusitis in males (Young's syndrome)

Clinical features
There is a history of chronic sputum production, which is often mucopurulent and accompanied by episodes of haemoptysis. Occasionally bronchiectasis can be dry with episodic haemoptysis and no sputum production. Exertional dyspnoea and wheeze may be associated. Patients complain of malaise and fatigue; one-third have symptoms of chronic sinusitis. There may be few abnormal clinical findings other than occasional basal crackles or wheeze on chest examination; clubbing may be present. Frequent infective exacerbations reduce the quality of life.

Investigations

- **Sputum microbiology**: most commonly shows *Haemophilus influenzae*, *Streptococcus pneumoniae* or *Pseudomonas aeruginosa*; mycobacteria and fungi may also be seen.
- **Chest radiograph**: may be normal or may show thickening of bronchial walls, and in cystic bronchiectasis, ring shadows ± fluid levels. The upper lobes are most frequently affected in ABPA, cystic fibrosis, sarcoidosis and tuberculosis.
- **Pulmonary function tests**: may be normal or show an obstructed/restricted pattern (or both).
- **High-resolution CT scanning**: is diagnostic in >90% of cases.
- **Immunoglobulin levels or antibody response following vaccination (eg *H. influenzae* or pneumococcal)**: may demonstrate deficiency of humoral immunity.

Treatment
As far as possible the aetiology of the bronchiectasis should be established in every case. If there is an underlying immune deficiency state, treatment with intravenous gamma globulin replacement therapy is beneficial. Regular physiotherapy with postural drainage and using 'The Active Cycle of Breathing'

helps to clear the airways. Inhaled bronchodilators are often used. Antibiotics are usually given in response to an exacerbation; however, some patients require continuous oral treatment, usually three antibiotics in monthly rotation. Nebulised antibiotics can be used to damp down the microbial load and are particularly useful when a patient is colonised with *Pseudomonas*. Good hydration is important but mucolytics are generally not helpful. Surgery is reserved for those with localised severe disease; lung transplantation has been successful.

Complications

Infective exacerbations are the principal problem. Antibiotic therapy should be tailored to sputum culture results. Prolonged courses and/or intravenous treatment often required. Haemoptysis usually settles with treatment of the infection but occasionally embolisation of the bleeding vessel is required. Chest pain over an area of bronchiectatic lung is not uncommon. In the long term, systemic amyloid may result.

3.5 Cystic fibrosis

Cystic fibrosis (CF) is the most common fatal autosomal recessive condition in the Caucasian population, affecting 1 in 2500 live births. One in 25 people are carriers. The gene for CF has been localised to the long arm of chromosome 7 and codes for the cystic fibrosis transmembrane conductance regulator protein (CFTR), which functions as a chloride channel. Over 800 mutations have been identified, the most common being δ508. The basic defect involves abnormal transport of chloride across the cell membrane; in the sweat gland there is a failure to reabsorb chloride and in the airway there is failure of chloride secretion. Diagnosis is made by detection of an abnormally high sweat chloride (>60 mEq/l) and by genetic analysis.

> **Essential note**
>
> CF is autosomal recessive, has an incidence of 1 in 2500 live births and a carrier frequency of 1 in 25

Pulmonary disease

A significant inflammatory infiltrate may be identified in the lungs at a very early age. The airways become obstructed by thick mucus due to decreased chloride secretion and increased sodium reabsorption, and so bacterial infection becomes established in early life.

Infection occurs in an age-related fashion: infants and young children become colonised with *Staphylococcus aureus* and subsequently *Haemophilus influenzae*. In the teenage years, infection with *Pseudomonas aeruginosa* occurs.

The other major pathogens involved are:

- *Streptococcus pneumoniae*
- *Burkholderia cepacia* complex
- *Mycobacterium tuberculosis*
- Atypical mycobacteria
- *Aspergillus fumigatus*
- Viruses.

Chronic infection and inflammation causes lung damage with bronchiectasis affecting predominantly the upper lobes. Patients have breathlessness and reduced exercise tolerance, cough with chronic purulent sputum production, and occasional haemoptysis. Physical signs include clubbing, cyanosis, scattered coarse crackles and occasional wheeze. Slight haemoptysis is often associated with infection but major haemoptysis may occasionally necessitate pulmonary artery embolisation.

- Pulmonary function tests show airflow obstruction; chest radiograph may show hyperinflation, atelectasis, visible thickened bronchial walls, fibrosis and apical bullae; pneumothorax occurs in up to 10% of patients.
- In the terminal stages of disease, respiratory failure develops; 90% of deaths are attributable to respiratory failure. The average life expectancy has increased into the fourth decade.

Gastrointestinal tract

Pancreatic insufficiency is present in over 90% of patients and malabsorption causes bulky offensive stools, with weight loss and deficiency of fat-soluble vitamins (A, D, E and K). Babies may present with meconium ileus and adults may develop an equivalent syndrome with obstruction of the small bowel due to poorly digested intestinal contents causing abdominal pain, distension, vomiting and severe constipation.

- Obstruction of the biliary ductules in the liver may eventually lead to cirrhosis with portal hypertension, splenomegaly and oesophageal varices.
- Gallstones (in 15% of patients), peptic ulcer and reflux oesophagitis are all more prevalent.
- Pancreatitis may develop in older patients.

Involvement of other systems

- **Diabetes**: eventually occurs in up to one-third of patients; there is a gradual loss of pancreatic islet cells with fibrosis developing. Ketoacidosis is very uncommon.
- **Upper airway disease**: nasal polyps occur frequently (up to one-third of patients) and chronic purulent sinusitis may develop.
- **Fertility**: virtually all males are infertile due to abnormal

development of the vas deferens and seminiferous tubules, but fertility in women is only slightly reduced. Although many women with CF have had successful pregnancies, pregnancy may lead to life-threatening respiratory complications.

- **Bones**: osteoporosis is more common with increased fractures risk.

Treatment

Antibiotics and respiratory treatments

Care is best given in a specialist CF unit with an extensive multidisciplinary team. In the UK most centres give antibiotics when sputum becomes increasingly purulent, PFTs are deteriorating or the patient is generally unwell with weight loss. Most patients become chronically colonised with *Pseudomonas aeruginosa* and so two different antibiotics (eg ceftazidime and tobramycin) are used in combination to prevent resistance developing.

- Up to 25% of patients become colonised with *Burkholderia cepacia*, an organism that is highly transmissible from one individual to another and associated with a worse prognosis. These patients are therefore segregated from patients colonised with *Pseudomonas*, in hospital, at outpatient clinics and socially.
- Most patients need continuous anti-staphylococcal treatment.

Nebulised antibiotics reduce the microbial load and are useful in those who need frequent courses of intravenous antibiotics; colomycin or tobramycin are used continuously in a twice daily regimen.

- DNase helps to liquefy viscous sputum and is helpful in some patients. Bronchodilators and inhaled steroid are given to treat airflow obstruction. Physiotherapy, using 'The Active Cycle of Breathing' technique, should be tailored to individual needs.

Pancreatic enzyme supplements

Given with main meals and snacks to those with pancreatic insufficiency. Meconium ileus equivalent is treated with vigorous rehydration and regular oral Gastrografin® (sodium amidotrizoate). Good nutritional status is associated with improved prognosis; supplementary overnight feeding with nasogastric tube or via gastroenterostomy can help to maintain body weight.

Transplantation

Either double-lung or heart-lung transplantation may be appropriate for some patients with terminal respiratory failure. Non-invasive positive pressure ventilation may be utilised to support a patient before transplantation. The timing of lung transplantation is difficult and must be assessed in each individual case. Liver and pancreas transplants are also frequently carried out.

Future

Newborn screening will soon be practised throughout the UK. Gene therapy, although a long way from clinical application, is being extensively researched.

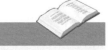

Further revision

The Cystic Fibrosis Trust at
http://www.cftrust.org.uk/index.jsp

3.6 *Aspergillus* and the lung

Aspergillus causes three distinct forms of pulmonary disease: allergic bronchopulmonary aspergillosis, colonising aspergillosis and invasive aspergillosis.

Allergic bronchopulmonary aspergillosis

(*See* section 2.1).

Colonising aspergillosis

Fungal colonisation of cavities in the lung parenchyma, of dilated bronchi or the pleural space.

A mass or ball of fungus develops known as an aspergilloma. *A. fumigatus* is usually responsible, but occasionally *A. niger*, *A. flavus* or *A. nidulans* may be implicated. Cavities due to TB, sarcoidosis, cystic fibrosis or neoplasms may be colonised. Cough and sputum production often occur and are features of the underlying disease. Haemoptysis is a common complication, and this may be massive.

Invasive aspergillosis

Fungal infection spreads rapidly through the lung causing granulomas, necrosis of tissue and suppuration. It occurs most commonly in the immunosuppressed host and may be rapidly fatal. Progressive chest radiograph shadowing (which may cavitate), associated with fever, chest pain and haemoptysis that do not settle promptly with antibacterial agents, suggests invasive aspergillosis.

- Cough with copious sputum production, often with haemoptysis, is usual.
- Examination of sputum or bronchoalveolar lavage fluid may demonstrate fungal hyphae. High resolution CT scanning shows pulmonary infiltrates with the 'halo' sign. Treatment is with systemic antifungal agents.

4. OCCUPATIONAL LUNG DISEASE

4.1 Asbestos-related disease

Exposure to asbestos was previously commonplace in many occupations including shipbuilders, laggers, builders, dockers and factory workers engaged in the manufacture of asbestos products.

Effects of asbestos on the lung

Pleural plaques

These appear 20 years or more after low-intensity exposure. They develop on the parietal pleura of the chest wall, diaphragm, pericardium and mediastinum, and commonly calcify. Pleural plaques are usually asymptomatic but they may cause mild restriction.

Diffuse pleural thickening

This can extend continuously over a variable proportion of the thoracic cavity, but is most marked at the lung bases. It causes exertional dyspnoea and spirometry is restricted.

Pleural effusions may occur in asbestos-related disease, usually within 15 years of exposure. They often resolve spontaneously, leaving thickening of the visceral pleura.

Asbestosis

Asbestosis refers to the pneumoconiosis caused by inhalation of asbestos fibres. The onset of asbestosis is usually >20 years after exposure (but with higher levels of exposure fibrosis occurs earlier). Fibrotic changes are more pronounced in the lower lobes; patients present with slowly worsening exertional dyspnoea and clinical examination reveals fine inspiratory crackles in the lower zones. Clubbing may occur.

- Chest radiograph shows small irregular opacities, horizontal lines and, in more advanced disease, honeycomb and ring shadows.
- High-resolution CT confirms fibrosis associated with pleural disease.
- PFTs show a restrictive defect with reduced KCO.
- There is an increased risk of lung cancer (see below).
- The disease is untreatable and death is usually due to respiratory failure or malignancy.
- Elderly patients are not suitable for transplantation.

Lung cancer

Asbestos exposure is associated with a substantially increased risk of lung cancer (see section 5.1), and the predisposition is synergistic with smoking. The risk of mesothelioma is also markedly increased. Asbestos exposure, in the absence of smoking, increases the risk of lung cancer six-fold. For cigarette smokers with a history of asbestos exposure, the risk is increased 59 times. I.e. the effects of cigarette smoke on asbestos are multiplicative.

Compensation claims

Patients with all of the above asbestos-related diseases except pleural plaques are entitled to state compensation and a disability pension. Patients may also wish to make a claim against their employers for negligently exposing them to asbestos for any asbestos-related condition, including pleural plaques. They should be advised to begin legal action within 3 years of being told that they have an asbestos-related condition. The same applies for patients with coal workers' pneumoconiosis and occupational asthma and a small number of other industrial diseases.

4.2 Coal workers' pneumoconiosis (CWP)

The incidence of this pneumoconiosis is related to total dust exposure. Dust particles 2–5 µm in diameter are retained in the respiratory bronchioles and alveoli. Simple CWP is characterised by small rounded opacities (<1.5 mm in diameter) on chest radiograph, and is associated with focal emphysema. The lesions are asymptomatic.

- **Progressive massive fibrosis** (PMF) involves the development of larger opacities (>3 cm in diameter) on a background of simple CWP, usually in the upper lobes.
- Coal mining is recognised as a cause of COPD.

Caplan's syndrome is the development of multiple round pulmonary nodules in patients with rheumatoid arthritis and a background of CWP. They may be associated with pleural effusion and may ultimately calcify.

4.3 Silicosis

This is caused by inhaling silicon dioxide, a highly fibrogenic dust, and it affects quarry workers, hard rock miners, civil engineers, etc. Silicosis was commonly associated with TB in the first half of the 20th century.

4.4 Byssinosis

This is caused by exposure to cotton dust, flax and hemp. Acute exposure causes airways narrowing in one-third of affected individuals. However, chronic byssinosis develops after years of heavy exposure to cotton dust; symptoms are worse on the first day back after a break from work, and include chest tightness, cough, dyspnoea and wheeze.

4.5 Occupational asthma

This is now the commonest industrial lung disease in developed countries. A large number of agents encountered at work cause asthma and are officially recognised for industrial compensation.

Causes of occupational asthma

A large number of agents, including isocyanates (paint spraying), dyes, epoxy resins, flour and laboratory animals, are associated with occupational asthma. It develops after a period of asymptomatic exposure to the allergen, but usually within 2 years of first exposure. Detection depends on a careful history, and PEFR monitoring both at work and at home. Once occupational asthma has developed, bronchospasm may be precipitated by other non-specific triggers such as cold air, exercise, etc. Occupational asthma may develop in workers with previously diagnosed asthma. In order to identify the substance involved, specific IgE levels may be measured or occasionally bronchial provocation testing may be performed. Early diagnosis and removal of the individual from exposure to the allergen is essential if they are to make a full recovery. Asthma symptoms may persist despite termination of exposure.

Essential note

Occupational asthma is the commonest industrial disease in developed countries

---

4.6 Extrinsic allergic alveolitis (hypersensitivity pneumonitis)

This is a hypersensitivity pneumonitis caused by a specific immunological response (usually IgG-mediated) to inhaled organic dusts.

- **Farmers' lung** is due to the inhalation of thermophilic actinomycetes (usually *Micropolyspora faeni* and *Thermoactinomyces vulgaris*), when workers are exposed to mouldy hay.
- **Bird fanciers' lung** is caused by inhaled avian serum proteins, present in excreta, and in the bloom from feathers; it primarily affects those who keep racing pigeons and those keeping budgerigars as pets.
- **Ventilation pneumonitis** occurs in inhabitants of air-conditioned buildings where thermophilic actinomycetes grow in the humidification system.
- **Bagassosis** is due to exposure to *Thermoactinomyces sacchari* in sugar cane processors.
- **Malt workers' lung** is due to the inhalation of *Aspergillus clavatus*.
- **Mushroom workers' lung** is due to the inhalation of thermophilic actinomycetes.

  The clinical features depend on the pattern of exposure. An acute allergic alveolitis develops several hours after exposure to high concentrations of dust.

Breathlessness and 'flu-like' symptoms occur, sometimes associated with fever, headaches and muscle pains. The symptoms are short-lived and usually resolve completely within 48 hours. Inspiratory crackles may be heard on chest auscultation. The disease may present in a sub-acute or chronic form characterised by cough, breathlessness, fatigue and weight loss. Clubbing may occur in association with irreversible pulmonary fibrosis.

- **Chest radiograph** may show a generalised haze sometimes associated with nodular shadows. In chronic cases progressive upper zone fibrosis and loss of lung volume occur.
- **Spirometry** becomes restrictive and gas transfer factor is reduced.
- The diagnosis is made by establishing a history of exposure to antigen and the demonstration of precipitating antibodies in the patient's serum. Histology of lung biopsy samples shows a mononuclear cell infiltrate with the formation of granulomas. Fluid obtained from bronchoalveolar lavage shows a high lymphocyte count.
- Once the diagnosis is established the patient should be isolated from the antigen; if this is impossible respiratory protection should be worn. Corticosteroids accelerate the rate of recovery from an acute attack but are generally not helpful once established fibrosis develops.

Further revision

The Health and Safety Executive at http://www.hse.gov.uk/index.htm

---

5. TUMOURS

5.1 Lung cancer

Lung cancer is the most prevalent cancer worldwide and accounts for 1:3 cancer deaths in men and 1:6.5 cancer deaths in women. Female mortality rate from lung cancer now exceeds that from breast cancer. Twenty per cent of smokers will develop lung cancer. The prognosis is poor, with a mean survival of less than 6 months. The 5-year survival rate is 10–13%.

Causes of lung cancer

- **Smoking**
  Over 90% of lung cancers occur in current or ex-smokers
- **Atmospheric pollution**
  Persistently higher lung cancer rates in urban populations; passive smoking
- **Industrial exposures**
  Asbestos fibre, aluminium industry arsenic compounds, benzoyl chloride, beryllium
- Increased incidence in patients with cryptogenic fibrosing alveolitis and systemic sclerosis

Smoking is the leading cause of lung cancer. Although smoking rates have declined amongst adult men and to a lesser extent among women, there are an increasing number of teenage smokers, particularly girls.

Cell types

- **Squamous cell** (20–30%): usually arise from a central airway
- **Small cell** (20%): arise in central airways and grow rapidly producing both intra-thoracic and metastatic symptoms
- **Adenocarcinoma** (30–40%): may be peripheral and slow-growing. Now the commonest form of lung cancer
- **Undifferentiated** large cell (10%)
- **Bronchiolo-alveolar** cell carcinoma (5%).

Clinical features

Patients commonly present with cough, breathlessness, haemoptysis, chest pain or weight loss. Lung cancer should be suspected if a pneumonia fails to resolve radiologically. Occasionally an asymptomatic lesion will be noted on a routine chest radiograph.

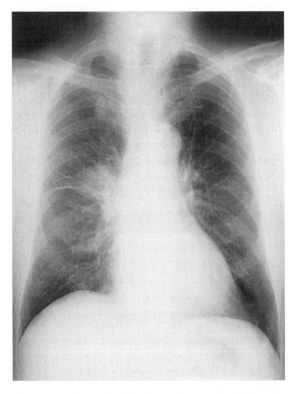

Figure 6 Radiograph of the chest of a patient with lung cancer

Credit SCIENCE PHOTO LIBRARY

Intra-thoracic complications of lung cancer

- Collapse of lung distal to obstructing tumour
- Recurrent laryngeal nerve palsy causing hoarseness
- Dysphagia due to compression of the oesophagus by enlarged metastatic lymph nodes or tumour invasion
- Pericarditis with effusion
- Phrenic nerve palsy with raised hemidiaphragm
- Pleural effusion
- Superior vena caval obstruction causing headache, distension of the veins in the upper body, fixed elevation of the JVP, facial suffusion with conjunctival oedema
- Rib metastases
- Spontaneous pneumothorax

Metastases can occur throughout the body but the most commonly involved sites are:

- Supraclavicular and anterior cervical lymph nodes, adrenal, bones, liver, brain and skin.

Essential note

Lung cancer is the most prevalent cancer worldwide, with >90% in current or ex-smokers

Further revision

Action on Smoking and Health U.K. at http://www.ash.org.uk/

Paraneoplastic syndromes

These include the following:

- **SIADH**: chiefly associated with small cell lung cancer. Treatment involves fluid restriction initially and demeclocycline for resistant cases.
- **Hypercalcaemia**: usually associated with multiple bony metastases from squamous cell carcinoma; ectopic parathyroid hormone (PTH) secretion occurs in a few squamous cell cancers.
- **Eaton–Lambert syndrome**: almost exclusively associated with small cell lung cancer; produces a proximal myopathy, reduced tendon reflexes and autonomic features.
- **Clubbing**: occurs in 10–30% of lung cancers; may resolve after resection.
- **Hypertrophic pulmonary osteoarthropathy (HPOA)**: produces periostitis, arthritis and gross finger clubbing. It involves the long bones (tibia/fibula, radius/ulna, femur/humerus). It is associated with subperiosteal new bone formation visible on plain radiograph and is often painful.

Pancoast's syndrome

This is due to a tumour of the superior sulcus. The most common presenting complaint is pain (due to involvement of the eighth cervical and first thoracic nerve roots) extending down the medial side of the upper arm to the forearm and hand, and the small muscles of the hand may atrophy. Horner's syndrome may develop (*see* Chapter 13, Neurology). Chest radiograph demonstrates a shadow at the extreme apex, and there may be destruction of the first and second ribs.

Diagnosis of lung cancer

- Sputum cytology – often not helpful
- CT thorax
- Percutaneous CT-guided biopsy of peripheral nodules
- Bronchoscopy
- Biopsy of metastatic deposit (including lymph nodes)
- Resection of peripheral nodules

Wherever possible the histological type should be confirmed and the patients should be staged, usually by CT scanning. Non small cell lung cancers are staged using the TNM (tumour/nodes/metastasis) classification whilst small cell lesions are classified as either limited stage (confined to one hemithorax) or extensive disease. An assessment of performance status is important prognostically.

Treatment

Surgery offers the best chance of cure. At the time of presentation only 10–20% of patients with non small cell lung cancer will be operable. The 5-year survival rate depends on the clinical stage: 60% for stage I tumours but as low as 7% for stage IIIb tumours (locally advanced disease). Patients whose tumour is technically operable, but who are unfit for surgery due to coexisting medical conditions or poor lung function, may be treated with **radical radiotherapy**.

- **Palliative radiotherapy** is very effective in relieving pain from bony metastases, controlling haemoptysis and cough. Dyspnoea and dysphagia due to oesophageal compression by lymph nodes respond well to radiotherapy.
- **Superior vena caval obstruction** can also be treated with radiotherapy; however, stenting provides more immediate relief of symptoms.
- **Chemotherapy** for non small cell lung cancer offers only a very small survival benefit but has been shown to provide effective palliation.

Small cell lung cancer is associated with an extremely poor prognosis if left untreated, with a median survival of only 8 weeks. The tumour is, however, much more sensitive to chemotherapeutic agents than other types of lung cancer, and cycles of combination chemotherapy can result in remission in up to 80% of cases. Median survival is now 14–20 months for limited disease and 8–13 months for extensive disease. Once the disease has relapsed, mean survival is 4 months.

5.2 Mesothelioma

This is most common in men between the ages of 50 and 70 years. The lesion arises from mesothelial cells of pleura or, less commonly, the peritoneum. **Asbestos exposure** is responsible for at least 85% of malignant mesotheliomas, and the risk of mesothelioma increases with the dose of asbestos received. Crocidolite (blue) is more potent than amosite (brown) and both are more potent than chrysotile (white asbestos) in causing mesothelioma.

There is usually a latent period of >30 years between asbestos exposure and development of mesothelioma. The tumour arises from the visceral or parietal pleura, and expands to encase the lung. Pleural mesothelioma presents with chest pain, weight loss and dyspnoea and may cause pleural effusion.

Controls over asbestos exposure only came into force in the 1970s and the incidence of mesothelioma is rising and expected to peak around 2020. A detailed occupational history is essential.

- Chest radiograph and CT thorax usually show an effusion with underlying lobulated pleural thickening and contraction of the hemithorax.
- Diagnosis is made by pleural biopsy often done as a VATS procedure (*see* section 6.4); the main differential diagnosis is adenocarcinoma of the pleura or benign pleural thickening.
- Treatment is unsatisfactory. Radiotherapy is helpful for pain relief and for preventing seeding of the biopsy track. Randomised trials of chemotherapy for mesothelioma are currently ongoing. Pleural effusions should be drained and talc pleurodesis considered once a tissue diagnosis has been made. Involvement of the palliative care team is often helpful.
- Median survival from presentation is 8–14 months for pleural mesothelioma and 7 months for peritoneal mesothelioma.
- Patients with mesothelioma may be eligible for industrial compensation.

Pulmonary causes of clubbing

- Carcinoma of the bronchus
- Asbestosis
- Lung abscess
- Cystic fibrosis
- Tuberculosis
- Cryptogenic fibrosing alveolitis
- Bronchiectasis
- Empyema
- Mesothelioma

Causes of haemoptysis

- Common causes

  - Carcinoma of the bronchus
  - Pneumonia/acute bronchitis
  - Bronchiectasis
  - Pulmonary tuberculosis
  - Pulmonary embolus
  - Mitral valve disease
  - Infective exacerbation of COPD

Causes of haemoptysis

- Rarer causes

  - Vascular malformations
  - Mycetoma
  - Connective tissue disorders
  - Vasculitis
  - Goodpasture's syndrome
  - Cystic fibrosis
  - Bleeding diathesis
  - Idiopathic pulmonary haemosiderosis

6. GRANULOMATOUS AND DIFFUSE PARENCHYMAL LUNG DISEASE

6.1 Sarcoidosis

Sarcoidosis is a multisystem granulomatous disorder primarily affecting young adults. The aetiology is unknown. The prevalence varies among different populations but in the UK it is 20–30/100 000, being highest among West Indian and Asian immigrants. The characteristic histological lesion is the granuloma composed of macrophages, lymphocytes and epithelioid histiocytes, which fuse to form multinucleate giant cells. The disease may present acutely with erythema nodosum and bilateral hilar lymphadenopathy on the chest radiograph (good prognosis with most patients showing radiological resolution within a year) or insidiously with multi-organ involvement. Ninety per cent of patients have intra-thoracic involvement.

Chest radiograph changes are graded as:

- **Stage 0**: clear chest radiograph
- **Stage 1**: bilateral hilar lymphadenopathy (BHL)
- **Stage 2**: bilateral hilar lymphadenopathy and pulmonary infiltration
- **Stage 3**: diffuse pulmonary infiltration.

Patients may have no respiratory symptoms or complain of dyspnoea, dry cough, fever, malaise and weight loss. Chest examination is frequently normal; finger clubbing is rare.

Diffuse parenchymal lung involvement may progress to irreversible fibrosis; the mid and upper zones of the lungs are most frequently affected. Calcification of the hilar nodes or the lung parenchyma may occur with chronic disease. Pleural effusion is rare.

Upper airway involvement (infrequent): the nasal mucosa may become hypertrophied and cause obstruction, crusting and discharge; perforation of the nasal septum and bony erosion are rare.

Extra-pulmonary disease

- **Hypercalcaemia** – due to increased intestinal calcium absorption induced by high serum calcitriol concentrations. Hypercalciuria is often present, even when the serum calcium is normal.
- **Lymphadenopathy**: painless, rubbery lymph node enlargement is more common in Black patients; the cervical and scalene lymph nodes are most frequently affected.
- **Splenomegaly** (25%).
- **Liver involvement**: common, but usually subclinical. LFTs may be deranged and the liver enlarged; liver biopsy is of diagnostic value in 90% (typical sarcoid granulomata).
- **Skin**: erythema nodosum (most commonly in Caucasian females) in disease with BHL; skin plaques, subcutaneous nodules and lupus pernio (violaceous lesions on the nose, cheeks and ears) seen in chronic disease.
- **Acute anterior uveitis (25%)**: chronic iridocyclitis affects older patients and responds poorly to treatment.
- **Heerfordt-Waldenstrom syndrome**: consists of parotid gland enlargement, uveitis, fever and cranial nerve palsies.
- **Neurological manifestations** (uncommon): cranial nerve palsies (facial nerve most often affected), meningitis, hydrocephalus, space-occupying lesions and spinal cord involvement; granulomata infiltrating the posterior pituitary may produce diabetes insipidus, hypothalamic hypothyroidism or hypopituitarism.
- **Cardiac sarcoid** may result in cardiac muscle dysfunction or involve the conducting system, producing arrhythmias, bundle-branch block or complete heart block.
- **Bone cysts** with overlying soft tissue swelling occur most often in the phalanges, metacarpals, metatarsals and nasal bones; arthritis is common.

Diagnosis

The combination of BHL with erythema nodosum in a young adult is virtually diagnostic of acute sarcoidosis; associated with fever and arthralgia it is known as Lofgren's syndrome. Thoracic CT appearances are often characteristic, showing hilar and mediastinal lymphadenopathy, nodules along bronchi, vessels and, in subpleural regions, ground glass shadowing, parenchymal bands, cysts and fibrosis. In other cases, tissue biopsy (transbronchial and endobronchial biopsy samples positive for non-caseating granulomata) in 85–90% is useful. Elevated serum angiotensin-converting enzyme and calcium are consistent with the diagnosis but are non-specific. Twenty-four-hour urinary calcium excretion is often raised. The Kveim–Siltzbach test (intradermal injection of extract of spleen from a patient with active sarcoidosis with skin biopsy at 4–6 weeks demonstrating a granulomatous response) is no longer used. The main differentials are TB and lymphoma and every effort should be made to confirm the diagnosis histologically. Anergy to Heaf testing favours sarcoid but patients who are HIV positive or who have overwhelming TB may be anergic.

Treatment

The best prognosis is associated with acute sarcoidosis, which frequently undergoes complete remission without specific therapy. Stage 0 and 1 disease usually resolve spontaneously. Serial full lung function tests should be performed in patients with stage 2 disease and treatment instituted if they show progressive deterioration. Steroids are the mainstay of therapy for chronic disease but response is unpredictable. Steroid therapy is definitely indicated for hypercalcaemia and hypercalciurua, which persist despite dietary calcium restriction, and also for ophthalmological and neurological complications such as sarcoidosis. Other immunosuppressive agents (eg azathioprine and methotrexate) may be used as steroid-sparing agents.

6.2 Histiocytosis X

In adults histiocytosis is often confined to the lung. It is rare and most likely in young adults.

- Strongly associated with smoking

  - Patients present with non-productive cough and breathlessness; the chest examination is usually normal.

- Chest radiograph shows multiple ring shadows on a background of diffuse reticulo-nodular opacities mainly in the upper and mid-zones; the lung bases are spared.
- With disease progression larger cysts and bullae form and interstitial fibrosis develops. Lung volumes are preserved.
- Diagnosis is by high-resolution CT scanning and lung biopsy.
- Treatment includes smoking cessation and steroids; spontaneous remission occurs in 25% of patients; however, in a further 25% the disease may be rapidly fatal. Patients may progress to end-stage fibrotic lung disease. Spontaneous pneumothorax occurs in 25%.

6.3 Pulmonary fibrosis

Interstitial lung disease is associated with many conditions including the connective tissue diseases (particularly systemic lupus erythematosus and systemic sclerosis), rheumatoid arthritis and sarcoidosis. When pulmonary fibrosis develops without obvious cause it is known as idiopathic pulmonary fibrosis. Extrinsic allergic alveolitis also causes diffuse interstitial fibrosis.

6.4 Idiopathic pulmonary fibrosis (usual interstitial pneumonia – UIP)

This is a specific form of lung fibrosis characterised by UIP on lung biopsy. It accounts for around 80% of patients with interstitial lung fibrosis. The prevalence is increasing (currently 20–30 per 100 000 in some areas). It is a disease of the middle aged and elderly, more common in men, and is possibly the result of an inhaled environmental antigen; metal and wood dusts have been implicated but no causal relationship has been identified. There may be an association with Epstein–Barr virus (EBV). Patients present with a dry cough and breathlessness, and signs include cyanosis, finger clubbing and fine late inspiratory crackles.

- **Lung function tests**: small lung volumes, with reduction in gas transfer and restrictive spirometry.
- **Blood gas analysis**: typically shows type 1 respiratory failure with hypoxaemia and a normal or low pCO_2.
- **Chest radiograph**: reveals small lung volumes and interstitial shadowing most marked at the bases and peripheries, and high-resolution CT (HRCT) scanning is useful to determine the degree of inflammatory change and the likelihood of response to steroids.
- **VATS** (video-assisted thorascopic surgery) or open lung biopsy confirms the diagnosis and histology shows variable degrees of established fibrosis and acute inflammation.
- **Treatment**: steroids and other immunosuppressive agents have been used; patients with established honeycomb fibrosis on HRCT do not usually respond. Patients may benefit from pulmonary rehabilitation, oxygen therapy and in the later stages morphine to palliate their symptoms. Single lung transplantation should be considered in patients below the age of 60 years.

UIP is by far the most common type of pulmonary fibrosis but other categories of fibrosis including NSIP (non-specific interstitial pneumonitis) are recognised.

Extrinsic allergic alveolitis (EAA or hypersensitivity pneumonitis)

(*See* section 4, Occupational lung disease.)

Multiple episodes of acute exposure to agents causing EAA, or long-term low-grade exposure, as occurs in budgerigar owners, can lead to irreversible lung fibrosis. Patients present acutely with a flu-like syndrome including breathlessness, fever, cough and crackles on auscultation several hours after exposure to the antigen. More chronic cases present with progressive dyspnoea, weight loss and fatigue. Exposures include birds, moulds, fungi or grain dusts.

- **Chest radiograph**: shows diffuse alveolar shadowing and lung shrinkage; calcification or cavitation does not develop.
- **Spirometry**: as for cryptogenic fibrosing alveolitis (CFA).
- **Precipitins**: the demonstration of specific IgG antibodies in serum against the identified antigen; precipitins may be present without disease.
- **Histology**: shows poorly formed non-caseating granulomas and a mononuclear cell infiltrate.

Prompt diagnosis of EAA is important as the disease is reversible when diagnosed early.

See section 4.6 for diagnostic strategy.

Drugs causing pulmonary fibrosis

Many drugs are associated with pulmonary fibrosis. These include amiodarone, methotrexate and bleomycin.

Causes of reticular-nodular shadowing on chest radiograph

- **Upper zone**
  - Extrinsic allergic alveolitis
  - Sarcoidosis
  - Coal workers' pneumoconiosis
  - Silicosis

- **Basal zone**
  - Idiopathic pulmonary fibrosis
  - Lymphangitis carcinomatosis
  - Drugs
  - Connective tissue disorders

Causes of calcification on chest radiograph

- **Lymph node calcification**
  - Sarcoidosis
  - Silicosis
  - Tuberculosis

- **Parenchymal calcification**
  - There are many causes, including healed tuberculous lesion, chicken pox pneumonia and benign lung tumours.

7. PULMONARY VASCULITIS AND EOSINOPHILIA

7.1 Wegener's granulomatosis

Small/medium-sized arteries, veins and capillaries are involved with a granulomatous inflammation. Ninety per cent present with upper or lower respiratory tract symptoms. Upper airway involvement includes crusting and granulation tissue on the nasal turbinates producing nasal obstruction and a bloody discharge; collapse of the nasal bridge produces a saddle-shaped nose; antineutrophil cytoplasmic antibody (c-ANCA) is present in 90% of cases (*see also* Chapter 9, Immunology, and Chapter 16, Rheumatology).

- Symptoms include cough, haemoptysis, breathlessness and pleurisy.
- Large rounded shadows may be visible on the chest radiograph and these often cavitate; pleural effusions and infiltrates may develop.

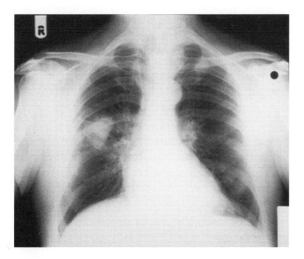

Figure 7 Radiograph of the chest of a patient with Wegener's granulomatosis

- Seventy-seven per cent develop glomerulonephritis and eye and joint involvement are common; mononeuritis multiplex may develop.
- Untreated the median survival is 5 months; cyclophosphamide and steroids can now induce lasting remission in 90%.

7.2 Churg–Strauss syndrome

A syndrome of necrotising vasculitis, eosinophilic infiltrates and granuloma formation; there is often a prior history of asthma, and sometimes allergic rhinitis. Peripheral blood eosinophilia occurs with eosinophilic infiltrates of the lungs and often the gastrointestinal tract. Vasculitic lesions appear on the skin (purpura, erythema or nodules).

7.3 Polyarteritis

This is a rare disease, which can occasionally cause pulmonary haemorrhage and haemoptysis.

7.4 Connective tissue disorders

- **Rheumatoid disease**: has many pulmonary associations which include bronchiectasis, obliterative bronchiolitis, pulmonary fibrosis, nodules and pleurisy.
- **Systemic lupus erythematosus (SLE)**: pulmonary fibrosis and pleural effusion.
- **Systemic sclerosis**: associated with bronchiectasis, pulmonary fibrosis and aspiration pneumonia (due to dysphagia).

All may cause pulmonary hypertension.

8. MISCELLANEOUS RESPIRATORY DISORDERS

8.1 Pleural effusion

Transudates are usually clear or straw-coloured, whereas exudates are often turbid, bloody and may clot on standing. Fluid protein content should be examined: protein levels >30 g/l (or fluid-to-serum ratio >0.5) and lactic dehydrogenase (LDH) levels >200 IU (fluid-to-serum ratio of >0.6) are consistent with an exudate; pH <7.1 also suggests an exudate.

- Low concentrations of glucose in the pleural fluid compared to serum glucose are found in infection and with rheumatoid arthritis.
- **Cell content should be examined**. A transudate is defined as having a protein content of <30 g/l with white cells made up of a mixture of polymorphs, lymphocytes and mesothelial cells. Exudates usually have a much higher white cell count. In bacterial infection this is usually polymorphs, but in established TB lymphocytes predominate.
- Malignant cells from a primary bronchial carcinoma or from metastatic disease may be found in approximately 60% of malignant pleural effusions.

Any patient with pneumonia who develops a pleural effusion should have the fluid analysed for pH. A pH of <7.2 suggests a developing empyema.

Causes of pleural effusion

Transudates

- **Common**

  LVF
  Cirrhosis of the liver
  Nephrotic syndrome
  Acute glomerulonephritis
  Other causes of hypoproteinaemia

- **Uncommon**

  Myxoedema
  Pulmonary emboli
  Peritoneal dialysis

Exudates

- **Common**

  Pulmonary embolism
  Bacterial pneumonia
  Carcinoma of the bronchus
  Metastatic carcinoma

- **Uncommon**

  Infections

  TB
  Fungal/fungal infection

  Malignancy

  Lymphoma
  Pleural tumours

  Connective tissue disorders

  Rheumatoid arthritis
  Systemic lupus erythematosus
  Wegener's granulomatosis
  Sjögren's syndrome

  Subdiaphragmatic

  Pancreatitis
  Subphrenic abscess
  Hepatic abscesses

  Trauma

  Haemothorax
  Chylothorax
  Ruptured oesophagus

Causes of pleural effusion

- **Other rare causes**

  Meigs syndrome
  Asbestos exposure
  Post-thoracotomy syndrome
  Dressler's syndrome

8.2 Pneumothorax

Pneumothorax may be classified as either primary or secondary, the latter complicating underlying lung disease. Presenting symptoms are of pleuritic chest pain and breathlessness and the degree of dyspnoea relates to the size of the pneumothorax. Primary spontaneous pneumothorax usually occurs at rest and the peak age of presentation is in patients in their early 20s. It is much more common in smokers. A tension pneumothorax implies mediastinal shift away from the side of the pneumothorax.

Clinical signs of pneumothorax

- Diminished breath sounds
- Decreased chest excursion on the affected side
- Hyper-resonance of percussion note
- Auscultatory 'clicks'

Clinical signs of tension pneumothorax

- Severe breathlessness
- Hypotension
- Mediastinal shift
- Cardiac arrest (often electro-mechanical dissociation)

Essential note

A tension pneumothorax is a medical emergency!

Diagnosis

This is made when a visceral pleural line is seen on chest radiograph. In patients with emphysema it must be differentiated from large, thin-walled bullae. In general, the pleural line is convex towards the lateral chest wall in pneumothorax, whereas a large bulla tends to be concave towards the lateral chest wall. CT scan can be used to differentiate between these two conditions.

Treatment

- In a patient who has no underlying lung disease and with no clinical distress accompanying a small pneumothorax, no specific therapy is required but follow-up chest radiography should be arranged to ensure lung re-expansion.
- In all other patients, aspiration of the pneumothorax should be attempted first, except if there are signs of a tension pneumothorax.
- If the pneumothorax recurs despite aspiration, a small-bore chest drain should be inserted.
- If the lung fails to re-expand within a few hours then suction should be applied to the drain. Chest drains should not be clamped. Once the lung has been fully re-inflated for 24 hours and bubbling has ceased the suction can be taken off, and the drain removed subsequently, provided the lung remains fully inflated. Removing the chest drain too early is likely to result in recurrence of the pneumothorax.
- If the lung does not re-expand with the chest drain and suction, then the patient should be referred for thoracic surgery.
- Patients with recurrent pneumothorax on the same side will also need thoracic surgical intervention.

8.3 Obstructive sleep apnoea/hypopnoea syndrome (OSAHS)

It is estimated that approximately 1–2% of adult men and 0.5–1% of women suffer from obstructive sleep apnoea. The cardinal symptom is daytime somnolence due to the disruption of the normal sleep pattern. This leads to poor concentration, irritability and personality changes and a tendency to fall asleep during the day. Road traffic accidents are more frequent in this group of patients. The problem is exacerbated by night-time alcohol intake and sedative medication.

Pathogenesis

During sleep, muscle tone is reduced and the airway narrows so that airway obstruction develops between the level of the soft palate and the base of the tongue. Respiratory effort continues but airflow ceases due to the obstructed airway; eventually the patient arouses briefly and ventilation is resumed. The cycle is repeated several hundreds of times throughout the night.

- Over 80% of men with OSAHS are obese (body mass index, BMI >30). Hypothyroidism and acromegaly are also recognised causes. Retrognathia can cause OSAHS, and large tonsils may obstruct the airway. Patients with OSAHS have higher blood pressure than matched controls.
- Patients (or their partners) give a history of loud snoring interrupted by episodes of apnoea. There may be a sensation of waking up due to choking. Sleep is generally unsatisfying.
- Patients suspected of suffering from OSAHS should have some measure of daytime somnolence made (eg using the Epworth scoring system). Concentration is impaired.
- Diagnosis is made by demonstration of desaturation (SaO_2 below 90%) associated with a rise in heart rate and arousal from sleep together with cessation of airflow. The frequency of apnoea/hypopnoea per hour is used to assess disease severity.

Treatment

- Nocturnal continuous positive airways pressure (CPAP) administered via a nasal mask
- Tonsillectomy if enlarged tonsils are thought to be the cause
- Correction of underlying medical disorders (eg hypothyroidism)
- Weight loss for individuals who are obese
- Anterior mandibular positioning devices are useful in some patients
- Tracheostomy (only as a last resort)

Uvulopalatopharyngoplasty is not generally of benefit.

Once a patient has been diagnosed as suffering from OSAHS and is suffering from excessive daytime somnolence, he/she should refrain from driving and inform the Licensing Authorities. Patients may resume driving once their OSAHS has been satisfactorily treated.

8.4 Adult respiratory distress syndrome (ARDS)

This is a syndrome comprising:

- Arterial hypoxaemia
- Bilateral fluffy pulmonary infiltrates on chest radiograph
- Non-cardiogenic pulmonary oedema (pulmonary capillary wedge pressure >18 cmH$_2$O, 1.76 kPa)
- Reduced lung compliance.

- Sepsis
- Burns
- Disseminated intravascular coagulation (DIC)
- Pneumonia
- Aspiration of gastric contents
- Near drowning
- Drug overdoses (eg diamorphine, methadone, barbiturates, paraquat)
- Trauma
- Pancreatitis, uraemia
- Cardiopulmonary bypass
- Pulmonary contusion
- Smoke inhalation
- Oxygen toxicity

Management

No specific treatment is available and management is essentially supportive. Supplemental oxygen is given and patients frequently require mechanical ventilation.

- Corticosteroids have been shown to be beneficial in the latter stages of ARDS that is characterised by progressive pulmonary interstitial fibro-proliferation.

Further revision

Kumar PJ, Clark ML. *Clinical medicine*, 5th edn. Philadelphia: WB Saunders, 2002.

Ramrakha P, Moore K. *Oxford handbook of acute medicine*. Oxford: Oxford University Press, 1997.

Sprigings D, Chambers JB. *Acute medicine: a practical guide to the management of medical emergencies*, 3rd edn. Oxford: Blackwell Science, 2001.

Warrell DA, Weatherall DJ, Cox TM, Benz EJ, Firth JD. (eds) *Oxford Textbook of Medicine*, 4th edn. Oxford: Oxford University Press, 2003.

Revision summary

1. Should have understood the basic function of the lung and the control of respiration. Should be aware of basic lung function tests and their interpretation.
2. Have developed a broad based understanding of the spectrum of conditions affecting the lung, including diseases of the airways, lung parenchyma and pleura.
3. Have understood the definitions of asthma and COPD and be able to categorise the severity of COPD according to spirometry criteria. Know how to treat asthma, including the emergency treatment of an acute attack. Have understood the spectrum of treatments of COPD including the indications for long-term oxygen therapy.
4. Be aware of the different types of pneumonia and the CURB-65 severity scoring system. Have understood the diagnosis and management of empyema and developed an overview of TB and opportunistic mycobacterial infections.
5. Know the different organ systems affected by cystic fibrosis; have developed an overview of management of this condition.
6. Have developed knowledge of occupational lung disease, particularly asbestosis-related disease and issues relating to compensation.
7. Be aware that lung cancer can present with a variety of different signs and symptoms, including paraneoplastic syndromes, and have an understanding of the management of this common cancer.
8. Know how to investigate a pleural effusion and the common causes. Understand the management of pneumothorax.
9. Be aware of some of the rarer conditions affecting the lung. Have developed a basic understanding of sleep apnoea.
10. Know where to look for guidelines for the management of respiratory disorders.

Rheumatology

CONTENTS

Revision objectives

You should be able to:

1. Classify the common types of arthritis
2. Describe the clinical features of rheumatoid arthritis
3. Describe the treatment of rheumatoid arthritis
4. Describe the clinical features of the spondyloarthropathies
5. Describe the clinical features of gout
6. Describe the clinical features of osteoarthritis
7. Classify the connective tissue disorders

1. ARTHRITIS

1.1 Classification

Arthritis may be classified by the number of joints involved, the duration of illness and the pathology.

Number of joints involved

Monoarthritis = one joint.
  Examples:

- Acute gout
- Septic arthritis
- Spondyloarthropathies.

Polyarthritis = more than one joint.
  Examples:

- Rheumatoid arthritis
- Chronic tophaceous gout
- Psoriatic arthritis.

Oligoarthritis = one to four joints.
  Examples:

- Spondyloarthropathies
- Diseases which usually cause monoarthritis can take this form.

Duration of illness

Inflammatory arthritis can be **transient**, **recurrent** or **persistent**. Most episodes (> 70%) are transient (possibly postviral). The duration of these self-limiting illnesses is quite variable; most will settle by 3 months but some may take 12 months to resolve. In clinical practice 3 months is used as the rule-of-thumb to identify persistent inflammatory arthritis.

Persistent inflammatory arthritis

Examples:

- Rheumatoid arthritis
- Psoriatic arthritis
- Spondyloarthritis
- Connective tissue diseases
- Chronic crystal arthritis

Recurrent inflammatory arthritis

Examples:

- Acute crystal arthritis
- Spondyloarthritis
- Palindromic rheumatism

Pathological type

Arthritis can be classified as **degenerative** (such as osteoarthritis) or **inflammatory** (such as rheumatoid arthritis). These can usually be distinguished by history and examination alone. Blood tests and radiographs are not usually needed for diagnosis.

1.2 Features of degenerative arthritis

- Insidious onset
- Short-lived morning stiffness (15 min)
- Pain with use
- Bony swelling
- Subchondral sclerosis on radiographs
- Normal C-reactive protein (CRP) and erythrocyte sedimentation rate (ESR).

1.3 Features of inflammatory arthritis

- Onset may be acute
- Prolonged morning stiffness (>60 min)
- Pain with use and at rest
- Nocturnal pain
- Soft tissue swelling
- Subchondral osteopenia on radiographs
- Elevated CRP and ESR.

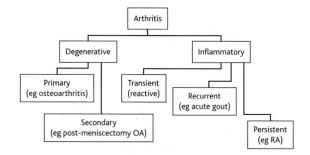

Figure 1 Classification of arthritis

2. RHEUMATOID ARTHRITIS (RA)

This is a persistent inflammatory polyarthritis with symmetrical involvement of small joints (metacarpophalangeal (MCP), proximal interphalangeal (PIP) or wrists). In clinical practice the diagnosis is made on these clinical features alone. The rheumatoid process can affect joints, soft tissues and organs outside the musculoskeletal system.

Essential note

Extra-articular features of rheumatoid arthritis include: nodules, keratoconjunctivitis sicca, scleritis/episcleritis, interstitial lung disease, pleural/pericardial disease and vasculitis

RA is the most common form of inflammatory arthritis. It affects 1–3% of the population in all racial groups, with a female:male ratio of 3:1. It may start at any age but onset is most commonly in the 40s. The cause is not known but both genetic and environmental factors are thought to play a part, with genetic factors accounting for 10–30% of the risk of developing rheumatoid arthritis (RA).

Prognosis is difficult to predict in individual cases but:

- 50% are too disabled to work 10 years after diagnosis
- 25% have relatively mild disease
- Associated with excess mortality.

The following are associated with a worse prognosis:

- Positive rheumatoid factor
- Extra-articular features
- HLA-DR4
- Early erosions
- Insidious onset
- Severe disability at presentation.

2.1 Clinical features of RA

Joints involved in RA

- Symmetrical MCP and wrist arthritis is characteristic
- Any synovial joint can be involved eventually
- Cervical spine is commonly affected
- Hip or distal interphalangeal (DIP) joint involvement is unusual in early disease.

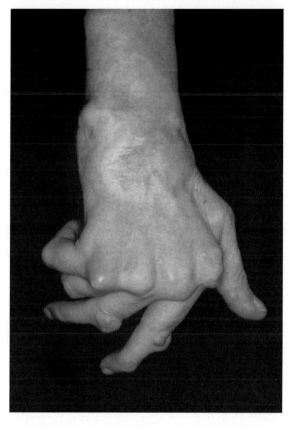

Figure 2 The hand of an elderly woman suffering from rheumatoid arthritis

Credit SCIENCE PHOTO LIBRARY

Characteristic deformities of RA

- Ulnar deviation of MCP joints (Figure 2)
- Boutonnière deformities of fingers
- Swan-neck deformities of fingers
- Z deformity of thumbs

Soft tissue involvement in RA

- Carpal tunnel syndrome (very common)
- Tenosynovitis
- Tendon rupture
- Cervical (atlanto-axial) subluxation
- Lymphoedema (rare)

Extra-articular manifestations

Extra-articular features arise in several ways:

- **True extra-articular manifestations** of the rheumatoid process
- **Non-articular manifestations** of joint/tendon disease (not specific to RA)
- **Systemic effects** of inflammation (not specific to RA) (eg amyloidosis).

True extra-articular manifestations of rheumatoid disease

- Present in 30% of RA patients
- Rheumatoid factor is always positive
- Arthritis tends to be more severe
- **Rheumatoid nodules** are the most characteristic extra-articular feature.

Rheumatoid nodules

Rheumatoid nodules occur in 20–30% of cases, and rheumatoid factor is always positive in these patients. They are associated with more severe arthritis, and can be induced by methotrexate. They are found most commonly on extensor surfaces but can occur anywhere (they may mimic malignancy in the lung). Pathologically, there is a central area of fibrinoid necrosis surrounded by pallisading macrophages and an outer fibrous capsule.

Eye involvement

Keratoconjunctivitis sicca (Sjögren's syndrome) occurs in 20–30% of cases. Episcleritis (a painless reddening of the eye lasting about a week) is common, but often goes unnoticed. Scleritis (reddening and pain) is a manifestation of vasculitis and is uncommon. Repeated attacks of scleritis produce scleromalacia (blue sclera) or perforation (scleromalacia perforans); this is very rare. In contrast to the spondyloarthropathies, iritis is not a feature.

Vasculitis

Nail fold infarcts and mild sensory neuropathy (benign) can occur. Systemic rheumatoid vasculitis has a significant mortality. Its features include cutaneous ulceration, mononeuritis multiplex and involvement of the mesenteric, cerebral and coronary arteries. Renal vasculitis is unusual.

Cardiorespiratory manifestations

- Asymptomatic pleural and pericardial effusions are common
- Interstitial lung disease (rare)
- Obliterative bronchiolitis (rare)
- Caplan's syndrome (massive lung fibrosis in RA patients with pneumoconiosis) is very rare

Felty's syndrome

This is a rare syndrome featuring splenomegaly, neutropenia and RA. Patients with Felty's syndrome usually have a positive antinuclear antibody (ANA) and may have leg ulcers, lymphadenopathy and anaemia.

Non-articular manifestations of joint/tendon disease

- Carpal tunnel syndrome: common, but usually mild
- Cervical myelopathy due to atlanto-axial subluxation (rare, but high mortality)
- Hoarseness and stridor due to cricoarytenoid arthritis (rare, but dangerous).

Systemic effects of inflammation

- Malaise
- Fever
- Weight loss
- Myalgia
- Lymphadenopathy
- Anaemia of chronic disease
- Amyloidosis
- Osteoporosis (immobility also contributes)

Other extra-articular features/associations of RA

- Palmar erythema (common)
- Pyoderma gangrenosum
- Recurrent respiratory infections
- Depression (30%).

2.2 Investigations

In practice the diagnosis of RA is based on the history and examination. Laboratory tests and radiographs are rarely diagnostic in early disease. In research settings the American College of Rheumatology (ACR) criteria are used to classify patients as having RA when four or more of the following are present:

- Morning stiffness >1 h for more than 6 weeks
- Arthritis of three or more joints for more than 6 weeks
- Arthritis of hand joints (wrist, MCP or PIP) for more than 6 weeks
- Symmetric arthritis for more than 6 weeks
- Subcutaneous nodules
- Positive rheumatoid factor
- Characteristic X-ray findings.

Radiological features

- Soft tissue swelling
- Juxta-articular osteopenia
- Joint space narrowing
- Erosions
- Subluxation
- Ankylosis (rare nowadays).

Essential note

Radiological changes in RA include soft tissue swelling, osteopenia, loss of joint space, erosions, subluxation and ankylosis (rare)

Laboratory studies

Rheumatoid factor is positive in 70%. Most laboratory abnormalities are secondary to active inflammation or drug effects and are not specific to RA. They are used to monitor disease activity and screen for adverse drug effects:

- ESR, CRP and plasma viscosity reflect disease activity
- Alkaline phosphatase is often mildly raised in active disease
- Anaemia is common
- Synovial fluid examination is rarely helpful in diagnosis but is often done to exclude other diagnoses (eg sepsis, gout).

2.3 Treatment

Patients should be educated about RA, its clinical course and treatment. Although symptom-modifying and disease-modifying drug therapies form the mainstay of treatment, physiotherapy and occupational therapy are essential components and have a major bearing on prognosis. Podiatry and orthopaedic surgery are also treatment options.

Drug therapy

Drugs used in the treatment of RA fall into two categories: **symptom-modifying** and **disease-modifying**. The disease-modifying drugs are also referred to as slow-acting anti-rheumatic drugs or second-line drugs; the newer anti-tumour necrosis factor alpha (TNFα) therapies fall into this category.

Symptom-modifying drugs: will reduce pain, stiffness and swelling (eg NSAIDs).

Disease-modifying drugs have additional actions and will:

- Reduce pain, swelling and stiffness
- Reduce ESR and CRP
- Correct the anaemia of chronic disease
- Slow disease progression.

Other extra-articular features do not respond to disease-modifying drugs, though nodules may regress.

Corticosteroids are widely used to control acute inflammatory episodes or when the response to treatment is inadequate. They can be used orally, injected directly into joints and soft tissues or as depot intramuscular injections. Although effective at reducing the acute phase response and synovitis they are not thought to be truly 'disease-modifying'.

Disease-modifying drugs in common use

- Methotrexate
- Sulfasalazine
- Leflunomide
- Hydroxychloroquine
- Anti TNFα therapies (infliximab, adalimumab, etanercept)

*Gold, penicillamine, azathioprine and ciclosporin are occasionally used

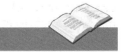

Further revision

The musculoskeletal section of Prodigy NHS guidance at http://www.prodigy.nhs.uk/ClinicalGuidance/ReleasedGuidance/GuidanceList.asp?specialityGuidanceList=13 and http://www.prodigy.nhs.uk/ClinicalGuidance/ReleasedGuidance/GuidanceList.asp are excellent sources of information on the background, diagnosis and treatment of several rheumatological conditions.

British Society for Rheumatology at http://www.rheumatology.org.uk/

Rheumatology (at http://rheumatology.oxfordjournals.org/) is the official journal for the British Society for Rheumatology

Other journal links from http://www.rheumatology.org.uk/link/journals_links

Clinical guidelines from http://www.rheumatology.org.uk/guidelines/clinicalguidelines

Training and provision guidelines at http://www.rheumatology.org.uk/guidelines/trainingprovisionguidelines

Continued over

Further revision (*continued*)

Links to other professional bodies and resources from http://www.rheumatology.org.uk/link/professional_bodies_links/

Links to patient support groups from http://www.rheumatology.org.uk/link/patient_support_links

Harris E D Jr., Budd R C, Firestein G S, Genovese M C, Sergent J S (eds) *Kelley's textbook of rheumatology.* Philadelphia: Saunders, 2004.

Isenberg D A, Maddison P, Woo P, Glass D, Breedveld F (eds) *Oxford textbook of rheumatology.* Oxford: Oxford University Press, 2004.

2.4 Rheumatoid factor

Rheumatoid factors (RF) are antibodies to human IgG, usually reacting with the Fc portion.

Routine hospital tests detect IgM rheumatoid factors, but RF may be of any immunoglobulin isotype (IgM/IgG/IgA). In rheumatoid arthritis, the RF is an assessment of prognosis rather than a diagnostic test.

Conditions with rheumatoid factors

- Normal population (4% overall; 25% of the elderly)
- Rheumatoid arthritis (70%)
- Connective tissue disorders (systemic lupus erythematosus (SLE) 20–40%)
- Chronic infections (eg bacterial endocarditis 25%)
- Other 'immunological' diseases (autoimmune liver disease, sarcoidosis)
- Paraproteinaemias and cryoglobulinaemia
- Transient during acute infections

3. SPONDYLOARTHROPATHIES (HLA-B27-ASSOCIATED DISORDERS)

The spondyloarthropathies include:

- Ankylosing spondylitis
- Psoriatic arthritis
- Reiter's syndrome/reactive arthritis
- Enteropathic arthritis (with ulcerative colitis or Crohn's disease).

This group of disorders is characterised by inflammatory arthritis and/or spondylitis. The peripheral arthritis is typically asymmetrical, involving larger joints, especially the knees and ankles. Characteristic articular features include enthesitis (inflammation at sites of tendon insertion), sacroiliitis and dactylitis. Rheumatoid factor is not present. These arthropathies should not be confused with seronegative RA, which is a symmetrical small joint arthritis.

Associated conditions:

- Psoriasis
- Inflammatory bowel disease
- Anterior uveitis
- Erythema nodosum
- HLA-B27.

Prevalence of HLA-B27

- Normal Caucasian population   8%
- Ankylosing spondylitis   90%
- Reiter's syndrome   70%
- Enteropathic spondylitis   50%
- Psoriatic arthritis   20%
- Psoriatic arthritis with sacroiliitis   50%

3.1 Ankylosing spondylitis

Typically begins with the insidious onset of low back pain and stiffness in a young man. The age of onset is usually between 15 and 40 years and the male:female ratio is about 5:1. It is less common than RA, with a prevalence of about 0.1%. The prognosis is good.

Clinical features of ankylosing spondylitis

- Articular

  - Inflammatory back pain (insidious onset, worse with rest, eases with use)
  - Spinal stiffness (worse in the morning)
  - Restricted spinal movements
  - Restricted chest expansion
  - Inflammatory arthritis, usually asymmetrical affecting large joints (35%)

- Extra-articular

  - Anterior uveitis (25%)
  - Aortic incompetence (4%)
  - Apical lung fibrosis (rare)
  - Aortitis (rare)

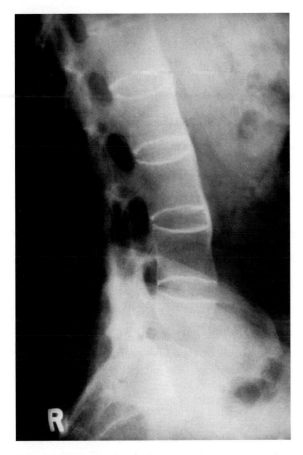

Figure 3 The spine of a patient with ankylosing spondylitis

Source Wellcome Trust Medical Photographic Library

Investigations

Laboratory investigations are not diagnostic and merely reflect inflammation.

- ESR/CRP may be elevated
- Normochromic anaemia
- Alkaline phosphatase often mildly elevated.

HLA-B27 in diagnosis

This should not be a routine test in back pain. Although a negative result makes ankylosing spondylitis unlikely, a positive result is of little help.

Radiological features

Sacro-iliitis is characteristic but radiological changes take several years to become evident.

- Loss of lumbar lordosis
- Squaring of vertebrae
- Enthesitis (calcification at tendon/ligament insertions into bone)
- Bamboo spine (calcification in anterior and posterior spinal ligaments) is a late feature

Treatment

- Physiotherapy and regular home exercises
- NSAIDs
- Disease-modifying drugs (eg sulfasalazine, methotrexate) help peripheral arthritis but are less effective for spinal disease
- Anti-TNFα therapy for disease that is refractory to other treatment
- Surgery (joint replacement, spinal straightening) in end-stage disease.

Essential note

Associations of the spondyloarthropathies include psoriasis, inflammatory bowel disease, anterior uveitis, aortic valve disease/aortitis, erythema nodosum and HLA-B27

3.2 Reiter's syndrome

Reiter's syndrome is a form of reactive arthritis characterised by a triad of arthritis, conjunctivitis and urethritis. A reactive arthritis usually begins 1–3 weeks after infection at a distant site. Antigenic material from the infecting organism may be identified in affected joints but complete organisms cannot be identified or grown. The arthritis does not respond to treatment with antibiotics.

Reiter's syndrome is said to be 20 times more frequent in men than in women. This is likely to be an overestimate because cervicitis may go unrecognised. The true male:female ratio is more likely to be 5:1. Post-dysenteric reactive arthritis has an equal sex distribution. The age of onset is 15–40 years.

Recognised precipitating infections:

- **Post-urethritis** (*Chlamydia trachomatis* – 50%)
- **Post-dysenteric** (*Yersinia, Salmonella, Shigella, Campylobacter*).

Clinical features of Reiter's syndrome

Classical triad

- Arthritis
- Conjunctivitis
- Urethritis.

Other common features

- Iritis (30%)
- Circinate balanitis (25%)
- Buccal/lingual ulcers (10%)
- Keratoderma blenorrhagica (10%).

Prognosis

There is complete resolution with no recurrence in 70–75% of cases. Complete resolution with recurrent episodes is found in 20–25%, usually HLA-B27 positive patients. Chronic disease occurs in < 5% of patients, who are usually HLA-B27 positive.

Treatment

- Mild disease: NSAIDs
- Disease-modifying drugs for persistent arthritis
- Systemic symptoms may need corticosteroids.

3.3 Psoriatic arthritis

Chronic inflammatory arthritis occurs in about 8% of patients with psoriasis. The arthritis may precede the diagnosis of psoriasis. Males and females are equally affected.

Patterns of psoriatic arthritis

- Polyarthritis similar to RA (most common type)
- Sacroiliitis and spondylitis (20–40%)
- Asymmetric oligoarthritis (20–40%)
- Distal interphalangeal joints (5–10%)
- Arthritis mutilans (<5%)

Characteristic features of psoriatic arthritis

- Nail pitting and onycholysis
- DIP joint arthritis
- Dactylitis
- Paravertebral calcification
- Telescoping fingers in arthritis mutilans

Essential note

Characteristic features of psoriatic arthritis include nail pitting and onycholysis, DIP joint arthritis, dactylitis, paravertebral calcification and telescoping fingers in arthritis mutilans

Drug treatment

The same approach is adopted as for treatment of rheumatoid arthritis:

- Symptom-modifying drugs (analgesics, NSAIDs)
- Disease-modifying drugs (eg sulfasalazine, methotrexate)
- Anti-TNFα therapy for refractory disease.

4. CRYSTAL ARTHROPATHIES

4.1 Gout

Uric acid is a breakdown product of purine nucleotides. Hyperuricaemia arises because of an imbalance in uric acid production/ingestion and excretion. Hyperuricaemia is common and usually asymptomatic, but in some individuals uric acid crystals form within joints or soft tissues to produce a variety of diseases.

Clinical features of gout

Acute crystal arthritis

This is characterised by acute recurrent inflammatory arthritis which can be extremely painful. The MTP of the big toe is the commonest joint involved.

Chronic tophaceous arthritis

There is a persistent inflammatory polyarthritis which can mimic RA and is usually associated with tophi (solid aggregations of urate crystals in articular, periarticular and non-articular cartilage (eg ears)).

Renal disease

Several patterns of renal disease are recognised in gout:

- Tubulo interstitial disease due to parenchymal crystal deposition
- Acute intratubular precipitation resulting in acute renal failure (either of these constitute gouty nephropathy)
- Urate stone formation (radiolucent).

Causes of gout

Primary (innate)

- Idiopathic (90% are due to under-excretion of uric acid)
- Rare enzyme deficiencies: eg hypoxanthine-guanine phosphoribosyltransferase (HGPRT) deficiency (Lesch–Nyhan syndrome).

Secondary hyperuricaemia

- Increased uric acid production/intake

  - Myeloproliferative and lymphoproliferative disorders
  - Cytotoxic therapy
  - Acidosis, eg the ketosis of starvation or diabetes
  - Extreme exercise, status epilepticus
  - Severe psoriasis.

- **Decreased uric acid excretion**

  - Renal failure
  - Drugs (diuretics, low-dose aspirin, ciclosporin, pyrazinamide)
  - Alcohol
  - Lead intoxication (saturnine gout)
  - Down's syndrome

Diagnosis of gout

In clinical practice, a characteristic history with hyperuricaemia is often thought sufficient for diagnosis, but there are pitfalls: uric acid may fall by up to 30% during an acute attack; hyperuricaemia is common and may be coincidental.

- Negatively birefringent needle-shaped crystals must be identified in joint fluid or other tissues for a definitive diagnosis
- In chronic tophaceous gout the X-ray appearances (large punched-out erosions distant from the joint margin) are characteristic and may allow diagnosis.

Treatment of gout

Acute attack

- NSAIDs, (colchicine or steroids used if NSAID intolerant).

Prophylaxis

Allopurinol, a xanthine oxidase inhibitor, is the drug of first choice. It may precipitate acute attacks at the outset of treatment unless an NSAID or colchicine is given. Probenecid and sulfinpyrazone are less effective.

Indications for prophylaxis

- Recurrent attacks of arthritis
- Tophi
- Uric acid nephropathy
- Nephrolithiasis
- Cytotoxic therapy
- HGPRT deficiency

Essential note

Indications for treatment with allopurinol are recurrent attacks of acute gout, tophi, uric acid nephropathy/nephrolithiasis, cytotoxic therapy and HGPRT deficiency

4.2 Calcium pyrophosphate deposition disease (CPDD)

This is a spectrum of disorders ranging from asymptomatic radiological abnormalities to disabling polyarthritis. The underlying problem is the deposition of calcium pyrophosphate crystals in and around joints. Usually idiopathic and age-related, but may occur in metabolic disorders especially those with hypercalcaemia or hypomagnesaemia. Calcium pyrophosphate forms positively birefringent brick-shaped crystals – 'pseudogout'.

Variants:

- **Asymptomatic**: radiological chondrocalcinosis (30% of over 80s)
- **Acute monoarthritis**: pseudogout (usually knee, elbow or shoulder)
- **Inflammatory polyarthritis**: mimicking RA (10% of CPDD)
- **Osteoarthritis**: often of hips and knees but with involvement of the index and middle MCP joints (rarely seen in primary osteoarthritis).

Causes of CPDD

- Hyperparathyroidism
- Wilson's disease
- Bartter's syndrome
- Hypomagnesaemia
- Haemochromatosis
- Hypophosphatasia
- Ochronosis

Treatment of CPDD

- Chondrocalcinosis alone needs no treatment
- NSAIDs for arthritis
- Correction of metabolic disturbances (if possible).

5. SEPTIC ARTHRITIS

Septic arthritis is the most serious of the acute inflammatory arthropathies. Joint destruction can occur within hours and the disease can be fatal. Ninety per cent of cases are monoarticular, with the knee the most commonly involved joint. In most cases the micro-organism reaches the joint via the bloodstream during an episode of bacteraemia, but infection can occur by direct inoculation or spread from adjacent tissues.

Septic arthritis is more common in the immunosuppressed and in arthritic joints. The diagnosis should always be considered when a patient with rheumatoid arthritis has a flare in a single joint.

Septic arthritis occurs most commonly in the very young and the elderly. In these groups *Staphylococci* are the most frequent cause, accounting for up to 75% of cases. Streptococci and Gram-negative bacilli account for most of the remainder. In young sexually active adults *Neisseria gonorrhoeae* is the commonest organism.

5.1 Clinical features

Non-gonococcal septic arthritis

The joint is hot and swollen, and usually very painful. The condition is monoarticular in 90% of patients, with the knee being the commonest site. There may be a known focus of extra-articular infection.

Gonnococal arthritis

Disseminated gonococcal infection occurs in 1–3% of cases. It is more common in women. There are two clinical patterns:

1. Triad of dermatitis, tenosynovitis and polyarthralgia
This is usually acute in onset. The skin lesions are small, red, maculopapular and sometimes painful. There are no purulent joint effusions.

2. Purulent arthritis, usually monoarticular, most commonly the knee

5.2 Investigation

The most important investigation is aspiration of synovial fluid for microscopy and culture. The white cell count in synovial fluid will be markedly elevated ($>50\,000/mm^3$) and organisms may be seen on Gram stain. The finding of frankly purulent fluid strongly suggests septic arthritis but similar appearances can occur in crystal arthritis.

- The next step is to search for the site of primary infection, including cultures of blood and urine.
- There will usually be non-specific signs of inflammation such as fever, raised C-reactive protein (CRP) and peripheral neutrophil counts. Radiological changes of septic arthritis do not become evident on plain films for 2–3 weeks.
- If gonocoocal disease is suspected it is important to obtain cultures from the urethra, cervix, pharynx and rectum as appropriate since synovial fluid cultures are rarely positive.

5.3 Treatment

Non-gonococcal septic arthritis will usually require a combination of drainage (by needle aspiration or arthroscopic washout) and prolonged antibiotic therapy for 4–6 weeks. There may still be significant morbidity and mortality.

Gonococcal arthritis responds to 1–2 weeks of antibiotic therapy and has an excellent prognosis.

6. DEGENERATIVE ARTHRITIS

6.1 Osteoarthritis

Osteoarthritis (OA) is the most common joint disease. It is characterised by softening and disintegration of articular cartilage, with secondary changes in adjacent bone. The prevalence of OA on X-ray rises with age and affects 70% of 70-year-olds. Many individuals with radiological OA, however, are asymptomatic.

Joints commonly involved are:

- Distal interphalangeal joints (Heberden's nodes)
- Proximal interphalangeal joints (Bouchard's nodes)
- Base of thumb (first carpometacarpal joint)
- Hips
- Knees
- Spine.

MCP joint OA suggests a secondary cause (eg trauma or CPDD disease).

Radiological changes in osteoarthritis

- Normal mineralisation
- Loss of joint space
- Subchondral new bone formation
- Osteophytes
- Subchondral cysts but no erosions

Essential note

Joints characteristically involved in osteoarthritis include distal interphalangeal joints (Heberden's nodes), proximal interphalangeal joints (Bouchard's nodes), base of thumb (first carpometacarpal joint), hips, knees and spine

OA subsets

- **Primary**

  - Localised (one principal site, eg hip)
  - Generalised (eg hands, knees, spine)

- **Secondary**

  - Dysplastic disorders
  - Mechanical damage (eg osteonecrosis, post-meniscectomy)
  - Metabolic (eg ochronosis, acromegaly)
  - Previous inflammation (eg sepsis, gout, RA)

Essential note

Radiological changes in OA include normal mineralisation, loss of joint space, subchondral new bone formation, osteophytes and subchondral cysts but no erosions

Treatment of osteoarthritis

Treatments for OA include exercise, physiotherapy and occupational therapy. Drug treatment should be with analgesics, including NSAIDs. Intra-articular injection of steroid or hyaluronic acid and joint replacement surgery are further treatment options.

7. FIBROMYALGIA

This is a common chronic disorder characterised by widespread musculoskeletal pain, fatigue and unrefreshing sleep. Female:male ratio 9:1. Prevalence 2–3%. The cause is uncertain but physical injury or psychological stress may be triggers.

Diagnostic features (all are required):

- Widespread pain for at least 3 months
- Pain on both sides of the body, above and below the waist
- Axial (spinal) pain
- Pain in 11 of 18 tender point sites

Other features of fibromyalgia

- Fatigue
- Stiffness
- Unrefreshing sleep
- Loss of delta-wave sleep (in which muscles completely relax)

Patients with fibromyalgia have an increased incidence of:

- Irritable bowel syndrome
- Temporomandibular dysfunction syndrome
- Headache.

Treatment

Fibromyalgia can be treated with amitryptyline and analgesics. Aerobic exercise is also beneficial.

8. INFLAMMATORY CONNECTIVE TISSUE DISORDERS

8.1 Systemic lupus erythematosus (SLE)

This is a multi-system inflammatory connective tissue disorder with small vessel vasculitis and non-organ-specific autoantibodies. It is characterised by skin rashes, arthralgia and antibodies against double-stranded DNA. Young women are predominantly affected with a female:male ratio of 10:1. It is more common in West Indian populations. SLE increases cardiovascular risk. Ten-year survival exceeds 90%.

Clinical features of SLE

- **Common** (>80% of cases)

  - Arthralgia or non-erosive arthritis
  - Rash (malar, discoid or photosensitivity)
  - Fever

Continued over

Clinical features of SLE

Continued

- **Others**

  - Serositis (30–60%): pericarditis, pleurisy, effusions
  - Renal: proteinuria (30–60%), glomerulonephritis (15–20%), nephrotic syndrome
  - Neuropsychiatric (10–60%): psychosis, seizures
  - Haematological (up to 50%): leucopenia, thrombocytopenia, haemolysis
  - Alopecia (up to 50%)
  - Raynaud's (10–40%)
  - Oral or nasal ulcers (10–40%)
  - Respiratory (10%): pneumonitis, shrinking lung syndrome
  - Cardiac (10%): myocarditis, endocarditis (Libman–Sacks)

Laboratory features of SLE

- Cytopenias (neutropenia, lymphopenia, thrombocytopenia)
- ESR reflects disease activity, whereas CRP may not. This discrepancy can be used to differentiate between a flare of SLE and intercurrent infection
- Haemolytic anaemia
- Anaemia of chronic disease
- Low complement C3 and C4 suggests lupus nephritis.

Antibodies

- ANA-positive in 95% of cases, usually with a homogeneous staining pattern
- Anti-double-stranded DNA antibodies in high titre are very specific for SLE
- Anti-Sm antibodies (present in 20% but very specific for lupus)
- Anti-Ro or anti-La are found in ANA-negative subacute cutaneous lupus
- Antiphospholipid antibodies (or false-positive VDRL) occur in 40%

Drug-induced lupus is more common in men than in women. It is usually mild and always resolves on stopping the drug. CNS and renal disease are rare. ANA is positive but antibodies to double-stranded DNA are not usually present. The drugs commonly implicated (procainamide, isoniazid and hydralazine) all have active amido groups.

Treatment of SLE

The treatment of lupus depends on severity and organ involvement. The goals are to control symptoms, limit organ damage and reduce cardiovascular risk factors.

- **Sunscreens** Sunburn can provoke a generalised flare in disease
- **Corticosteroids, immunosuppressive drugs or plasma exchange** for vital organ involvement
- **Anticoagulation** for thrombotic features
- **NSAIDs and hydroxychloroquine** for arthritis and skin-limited disease
- **Cardiovascular risk reduction** (blood pressure, lipids, weight).

8.2 Dermatomyositis and polymyositis

Polymyositis is an idiopathic inflammatory disorder of skeletal muscle. When associated with cutaneous lesions it is called dermatomyositis. These conditions are rare (5 cases per million). Five-year survival is 80% with treatment. Myositis may also occur with other connective tissue disorders.

Clinical features of dermatomyositis and polymyositis

Muscle disease

Weakness is usually most evident in the larger muscle groups of the shoulder and pelvic girdles. Patients experience difficulties rising from chairs, getting out of baths and lifting weights above their heads. Muscles are usually painful and stiff and may be swollen.

Skin features

- Heliotrope discoloration of the eyelids
- Gottron's papules (raised scaly areas over MCP/PIP joints)
- Erythematous macules

Other features

- Periungual telangiectasia
- Respiratory muscle weakness
- Interstitial lung disease
- Oesophageal dysfunction
- Arthralgia
- Weight loss
- Fever

Malignancy

The elderly with dermatomyositis and polymyositis have a higher prevalence of malignancy than would be expected by chance and this is most pronounced in dermatomyositis. There is no association between dermatomyositis/polymyositis and malignancy in children or adults of young and middle age.

Juvenile dermatomyositis differs from the adult form. Vasculitis, ectopic calcification and lipodystrophy are commonly present.

Laboratory tests in dermatomyositis/polymyositis

Diagnosis requires two of the following:

- Elevated muscles enzymes (CK)
- Positive muscle biopsy
- Abnormal EMG.

Antinuclear antibodies are positive in most (80%). Anti-Jo-1 antibodies are associated with a specific syndrome of myositis, interstitial lung disease, fever, arthritis and mechanics' hands (fissuring of the digital pads).

Treatment

- **Corticosteroids**: CK falls rapidly but muscle power takes many weeks to improve
- **Immunosuppressives**: methotrexate or cyclophosphamide are used in resistant cases.

8.3 Systemic sclerosis

Systemic sclerosis is a connective tissue disorder characterised by thickening and fibrosis of the skin (scleroderma) with distinctive involvement of internal organs. It is a rare condition, occurring in all racial groups, with an incidence of 4–12/million per year. It is more common in women (female:male ratio 4:1) and may start at any age. Some cases may be due to exposure to substances such as vinyl chloride.

Clinical features of systemic sclerosis

- Scleroderma
- Raynaud's phenomenon
- Musculoskeletal symptoms
- Gastrointestinal motility disorders
- Interstitial lung disease
- Pulmonary hypertension
- Renal crisis

Scleroderma

After an initial oedematous phase the skin become thickened and eventually hidebound (fixed to deeper tissues). Subcutaneous tissues can become atrophied. When the fingers are involved it is known as sclerodactyly and can produce severe flexion deformities. Facial involvement produces a characteristic beaked nose, difficulty opening the mouth and vertical furrows around the mouth.

Raynaud's phenomenon

The initial complaint in 70%. It can be severe and lead to ulceration of the skin, pitting and scarring of the finger pulps or even loss of digits.

Musculoskeletal

Arthralgia is common, 30% have erosive arthritis; myositis may occur with elevated CK but is usually asymptomatic.

Gastrointestinal

Motility can be impaired at any level:

- Oesophagus (reflux, dysphagia, strictures)
- Stomach (gastric stasis)
- Small bowel (bacterial overgrowth, malabsorption, pseudo-obstruction)
- Colon (constipation).

Cardio respiratory

- Fibrotic interstitial lung disease
- Pulmonary hypertension (poor prognosis).

Renal crisis

Scleroderma renal crisis (malignant hypertension, rapid renal impairment).

Disease patterns

Skin disease may occur with or without internal organ involvement and may be limited or diffuse.

Limited scleroderma with systemic involvement – CREST
Scleroderma is limited to the face, neck and limbs distal to the elbow and knee, and usually begins with Raynaud's phenomenon. It was previously known as CREST (**C**alcinosis, **R**aynaud's, o**E**sophageal dysmotility, **S**clerodactyly, and **T**elangiectasia). Most patients are positive for anti-centromere antibody. Renal crisis is rare, but pulmonary hypertension is more common. It has a better prognosis (70+% 10-year survival).

Diffuse scleroderma with systemic involvement

In these patients, scleroderma involves the trunk and proximal limbs as well as the face and distal limbs. It usually begins with swelling of the fingers and arthritis. Anti-Scl-70 antibodies are found in 20–40% of cases. Pulmonary hypertension is rare, but renal crisis is more common. There is a worse prognosis (50% 10-year survival).

Scleroderma without internal organ disease

- Plaques: morphoea
- Linear: coup de sabre.

Investigation

Diagnosis is based on clinical findings but detailed investigation is required to assess the degree of organ involvement.

- Echocardiography (pulmonary hypertension)
- Pulmonary function tests and chest CT (interstitial lung disease)
- Barium studies (motility disorders)
- Renal function assessment
- Muscle enzymes (CK)
- Nailfold capillary microscopy
- Autoantibodies.

Autoantibodies

- Rheumatoid factor positive in 30%
- Antinuclear factor positive in 90% (speckled or nucleolar staining)
- Anticentromere and anti-Scl-70 are quite specific
- Anticentromere positive in 50–90% of limited and 10% of diffuse scleroderma
- Anti-Scl-70 positive in 20–40%

Treatment

Presentation	Treatment
Skin involvement	Penicillamine
Raynaud's phenomenon	Vasodilators
Severe Raynaud's with digital ischaemia	Iloprost infusions
Arthralgia/arthritis	NSAIDs
Reflux	Proton pump inhibitors
Bacterial overgrowth in the small bowel	Intermittent antibiotics

Presentation	Treatment
Renal crises	ACE inhibitors
Pulmonary hypertension	Iloprost infusion, vasodilators
Interstitial lung disease	Steroids and immunosuppressives

Steroids do not help the skin.

8.4 Sjögren's syndrome

This is a connective tissue disorder characterised by lymphocytic infiltration of exocrine glands, especially the lacrimal and salivary glands. The reduced secretions produce the dry eyes and dry mouth of the sicca syndrome. Secondary Sjögren's syndrome describes the presence of sicca syndrome and either RA or a connective tissue disorder. About 30% of rheumatoid patients have secondary Sjögren's syndrome.

Clinical features of Sjögren's syndrome

Atrophy of exocrine glands

- Dry eyes (xerophthalmia)
- Dry mouth (xerostomia) with increased dental caries
- Dry skin
- Reduced vaginal secretions (dyspareunia)
- Reduced respiratory secretions (hoarseness)

Other features:

- Gland swelling (especially the parotids)
- Lymphadenopathy
- Vasculitic purpura
- Neuropathies
- Renal tubular acidosis (30%)
- Arthralgia or arthritis
- Pancreatitis
- Raynaud's phenomenon

Laboratory tests

Diagnosis is based on clinical features with objective evidence of reduced secretions (Schirmer's test for tear production, or reduced salivary flow by scintigraphy). Biopsy of minor salivary glands can be helpful in difficult cases.

- Anaemia and leucopenia (common)
- ESR and CRP reflect disease activity
- Rheumatoid factor is positive in most

- ANA frequently present
- Anti-Ro or anti-La are present in primary Sjögren's syndrome
- Polyclonal hypergammaglobulinaemia.

Treatment

- **Artificial tears**: plugging of lacrimal punctae in severe cases
- **Moistening sprays**: for the mouth
- **NSAIDs**: and sometimes hydroxychloroquine for arthritis.

8.5 Mixed connective tissue disease/overlap syndromes

Some patients have features of more than one connective tissue disorder and are said to have overlap syndromes. One specific overlap syndrome, mixed connective tissue disease, is associated with anti-RNP antibodies. The clinical features are Raynaud's phenomenon, swollen hands and other features from at least two other connective tissue disorders (SLE, scleroderma or polymyositis). The 10-year survival is 80% but patients who have features mainly of scleroderma and polymyositis fare much worse, with a 10-year survival as low as 30%.

9. VASCULITIS

9.1 Overview of vasculitis

Systemic vasculitis usually presents with constitutional symptoms such as general malaise, fever and weight loss, combined with more specific signs and symptoms related to specific organ involvement. The diagnosis is based on a combination of clinical and laboratory findings, and is usually confirmed by biopsy and/or angiography.

Aetiology

Infections, malignancy and drugs may all produce vasculitic illness but, in most cases, the trigger is unknown.

Clinical features of vasculitis

Constitutional

- Fever
- Weight loss
- Fatigue
- Anorexia

Clinical features of vasculitis

Related to specific organ involvement

- **Renal**: proteinuria, hypertension, glomerulonephritis
- **Respiratory**: alveolitis, haemorrhage, sinusitis
- **Skin**: livedo reticularis, urticaria
- **Musculoskeletal**: arthralgia, arthritis, myalgia
- **Neuropathy**: mononeuritis multiplex, sensory neuropathy
- **Gastrointestinal**: diarrhoea, abdominal pain, perforation, haemorrhage
- **Cardiovascular**: jaw or extremity claudication, myocardial infarction
- **Central nervous system**: headache, visual loss, stroke, seizures

Classification of vasculitis

The vasculitides are classified according to the size of vessel involved and the pattern of organ involvement.

Large vessels

- Takayasu's arteritis
- Giant cell/temporal arteritis
- Aortitis.

Small/medium-sized vessels

- Wegener's granulomatosis
- Microscopic polyangiitis (MPA)
- Churg–Strauss syndrome
- Polyarteritis nodosa
- Kawasaki disease
- Arteritis/vasculitis of RA, SLE, Sjögren's syndrome.

Small vessel vasculitis

- Vasculitis of RA, SLE, Sjögren's syndrome
- Henoch–Schönlein syndrome
- Cryoglobulinaemia
- MPA
- Allergic or hypersensitivity vasculitis
- Drug-induced vasculitis.

Others

- Behçet's syndrome (vasculitis and venulitis).

Laboratory tests

ESR and CRP are invariably elevated in active disease. Normochromic anaemia and leukocytosis (usually neutrophilia) are common. Eosinophilia is characteristic of Churg–Strauss syndrome but may occur in any vasculitis. Serum creatinine and urinary protein assessments are essential if vasculitis is suspected since renal involvement is one of the most important factors affecting prognosis.

Autoantibodies

- cANCA (anti-PR3) is useful in identifying Wegener's disease and microscopic polyangiitis
- pANCA (anti-MPO) may be positive in any vasculitis
- ANCA titres may reflect the activity of vasculitis and titres may begin to rise before a flare in disease activity.

Treatment

- **Large vessel group**: corticosteroids only for most cases
- **Medium/small vessels**: corticosteroids and immunosuppressives (cyclophosphamide and/or azathioprine)
- **Small vessel group**: some conditions benign, corticosteroids and immunosuppressives in some cases.

Prognosis

The size of vessel involved and presence of renal involvement are the most important factors determining prognosis. Despite treatment with immunosuppressive agents and steroids, up to 20% of patients with systemic vasculitis of the small/medium vessel group die within 1 year of diagnosis. Patients with large or small vessel vasculitis have a much more favourable outlook.

9.2 Polymyalgia rheumatica, giant cell and other large vessel arteritis

Giant cell arteritis is a vasculitis of large vessels, usually the cranial branches of arteries arising from the aorta. Polymyalgia rheumatica is not a vasculitis, but is found in 40–60% of patients with giant cell arteritis. Both are disorders of the over 50s and both are relatively common. Polymyalgia has an incidence of 52/100 000 people aged over 50, and giant cell arteritis of 18/100 000 people over 50. Treatment is with corticosteroids.

Features of polymyalgia rheumatica and giant cell arteritis

Polymyalgia rheumatica

- Female:male ratio 3:1
- Age >50 years
- Proximal muscle pain (shoulder or pelvic) *without* weakness
- Early morning stiffness
- Raised acute phase response (ESR/CRP)
- Abnormal liver function tests (alkaline phosphatase/gammaGT)
- CK normal
- Synovitis of knees, etc may occur
- Response to corticosteroids is dramatic and prompt (within 24–48 hours)

Giant cell arteritis

- General malaise, weight loss, fever
- Temporal headache with tender enlarged non-pulsatile temporal arteries
- Scalp tenderness
- Jaw claudication
- Visual disturbance/loss
- Polymyalgia rheumatica
- Positive temporal artery biopsy (patchy granulomatous necrosis with giant cells)

9.3 Takayasu's arteritis (pulseless disease)

This rare condition presents with systemic illness such as malaise, weight loss and fever. The main vasculitic involvement is of the aorta and its main branches, producing arm claudication, absent pulses and bruits. Thirty per cent of patients have visual disturbance. Diagnosis is by angiography and treatment is with corticosteroids.

9.4 Wegener's granulomatosis

This is a rare disorder (incidence 0.4/100 000) characterised by a granulomatous necrotising vasculitis. Any organ may be involved but the classical Wegener's triad is:

- **Upper airways (sinuses, ears, eyes):** saddle nose, proptosis
- **Respiratory**: multiple pulmonary nodules
- **Renal**: focal proliferative glomerulonephritis with segmental necrosis.

cANCA is present in 90% of cases. Treatment is with corticosteroids and immunosuppressives.

9.5 Churg–Strauss syndrome (allergic angiitis and granulomatosis)

This is a rare systemic vasculitis with a similar pattern of organ involvement to polyarteritis nodosa but with associated eosinophilia and asthma. Though corticosteroids are required, the condition of most patients can be controlled without immunosuppressives.

9.6 Polyarteritis nodosa (PAN)

This features necrotising vasculitis of medium-sized vessels with formation of microaneurysms.

It is uncommon with an incidence of 5–9 per million, but it may be as much as 10 times more frequent in areas where hepatitis B is endemic. Presentation is usually with constitutional symptoms. Skin, peripheral nerves, kidney, gut and joints are commonly affected. Treatment is with corticosteroids and immunosuppressives.

- Hepatitis B surface antigen is present in 30% of cases worldwide, but <10% in the UK
- Mild eosinophilia may be present
- Liver function tests (LFTs) often abnormal
- ANCA is positive in <10%
- Renal disease is manifest by accelerated phase hypertension, but not typically with glomerulonephritis.

9.7 Microscopic polyangiitis (microscopic polyarteritis)

This usually presents between the ages of 40 and 60 with constitutional illness and renal disease. Though classified with the medium/small vessel disorders, microscopic angiitis tends to affect small arteries and arterioles of the kidney. Organs involved include:

- **Kidney**: glomerulonephritis as for Wegener's disease
- **Skin**: palpable purpura
- **Lung**: infiltrates, haemoptysis, haemorrhage
- **Gut, eye or peripheral nerves** can also be involved.

ANCA is positive in most cases: pANCA in 60% and cANCA in 40%.

9.8 Kawasaki disease

This is an acute febrile illness of children less than 5 years old, with systemic vasculitis. The peak onset is at 1.5 years and it has an incidence of about 6/100 000 in the under fives. It is more common and more severe in males. The cause is not known but its occasional occurrence in mini-epidemics suggests an infectious agent.

Clinical features of Kawasaki disease

- **Fever** (followed by thrombocytosis)
- **Vasculitis** with coronary aneurysm formation, Myocardial infarctions in 2.5%
- **Mucocutaneous**: rashes, red cracked lips, strawberry tongue, conjunctivitis
- **Lymphadenopathy** (especially cervical)

Treatment differs from most other vasculitides. Corticosteroids are contraindicated since they increase coronary aneurysms. Anti-inflammatory doses of aspirin are used during the acute febrile phase and anti-platelet doses once the fever resolves and thrombocytosis occurs. Intravenous immunoglobulin is also effective.

9.9 Behçet's syndrome

Behçet's syndrome is a rare condition most commonly found in Turkey and the eastern Mediterranean where there is a strong association with HLA B5. There is an equal sex ratio but the disease is more severe in males. The pathological findings are of immune-mediated occlusive vasculitis and venulitis. The diagnosis is based on clinical features.

Main clinical features

- Recurrent oral ulceration (100%)
- Recurrent painful genital ulceration (80%)
- Recurrent iritis (60–70%)
- Skin lesions (60–80%)

Other features

- Cutaneous vasculitis
- Thrombophlebitis
- Erythema nodosum
- Pathergy reaction (red papules >2 mm at sites of needle pricks after 48 hours)
- Arthritis (usually non-erosive, asymmetrical, lower limb)
- Neurological involvement (aseptic meningitis, ataxia, pseudobulbar palsy)
- Gastrointestinal involvement

Rheumatology

10.1 Classification
This can take the form of:

- Juvenile idiopathic arthritis (previously termed 'juvenile chronic arthritis' (JCA))
- Systemic connective tissue disease
- Reactive arthritis (eg rheumatic fever)
- Other (psoriatic, viral, leukaemic).

10.2 Juvenile idiopathic arthritis
Juvenile idiopathic arthritis is persistent arthritis of more than 3 months' duration in children under the age of 16. It is one of the more common chronic disorders of children and is a major cause of musculoskeletal disability and eye disease. The cause is not known. A number of distinct clinical patterns of onset are recognised.

Polyarticular
Arthritis of more than four joints. Polyarticular juvenile arthritis probably describes two distinct disorders. Younger children with negative rheumatoid factor have a symmetrical arthritis of large joints (especially the knees), though the small joints can be affected. Older children (usually teenagers) with a positive rheumatoid factor have, in fact, early-onset rheumatoid arthritis.

Pauciarticular
Arthritis of between one and four joints. Again there are two distinct groups. Older boys with sacroiliitis and HLA-B27 probably have juvenile-onset ankylosing spondylitis, and younger girls, usually ANA positive, may have uveitis. Regular ophthalmological screening is required in this group.

Clinical patterns of onset of juvenile idiopathic arthritis			
	Systemic	Polyarticular	Pauciarticular
Frequency (%)	10	30	60
Number of joints	Variable	Five or more	Four or less
Female:male ratio	1:1	3:1	5:1
Extra-articular	Prominent	Moderate	Rarer
Uveitis (%)	Rare	5	20
Rheumatoid factor (%)	Rare	15	Rare
Antinuclear factor (%)	10	40	85
Prognosis	Moderate	Moderate	Good

10.3 Systemic (classical Still's disease)
The hallmark is a high spiking fever, which, with the salmon pink rash, is virtually diagnostic. There is usually visceral involvement with hepatosplenomegaly and serositis. Initially the arthritis may be flitting (as in rheumatic fever), but in 50% of cases this develops into a chronic destructive arthropathy. This is usually a disease of the under-fives, but adult cases do occur.

Treatment of arthritis in children

- Physiotherapy
- Splintage
- NSAIDs
- Disease-modifying drugs (eg methotrexate) in persistent polyarticular disease
- Corticosteroids may be needed for systemic disease
- Anti-TNFα therapy for refractory cases

You should know that:

1. The common types of arthritis are classified as:

- Degenerative or inflammatory
- Primary osteoarthritis (OA) or secondary OA
- Persistent or transient inflammatory arthritis

2. The clinical features of rheumatoid arthritis are:

- Persistent inflammatory arthritis with symmetrical involvement of small joints
- Extra-articular features (nodules, eye involvement, cardiorespiratory features, vasculitis, Felty's syndrome)

3. The treatment of rheumatoid arthritis includes:

- Education
- Symptom-modifying medication (eg NSAIDs)
- Disease-modifying medications (eg methotrexate)
- Corticosteroids
- Biological treatment
- Physiotherapy and occupational therapy
- Surgery

4. The clinical features of the spondyloarthropathies include:

- Persistent inflammatory arthritis with asymmetrical involvement of large joints and the spine; sacroiliitis is characteristic

- Associations (psoriasis, uveitis, inflammatory bowel disease, HLA-B27)

5. The clinical features of gout include:

- Acute recurring inflammatory monoarthritis
- Chronic inflammatory arthritis with tophi
- Urate nephropathy

6. The clinical features of osteoarthritis include:

- Persistent degenerative arthritis
- Typically involves DIP joints, PIP joints, 1st CMC joint, knees, hips or spine

7. The characteristic features of the connective tissue disorders are:

- SLE: skin involvement, photosensitivity, arthritis, haematological abnormalities, renal involvement, anti-DNA antibodies
- Dermato/polymyositis: inflammatory myositis, skin involvement, elevated CK
- Systemic sclerosis: scleroderma, involvement of the GI tract and lung, anti-centromere antibodies or anti-SCL70 antibodies
- Sjögren's syndrome: exocrine gland failure (dry eyes, mouth), anti-Ro and anti-La antibodies